UCPA
2141 Overlook Rd.

PSYCHOLOGICAL APPRAISAL OF CHILDREN WITH CEREBRAL DEFECTS

Psychological Appraisal
of Children with Cerebral Defects

By EDITH MEYER TAYLOR

PUBLISHED FOR
THE COMMONWEALTH FUND

Harvard University Press, Cambridge, Massachusetts

1959

Published for
The Commonwealth Fund
By Harvard University Press
Cambridge, Massachusetts

For approximately a quarter of a century THE COMMONWEALTH FUND, through its Division of Publications, sponsored, edited, produced, and distributed books and pamphlets germane to its purposes and operations as a philanthropic foundation. On July 1, 1951, the Fund entered into an arrangement by which HARVARD UNIVERSITY PRESS became the publisher of Commonwealth Fund books, assuming responsibility for their production and distribution. The Fund continues to sponsor and edit its books, and cooperates with the Press in all phases of manufacture and distribution.

Distributed in Great Britain
By Oxford University Press
London

LIBRARY OF CONGRESS CATALOG CARD NO. 59–7647

MANUFACTURED IN THE UNITED STATES OF AMERICA

Foreword

It is a great pleasure to me to be asked to write a preface to Dr. Taylor's book, *Psychological Appraisal of Children with Cerebral Defects*. I have had the pleasure of close professional association with her, and have come to rely with great confidence on her understanding of the psychological aberrations and problems of children suffering from cerebral injuries.

These problems can for descriptive purposes be divided into two groups. The first concerns the differences in experience of the developing child impaired by sensory-motor handicap compared with the averagely competent child. These differences encompass all the fields important in personality development; for example, the satisfaction of parents, the exploration of the physical world, motor achievement—such an important source of personal satisfaction to children—and finally the very meaning of words learned without the template of experience. These disabling factors make themselves felt in the development of personality in various children in various ways at different ages and are modified, if at all, only when thoroughly understood by the involved adults.

In addition to the abnormalities of experience encountered by infants and children impaired by cerebral handicaps, learning ability in many of these children functions inadequately and thereby distorts their social and emotional as well as their intellectual development.

In the recent past these deficits have been increasingly recognized by many. However, when appraising competence, medical men and psychologists alike have tended to rely too much either on global scores (which average together accomplishments as related to age into an

I.Q.) or on the presence or absence of some specific isolated signs often known to be characteristic of brain injury in adults.

Dr. Taylor has in the past presented many arguments demonstrating the fallacy of such procedures and has stressed the importance of recognizing the many variations and relationships of symptoms occurring in children who have sustained cerebral injuries from various causes at different developmental stages.

In the present volume she has assembled a series of rather typical portraits of children affected by injuries of various etiologies involving topographically diverse portions of the nervous system. The effects of impaired sensory-motor and emotional experiences on developmental processes at various ages are described; concessions directed toward making life rewarding for the children are suggested; and relevant academic plans are implied.

Dr. Taylor has described in considerable technical detail her methods of appraising this most baffling group of children. Combining developmental tests and acute, detailed, clinical observation with psychological understanding of the child and his special situation has allowed her to make a reliable survey of existing intellectual and emotional assets and liabilities. Such a descriptive diagnosis not only gives a basis of functional understanding to immediate plans and projected expectations, but may also in the long run be translatable into terms of cerebral physiology.

RANDOLPH K. BYERS, M.D.

Preface

The reader of this book will need no special statement to know how much I owe to my former teachers, colleagues, and patients. Their influence and help should be obvious all through. In addition to those named in the text, a small group of assistants and interns in psychology at the Children's Hospital in Boston should be mentioned because it was their interest and participation in our particular type of work which prompted the plan to write. They are in chronological order: Marianne Simmel, Harriet Hyde Sands, Dorothy Pope, Ellen Drori, Selma Rappaport, George Roth, Ruth Friedman, Paul Sapir, Kenneth and Carol Dinklage. Amongst the many friends and colleagues who read all or parts of the manuscript, I am especially grateful to Dr. Tamara Dembo and Dr. John Eberhart, whose helpful suggestions should add to the clarity of the content. My heartfelt thanks goes to The Commonwealth Fund which sponsored the writing of this book. Before my days it had already contributed substantially to the support of the psychological work at the Children's Hospital and the publication of Dr. Elizabeth Lord's findings. Since then our nonmedical discipline had been partly maintained within the pediatric framework through gratefully acknowledged successive contributions by organizations such as the National Foundation for Infantile Paralysis, Inc., the Heckscher Foundation for Children, the Bay State Society for Crippled and Handicapped, Inc., the United Cerebral Palsy Association, the National Institute of Neurological Disease and Blindness.

The progress of our work and the modest insights we may have acquired owe the most to the constant moral and scientific support and the opportunities provided by the two successive heads of the neurological division, Dr. Bronson Crothers and Dr. Randolph K. Byers. Besides my lasting gratitude to each of them, I should like to acknowledge the friendship and good will of the members of the medical department, under Dr. Charles A. Janeway's direction, to which I proudly belonged until reorganization of the hospital services in 1953.

E. M. T.

Cambridge, Massachusetts
January 1959

Acknowledgments

I wish to acknowledge the cooperation of the following persons and organizations in granting permission to use certain materials in this book:

Houghton Mifflin Company for permission to reproduce material from the Revised Stanford-Binet Scale, published in Lewis M. Terman and Maud A. Merrill, *Measuring Intelligence* (Boston: Houghton Mifflin, 1937)

Dr. David Wechsler for permission to use material from the Wechsler-Bellevue Intelligence Scale, published in David Wechsler, *The Measurement of Adult Intelligence* (Baltimore: Williams and Wilkins, 1944)

Dr. Wechsler and the Psychological Corporation for permission to use material from the Wechsler Intelligence Scale for Children, published in David Wechsler, *The Wechsler Intelligence Scale for Children* (New York: Psychological Corporation, 1949)

Appleton-Century-Crofts, Inc. for permission to reprint age norms and scoring system for assembling a manikin, published in Rudolf Pintner and Donald G. Paterson, *A Scale of Performance Tests* (New York: Appleton, 1923)

Warwick and York, Publishers, for permission to reproduce figures from Frederick Kuhlmann, *A Handbook of Mental Tests* (Baltimore: Warwick and York, 1922)

Warwick and York, Publishers, and C. H. Stoelting Company for permission to reproduce the Ellis visual designs and the samples of half-point credits for these designs, appearing in Louise Wood and Edyth Shulman, "The Ellis Visual Designs Test," *Journal of Educational Psychology* 31:592, 595, 1940

C. H. Stoelting Company for permission to reproduce some of the designs from the Kohs block designs test

Dr. Arnold Gesell and Harper and Brothers Publishers for permission to reproduce some of the blockbuilding models published in Arnold Gesell, *The First Five Years of Life* (New York: Harper, 1940)

American Psychological Association for permission to use adaptations of some of the designs made with the Goldstein-Scheerer sticks, from Kurt Goldstein and Martin Scheerer, *Abstract and Concrete Behavior,* Psychological Monographs, Volume 53, Number 2 (Evanston, Illinois: American Psychological Association, 1941)

Dr. Augusta F. Bronner and Dr. Edward A. Lincoln for permission to reproduce the drawing of the Lincoln hollow square formboard, published in Augusta F. Bronner, William Healy, Gladys M. Lowe, and Myra E. Shimberg, *A Manual of Individual Mental Tests and Testing,* Judge Baker Foundation Publication Number 4 (Boston: Little, Brown, 1927)

Dr. Arthur L. Benton for permission to reproduce designs published in Arthur L. Benton, *The Revised Visual Retention Test: Clinical and Experimental Application* (New York: Psychological Corporation, 1955)

Dr. Lauretta Bender and the *American Journal of Orthopsychiatry* for permission to reproduce designs published in Lauretta Bender, *A Visual Motor Gestalt Test and Its Clinical Use* (New York: American Orthopsychiatric Association, 1938)

Delachaux et Niestlé for permission to use the age norms, scoring system, and drawings of the Rey-Osterrieth complex figure, which appeared in Paul A. Osterrieth, "Le test de copie d'une figure complexe," *Archives de psychologie* 30:206–356, 1944; the drawing showing the materials of the Rey nonverbal learning test, which appeared in André Rey, "D'un procédé pour évaluer l'éducabilité," *Archives de psychologie* 24:287–337, 1934; and the age norms and scoring system for "Lady Walking in the Rain," from André Rey, *Monographies de psychologie appliquée,* Number 1 (Paris: Delachaux et Niestlé, 1947)

Bettendorff, Editeurs, and Dr. Rey for permission to reprint the age norms for the nonverbal learning test, published in André Rey, *Six épreuves au service de la psychologie clinique* (Brussels: Bettendorff, 1951)

Dr. André Rey for permission to use the original, unpublished age norms developed by him for the test of learning fifteen words

Presses Universitaires de France for permission to use the revised age norms for the test of learning fifteen words, published in André Rey, *L'examen clinique en psychologie* (Paris: Presses Universitaires, 1958)

Benno Schwabe and Company for permission to use the age norms and scoring system for "Lady Walking in the Rain," from J. Wintsch, "Le dessin comme témoin du développement mental," *Zeitschrift für Kinderpsychiatrie* 2:33 June; 2:69 August 1935

World Book Company for permission to reprint the age norms and scoring system for "Drawing a Man," published in Florence L. Goodenough, *The Measurement of Intelligence by Drawings* (Chicago: World Book Company, 1926)

Contents

INTRODUCTION

Introduction

This is a psychologist's book on childhood conditions involving the nervous system. It is the result of many years of experience with large numbers of children with cerebral difficulties and is designed to help in the understanding and management of some of the serious problems arising from such conditions.

Certain methods will be described that have proved useful to me and my collaborators when evaluating the potentialities of these children. Certain typical child patients will be portrayed at various age levels to show how certain psychological traits, tendencies, and problems continue but change form in the course of the child's development. Interrelationships will be briefly outlined between the child's behavior picture and the emotional climates that surround him at various stages. Some of the findings obtained in a follow-up study of patients with cerebral palsy will be presented to help validate some of the descriptions.

It is well known that children with neurological impairment seem to be difficult to assess psychologically. Often it is claimed that only psychologists with unusual opportunities for accumulating experience are able to be successful. The fact remains that with increasing demands in the field, more and more people learn how to evaluate these children skillfully and reliably. Still, when facing their colleagues who seem to have easier tasks, many of these clinicians feel that they have to apologize for the many adjustments, considerations, and shortcuts they use. One of the hopes that accompanies this book is that it may help to modify this attitude somewhat and to elicit pride in some and respect in others for the resourceful and serious efforts of the perceptive clinician who tries to meet the demands of very difficult and special situations. There will be at no point any claim that ours is the only way of seeing or handling the varied problems that arise in our field. The only justification for our particular approach is that it has proved practical, economical, reliable, and helpful.

This book may interest various professional workers in different ways. Primarily, it is meant for clinical psychologists concerned with differential diagnosis in children with cerebral defects. It may be useful also to psychologists who work in pediatric and psychiatric clinics mostly as diagnosticians. Those chiefly interested in psychotherapy may see new methods of treatment through increased awareness of the complex deviations of functioning common in many cases. To doctors, teachers, therapists, nurses, social workers, and other persons working with children with cerebral defects, some of our descriptions may be generally useful. However, the technical details of diagnosis should not and could not be of use to nonpsychologists or to those trained in the use of standard psychometric tools only.

Here is the background that may help to explain some of the practical and theoretical aspects of this book.

In 1943 I joined Dr. Crothers' unit in the neurological division of the Children's Hospital in Boston. The post of psychologist had been vacated through the death of Dr. Elizabeth Lord, who had worked in this unit since its beginnings in 1929. Dr. Crothers' early interest in childhood conditions of the nervous system attracted large numbers of patients for diagnosis and guidance. Usually the psychologist was asked to collaborate in both phases; she evaluated the developmental status of the child and consulted at length with the parents. Supported by the pediatrician, she usually helped to formulate some tentative plan.

Dr. Crothers and Dr. Lord had worked as a highly successful team; their long-time collaboration had established certain valuable traditions. The psychologist's emphasis was on the study of the educational potentialities of the patients. Study and manipulation of emotional factors *per se* seemed to her less important than provisions for an emotionally serene environment which would assure the best educational opportunities. She warned teachers and parents about the inefficacy and danger of exerting pressure on a child who is unable to comply. Shrewd observation and psychological understanding led her to be amongst the first to become aware of typical learning disabilities in children with organic brain damage. In her pioneer work on testing children with cerebral palsy,[1] she attached great importance to the areas of perception, reasoning, and learning. Keenly interested in individual variation of abilities in these areas, she recognized early the limitations of global test results in the psychological appraisal of children with neurological difficulties. Like various authors after her, she found that intelligence quotients have a restricted significance only and may actually be misleading. I.Q. ratings may be used to classify children in distinct but broad groups. They also may enable one to judge how "intelligent" an individual child is compared with the wide range of normal children. However, they often fail to do justice to the many individual variations in functioning that seem directly or indirectly determined by the multiple handicapping deviations connected with physical conditions. In their work with children with neurological difficulties, Dr. Lord and her collaborators used a number of the then-current clinical instruments, such as the 1916 edition of the Stanford-Binet Scale,[2] the Kuhlmann tests,[3] Gesell's Developmental Schedules,[4] and later the Revised Stanford-Binet Scale[5] and the Wechsler-Bellevue Intelligence Scale.[6] She supplemented these with special tests of her own choice, often using her own adaptations. She used the Kohs block designs,[7] the Ellis visual designs,[8] the Seguin formboard,[9] the Wood picture completion test,[10] and many others. Instead of expressing results of one examination in total scores, she frequently plotted numerical results in a profile. Its lows and highs then gave an expressive picture of a patient's potential assets and liabilities.

For the medical men she condensed her findings in concise re-

[1] Elizabeth Lord, *Children Handicapped by Cerebral Palsy* (New York: The Commonwealth Fund, 1937). Out of print.

[2] Lewis M. Terman, *The Measurement of Intelligence* (Boston: Houghton Mifflin, 1916).

[3] Frederick Kuhlmann, *A Handbook of Mental Tests* (Baltimore: Warwick and York, 1922).

[4] Arnold Gesell, *The Mental Growth of the Pre-School Child* (New York: Macmillan, 1925).

[5] Lewis M. Terman and Maud A. Merrill, *Measuring Intelligence* (Boston: Houghton Mifflin, 1937).

[6] David Wechsler, *The Measurement of Adult Intelligence* (Baltimore: Williams and Wilkins, 1941).

[7] S. C. Kohs, *Intelligence Measurement* (New York: Macmillan, 1923).

[8] Louise Wood and Edyth Shulman, "The Ellis Visual Designs Test," *Journal of Educational Psychology* 31:591–602, 1940. Also Elizabeth Lord and Louise Wood, "Diagnostic Values in a Visuo-Motor Test," *American Journal of Orthopsychiatry* 12:414–428, 1942.

[9] H. H. Goddard, "The Form Board as a Measure of Intellectual Development in Children," *Training School Bulletin*, pp. 49–51, 1912.

[10] Louise Wood, "A New Picture Completion Test," *Journal of Genetic Psychology* 56:383–409, 1940.

ports. Usually she described the potential rate of children's mental development in terms of "superior, high or low average," etc., and added qualifications regarding educational potentialities. She accustomed her collaborators to know that with a few exceptions she was able to evaluate even those children who had serious physical impairment. She warned superficial observers of these patients not to underestimate them because they were unable to talk or to move properly. At the same time, she tried to show the fallacy of overestimating the same children by assuming undisclosed, unprovable, and often nonexisting potentialities. In cases of children with mild disabilities only, she pointed out the warning signs of potential learning difficulties. Her readers came to appreciate the predictive significance of signs such as visuo-motor difficulties, attention defects, and overdeveloped rote memory in children who, in spite of their brain injuries, seem at first sight alert and intelligent.

Dr. Lord's competence and psychological insight had been thoroughly accepted by her medical colleagues and had created unique opportunities for psychological work in a medical unit. As her successor, I had the chance to continue in her steps. At the same time, I had to preserve my own professional identity, which was based on different psychological background and experience.

My psychological beginnings were with Felix Krueger, whose *genetische Ganzheitspsychologie* had considerable impact in the 1920's and early 1930's on the development of child psychology at the University of Leipzig, Germany, from which I was graduated in 1933. From there I went to Geneva, Switzerland, where my psychological thinking was decisively and permanently influenced by close association with Jean Piaget. I worked under him for five years on problems concerning the development of children's reasoning. In Geneva also, André Rey taught me to combine theoretical psychological viewpoints with the demands of clinical work. Partly through his influence, I became much interested in the psychological deviations that result from physical abnormality in children and adults. These interests turned into more practical channels during the following years—my first in this country. During a year's stay at Gesell's clinic in New Haven, and later during several years' work as consultant to child-caring agencies in Connecticut, I became familiar with many aspects of psychological work as practiced in consulting clinics in this country. I had in these places much opportunity for contact with social conditions, parental attitudes, and com-

munity problems that affect the development of children in this culture. In view of my European background, these contacts were for me
especially enlightening. Arriving in Boston and seeing Dr. Bronson
Crothers at work multiplied these sociological experiences and deepened
my respect for the intricate relationships between physical growth, physiological condition, social environment, and psychological development.

The varied things I had learned and done in the different phases
of my professional life were all useful to me in the psychological work
at the Children's Hospital. There were all types of children of different
ages with varied problems of all degrees of severity. Many presented
behavior difficulties either alone or in combination with physical handicaps. Besides the regular patients of the neurological division, there
were many children who were to be studied in other departments of the
hospital. Since ours was the only psychological service available at the
hospital at that time, consultations were requested on many children
whose conditions raised questions of a psychological character. Like Dr.
Lord, I was asked primarily for a diagnosis of mental ability in the
majority of cases. These requests usually involved many other aspects,
such as emotional status, effect of physical condition, past experiences.

Patients at the Children's Hospital came from varied social and
cultural backgrounds, from different parts of this country or of the world.
Some stayed for weeks and months, some for a few days or even hours.
Medical study and corrective measures were for many cases the primary concern, whereas psychological study was incidental only. For
others, the focus of interest and main reason for admittance were behavior observation, appraisal, and future guidance.

Conditions for psychological study varied widely. Frequently, reasonably normal testing conditions could be arranged; often, however, some
or many disturbing factors interfered. Some children tended to be upset
by the strange surroundings, hospital atmosphere, and separation from
their families. Some had permanent and serious physical impairment;
some were temporarily incapacitated by illness or corrective procedures.
In many instances permanent physical and emotional conditions had
prevented ordinary background experiences. Some of the examinations
had to be made in a hurry. Often the examiner had to form some judgement reluctantly, on the basis of meager evidence, and trust that the
opinion would be either verified or corrected by future developments
and subsequent examinations.

Under these circumstances the psychologist had to be flexible and resourceful where it was possible, and cautious and resistant to pressure where it was not. In general, I tried to follow my predecessor's leads. Many of her methods proved as valuable to me as they had been to her; besides, they had the advantage of being familiar to our medical colleagues. Gradually, I added others of the current test scales and supplemented them by some of the less customary older and newer techniques. Like Dr. Lord, I centered much effort and interest on the study of perception, reasoning, and learning, characteristically of importance with the majority of our patients. As she had done, I tended to use test methods adaptively, picking and choosing what seemed most appropriate and expedient in each case.

Like most experienced examiners, I had to rely for judgement on many psychological signs besides numerical results of test items. Observation of a child's motility, his working methods, his attitude, his interest spans during the examination, were as important as his behavior manifestations in free observation, spontaneous play, or conversation. Ordinarily, many of these observations do not lend themselves to objective appraisal. Their interpretation often depends on the psychological knowledge and flair of the examiner. While he tries to understand them in their context, he has to decide for himself whether certain responses which he notices are altogether normal, whether they fit the age of the child, or whether they indicate deviation or immaturity. He is lucky if he knows well how normal children in similar circumstances act at varying age levels. Many of us possess a private set of unofficial norms which has been acquired in experiences with other children, be they friends, neighbors, or clients, nieces or sons. Tentatively—if not inadvertently—against these standards we are inclined to compare our fringe observations on patients.

However, many truly objective and legitimate norms can be found in the varied genetic studies that have been conducted at psychological research centers. To have these at one's disposal is especially important in the study of children whose special circumstances make short cuts in examining procedures necessary. My psychological experiences in Leipzig, Geneva, and New Haven were to me of great help in this direction.

Gesell's genetic schedules, with their minute descriptions of normal children's behavior patterns at various age levels, do not need explanation here.[11] It is assumed that most readers are familiar with this work, which has proved to have much practical value for those working with

[11] Arnold Gesell, *The First Five Years of Life* (New York: Harper, 1940).

the younger age groups. However, a few remarks may be in order about the two European centers of child psychology, which are likely to be less well known. These few brief comments will be confined to the description of those aspects only that seem most pertinent here and may help to explain some elements of my approach and method which will be discussed later on.

In the Psychological Institute of the University of Leipzig, in my days under Felix Krueger, much interest was devoted to the study of early psychological tendencies and emotional habits which determine the young child's awareness before he becomes dominated by the "intellectualizing" influences of his environment.[12] These studies centered on areas in which these original tendencies could manifest themselves in their purest form: children's creative art with blocks, crayons, plasticene, and other materials was scrutinized. Perceptual activity also was investigated thoroughly from various angles. My own doctor's thesis on sorting processes of very young children was an attempt to understand the principles that underlie the fitting together of heterogeneous objects before sorting by concepts becomes an intellectual necessity to the individual.[13] The findings of all these studies indicated that a child's sorting ability develops in orderly sequence from primitive awareness of diffuse, holistic entities to perception according to better organized, more differentiated, and better structured Gestalten. This apparent progress, while necessary for and inherent in intellectual and social development, nonetheless was thought to entail a rather regrettable transformation and reduction of the more spontaneous, more original, purer, and emotionally richer psychological tendencies.

For the clinician these studies were a gold mine of information about psychological attitude as well as of factual material. We learned to respect primitive solutions *per se* and saw the continuity between them and more mature forms of expression. We learned to appreciate tendencies and feelings common to children of similar developmental levels, and to distinguish between abnormal manifestations and normal individual variations. Most of all, we acquired a rather solid stock of factual material on normal development of young children in such areas as drawing, perception, form discrimination, sorting, and rhythm.

In Geneva, under Piaget, genetic problems were attacked from dif-

---

[12] Felix Krueger, "Über Entwicklungs-Psychologie, ihre sachliche und geschichtliche Notwendigkeit," *Arbeiten zur Entwicklungs-Psychologie,* Volume I, 1915; *Der Strukturbegriff in der Psychologie (1923–1931)* (Jena: Fischer, 1931).

[13] Edith Meyer, "Ordnen und Ordnung bei drei- bis sechsjährigen Kindern," *Neue Psychologische Studien,* Band X, Heft 3 (Munich: Beck, 1934).

ferent angles. Children's thought was investigated in order to get insight into the development of mental activity itself. Then as now, Piaget was primarily interested in theory of intelligence and problems of adaptation. This led to his many stimulating studies on reasoning processes of children.[14] With his collaborators he carefully studied how children learn to master the many problems which their physical, social, and intellectual environments present to them at varying age levels. The young child's early discoveries and adaptations are of considerable importance in Piaget's research and theory. As the child gradually comes to discover and to understand relationships around him, he also learns to understand his own relations to objects, persons, and events. This process is closely linked to the child's elaboration of permanent concepts of space, time, causality, and also leads to the development of moral judgement and emotional attitudes. Before he reaches the level at which adult logical thinking becomes possible for him, he goes through stages of partial comprehension. In some areas he arrives at full understanding earlier than in others. The steps of this development generally follow in orderly progression and interdependence. Objective stages are first reached in the field of action, later in practical comprehension, and still later in reflective reasoning. All normal children go through similar stages in the same succession at more or less similar age levels. This is being demonstrated by the Geneva group through many genetic studies on groups of children of varying age levels. My own studies during my Geneva days concerned the development of notions of space and time, and helped in that area to demonstrate the gap between children's comprehension as shown in their actions and as shown in their reflective thinking.[15]

For the clinician, these and other aspects of the studies of Piaget's group provide, first of all, many valuable viewpoints. Investigating and understanding the degree, quality, and rate of a child's comprehension enables the observer to interpret many behavior manifestations by his

[14] Jean Piaget, *The Psychology of Intelligence*, trans. (New York: Harcourt, Brace, 1950); *Judgement and Reasoning in the Child*, trans. (New York: Harcourt, Brace, 1928); *Language and Thought of the Child*, trans. (New York: Harcourt, Brace, 1926); *The Origins of Intelligence in Children*, trans. (New York: International Universities Press, 1953); *The Construction of Reality in the Child*, trans. (New York: Basic Books, 1954).

[15] Edith Meyer, "La représentation des relations spatiales chez l'enfant," *Cahiers de pédagogie expérimentale et de psychologie de l'enfant*, Number 8 (Geneva: Institut des Sciences de l'Education, 1935), pp. 1–16; also in Jean Piaget, *Le développement de la notion du temps chez l'enfant* (Paris: Presses Universitaires, 1946), Chapter VIII; and in Jean Piaget and Bärbel Inhelder, *The Child's Conception of Space*, trans. (London: Routledge, 1956), Chapter VIII.

level of maturity. How the child understands his environment, those around him, and his own relationships to them, often presents clues that explain some of his attitudes, feelings, and actions. The study of mental activity, then, acquires a broader meaning than investigation of intellectual status only. It helps toward comprehension of adjustment to present life situation and may allow some predictions for the future.

The factual material derived from these studies generally is expressed in descriptive terms. The successive stages of growing comprehension cover rather broad age ranges. Precise age norms are rarely available, since the data usually were obtained from small numbers of children only. Though none of Piaget's studies were primarily intended for clinical use, their factual content helps the clinician to determine a patient's approximate stage of mental development. He may discover a rather mature form of thinking in an otherwise inefficient child, or typically primitive concepts in another who appears bright and alert on the surface. These clues may help him to understand better some of the children's behavior or learning difficulties.

Some of André Rey's studies[16] on practical intelligence originated within this group of research projects. These were later systematically adapted as clinical tools and standardized on larger populations. Rey had a special interest in learning processes also. He combined the genetic and the clinical approach in a most stimulating way: in various studies he investigated how children of different ages learn sets of new facts either in practical or in purely verbal settings. He found that children's efficiency in such tasks increases with age as they become abler to organize various clues and to profit from their present and previous experiences. Norms were developed through precise and detailed descriptions of the learning processes of children of varying ages.

Some of these tests are of particular interest to the clinician who works with children and, therefore, frequently deals with learning problems. In many instances it is not easy to decide whether a child has difficulties because he cannot learn or because he has not been taught properly, or whether, owing to other reasons, he cannot profit from what he is exposed to. Often inability to learn at home or in school is much entangled with a whole set of emotional problems.

[16] André Rey, *L'intelligence practique chez l'enfant* (Paris: Alcan, 1935); "D'un procédé pour évaluer l'éducabilité," *Archives de psychologie* 24:287–337, 1934; *Six épreuves au service de la psychologie clinique* (Brussels: Bettendorff, 1951); *Etudes des insuffisances psychologiques* (Paris: Delachaux et Niestlé, 1947); *L'examen clinique en psychologie* (Paris: Presses Universitaires, 1958).

Rey's approach to learning problems, which separates the study of *how* a child learns from that of *what* he learns or has learned, often allows some insight into the causes of learning defects. It may help the psychologist to differentiate between an emotional and a constitutional basis or to distinguish varied kinds of organic causes.

Despite the difference of their theoretic approaches, both centers of genetic studies, Leipzig and Geneva, had a few important points in common: investigators in both places were primarily interested in those developmental stages that in children precede the level of full comprehension and correct performance from the adult's point of view. Whether reproduction of a perceived design was studied in Krueger's group, the interpretation of a physical event appraised or a new learning situation introduced in Geneva, the observers watched mostly for characteristically childlike manifestations. Primitive solutions were intriguing objects for inquiry instead of errors or peculiar behavior phenomena only.[17] The investigator tried to understand how they had come about, how they were explained and modified. Through such study he hoped to learn what factors underlie psychological development in children generally or individually.

The research involved in all studies that were described required special methods: in most of them, the process rather than its end result was under constant investigation. The overt end result becomes meaningful only through the way in which it comes about. A design, for instance, can be drawn in various manners, a mathematical problem can be solved or some facts remembered in different ways, some more efficient and mature than others. A perfect solution may turn out to be the result of a fortunate hazard, whereas mature approach may lead to a wrong solution because of lack of technical skill, tension, interruption, or the like. The observer needed always to be sensitive to events and moods that might influence the outcome. He took note of trials, hesitations, intermittent solutions. Depending on the subject of investigation, he played a more or less active part himself. In some of the Leipzig studies he introduced at proper moments certain questions and choices. In Rey's investigations he manipulated systematic suggestions, varied presentations, asked questions. Where beliefs and thought were under investigation, as in most of Piaget's studies, many decisions depended on the experimenter: there, for instance, it was essential that no verbal

---

[17] Similar viewpoints underlie many of Heinz Werner's studies. See among others, *Comparative Psychology of Mental Development* (New York: Harper, 1940).

response be taken at its face value without careful check and counter-check on the meaning of the response. The child was led to discuss the subject and to explain his thoughts. With the necessary practice, the examiner learned to recognize those statements in which children repeat things heard and to distinguish them from those that express underlying belief. A child's thought about a subject often reflects his partial understanding of what he has learned. By tracing back to how the belief developed, the examiner often comes to elucidate an otherwise obscure and seemingly senseless statement. In his early writings Piaget described his clinical method,[18] which consisted of individual interviews only. Later he and his collaborators started to combine purely verbal questions with practical experimental set-ups. The inquiry begins in standardized fashion with some uniform introductory questions. These lead to a free conversational exchange which is directed by the child's responses, expressions, and behavior. The essentially social climate of Piaget's methods adds a special dimension.

My early experiences helped later in many ways: the interest in perception, reasoning, and learning was especially useful. These areas have been recognized as fruitful for inquiry into the assessment of mental functioning. Their interrelationship and their role within the development of personality remains an intriguing and still incompletely solved question. Deficiencies in these areas may cause distortions in over-all adjustment that vary with age, environmental circumstances, and physical conditions, and that are reflected in behavior.

The methodological approach used in many experimental and clinical situations in my European days also proved well suited to work with handicapped children. The controlled flexibility of these methods, together with the emphasis on descriptive and qualifying findings, fitted into the framework of established procedures in our unit at Children's Hospital. Dr. Lord had used it in her way to meet the varying demands of test conditions; Dr. Crothers himself had developed most effective interview and examining procedures that transcended customary methods used in pediatrics or neurology. He knew how to discover and use many hardly perceptible clues in the evaluation of his patients and their conditions. The way in which he collected, besides physical signs, items of general psychological importance through more or less casual conversation with family or child was most stimulating and instructive to

---

[18] Jean Piaget, *The Child's Conception of the World,* trans. (New York: Harcourt, Brace, 1929), p. 8.

observe. Dr. Crothers' influence, with his interest in the combination of medical and social problems, gave to all those who worked with him much opportunity to widen their horizons and judgements.

Gradually our psychological studies, practiced first by myself and later by students and associates, assumed a certain style in accordance with our special emphases, viewpoints, and prejudices. Our methods were adapted and oriented for each case and were used this way not only in testing each child but also in interviewing his parents. Each psychological examination followed an individual plan, and often test items were modified systematically to reveal as much as possible. Briefly described, this works as follows.

The choice of procedures for the examination proper may depend on many factors, ranging from physical ability, age, and experience of the child, to time available or to specific questions that have been raised by parents, physicians, or others. An effort is made to avoid wherever possible the accumulation of cumbersome and possibly meaningless data, and instead to assemble as many pertinent and measurable findings as is feasible. Instead of using full test scales, the psychologist selects certain activities which in her judgement will yield the least equivocal results under the particular circumstances. Emphasis is placed on the unity of the examination process. Certain test situations will serve to canvass the various areas of functioning and enable the examiner to form some first tentative hypotheses about the child's personality and about his mental functioning. In the subsequent stages of the examination, initial hypotheses are checked and counterchecked; certain leads may be followed but may be verified, rejected, or replaced by others as the investigation goes on. The child's responses to specific situations give clues for further inquiry.[19] (Such selective examining procedures were used in similar ways more frequently than now, before the development of the now most popular test scales.)

Measurable findings can be obtained with items of the current scales or with special individual standardized test procedures. Norms derived from genetic studies help to evaluate and rate many spontaneous play activities. These prove informative, especially with younger or immature children. All numerical data are supplemented and, if indicated,

[19] Edith Meyer and Marianne Simmel, "The Psychological Appraisal of Children with Neurological Defects," *Journal of Abnormal and Social Psychology* 42:193–205, April 1947.

qualified by many other observations. In some areas, many different test situations and observations may be necessary for a detailed analysis; in others the examiner may get a satisfactorily clear picture by abbreviated investigation with one or another instrument designed to furnish data for evaluation.

Not only may the whole of the psychological examination resemble a psychological experiment, but also each individual test situation. The child himself, rather than the test that is being administered, is the subject of experimentation. Wherever possible each test item is presented in standard form first. This is a prerequisite wherever scoring with available norms is aimed at. Then the examiner introduces modifications, partial solutions, questions. These may help to show up how the child has understood the task. They may also uncover feelings and thoughts or demonstrate whether and how the child follows suggestions, adjusts to directions, changes. The skilled examiner avoids arbitrary modifications but manipulates with psychological insight.

Much emphasis is placed on the social atmosphere of the examination. Both the child and the examiner interact throughout the examination and together create its climate. This methodological approach makes considerable use of the examiner's personality within the plan of the examination; she responds and decides at each stage of the interview and has considerable freedom of action. She learns to count her own emotions and actions amongst the factors that shape the course of the examination. She also watches and notes carefully the child's emotional responses in and outside the examining room. She observes him in relation to his parents or to other people, places, or events. All these observations add up to show how, as a person, the child reacts in this specific situation. The findings that are collected through the examination or through observations around it are supplemented by information obtained from outside sources. Descriptions of activities at home or in school are compared with those seen in the interview. Occasionally, if there is conflict, the psychologist makes the choice whether to trust her own impressions or the opinion of those who have known the child longer than she has. Psychological judgement does not center on the patient alone but also on the sources of outside information. Facts about the child's development may in many cases be available in medical or other records. How much to rely on these may depend on who saw and recorded what. Behavior manifestations noticed by experienced pediatricians may be most revealing and informative from the psychological point of view. However, sometimes symptoms like irritability or passivity, may have been recorded by casual medical observers who failed to understand psychological factors that caused the symptom at the time.

The psychologist's own conversations with the parents can help to recreate a portrait of the child as he has developed up to the present. Efforts are made to estimate the rate of development prior to the time of the study. Questions may vary, depending on the child and his conditions. One may aim, for instance, to retrace the development of a child's motor or social independence through the years. One may ask about his gradual progress in communication or in comprehension of daily events. One may find out how the child participates now in everyday life, what he knows and does around the house, where he stays, plays, or cuddles.

Through the seemingly casual but well-planned interview with the family, one may come to see the child through the eyes of those around him. One may try to understand circumstances and personalities involved in a particular family setting. Often it is well to take into account how much the years may gradually change the conditions that surround a child, especially a handicapped one. Many parents' life situations change through the years, and so do their attitudes and feelings. Acquaintance with local conditions, sociological factors, and cultural prejudices may help in understanding the emotional and social implications of a child's specific problems. Many of the tensions and needs within a family may be at least partially explained if the clinician understands that the same degree of physical handicap or mental irregularity may seem appealing in a child in one social group or almost intolerable in another. Flexibility in one's loyalties is an asset for the psychologist who finds that her judgement may become obscured as she identifies exclusively either with the child or with the parents and their often most real difficulties.

Some understanding of the patient's medical condition with its outstanding symptoms and side effects comes naturally to the psychologist through her work in a medical setting, even though she may be untrained in things medical. Through more or less close contact with the medical men, bits of information are picked up and incorporated into one's frame of reference. These can help in judging what certain medical situations or events may mean in the life of a child or his family. Psychological reactions to hospital visits or operations, to corrective procedures, to convulsions, braces, etc., can become clues by which to understand more about the child, his parents, or both. One may learn about a mother's emotional situation, for instance, if one can check with the doctor on how real her anxieties about feeding difficulties or lack of weight gain are. Loyalty rather than hostility, to the medical efforts, is an important asset for the psychologist. It helps her to appreciate and to compromise in conflicts that may arise, for instance, between the orthopedic necessity for casts, braces, or other measures of immobilization and the psychological need for optimum freedom.

Experience with a physician's special manner sometimes enables the psychologist to understand how his advice or prognosis has affected the feelings that surround the child. Often the emotional climate in a family is at least partially determined by the physician's attitudes, which may be supportive or defeatist, geared toward vigorous treatment or to a laissez-faire policy.

The psychological judgement resulting from putting together all information obtained is based on evidence from many sources. Many items lend themselves to objective and even quantifiable treatment; many others may seem to depend on psychological experience and intuition. Familiarity with people in general and clinical cases in particular helps here, as it does in other psychological areas.

At the Children's Hospital the findings of each psychological study are usually discussed orally with those who had asked for them. They are also expressed in a written report that becomes part of the medical record. Short of definite Intelligence Quotients,[20] these psychological reports contain most details essential and common to many psychological résumés reporting on results of nonprojective methods. Usually an estimate of a child's level of maturity is given in terms of age norms; the approximate rate of development is indicated by ratings such as superior, average, borderline, defective. These statements are accompanied by remarks on attention spans, learning ability, reasoning power, and perceptual skills; motor situations and language habits are described, as are working habits, attitudes, moods, and emotional tension during the test situations. Usually a comment is made also about a child's level of knowledge—general information, vocabulary, school achievements, etc. To these descriptions is added what is known about attitudes and special stresses within the family, social conditions, past experiences. However,

---

[20] In a limited number of cases where an I.Q. rating is requested for administrative purposes, a note is added saying that in the estimation of the examiner this rating would correspond to an I.Q. range of, for example, 75 to 80.

for most readers no single psychological factor is meaningful unless it is shown in interaction with others in terms of a person's adjustment to the life situation in the past and present.

The report is aimed at conveying a plausible picture of the child as a person with his own distinct physical and psychological features, as he may act or develop in relation to his surroundings. Such descriptions in simple wording make the report more informative and interesting to more people than it would be if only those findings were reported that were obtained with methods of statistical precision. There are many clinical situations in the field we are dealing with where precise numerical ratings—even where obtainable—are less important than a reasonable estimate of a level of maturity qualified by descriptive details from varied viewpoints.

The work with handicapped children at the Children's Hospital usually involves varied professional workers to handle the specific difficulties and problems arising in connection with each case. The psychological report is used by many of them. Each is apt to read it from his own angle.

Some of the physicians may prefer to rely on one or another aspect of psychological evidence, the choice depending on their interests and special attitudes. Some pediatricians and some orthopedists are interested mostly in the estimated level of maturity and take it as a baseline from which to judge the child's rate of development now, and again later on. Some find psychological opinions or facts helpful in corroborating or refuting their own leads. Neurologists especially attach importance to psychological symptoms of sensory disturbances or of specific effects of brain injury. They seem convinced of the diagnostic importance and prognostic significance of factors such as perceptual distortions or attention defects. Frequently, the medical adviser may use other psychological evidence to steer him in his own conversations with the parents. Emotional factors that have come to light in the psychological interview may in many ways determine how and what he discusses with the parents regarding their plans and attitudes. If psychiatrists are dealing with specific behavior problems, they may use information regarding the child's level of maturity as a baseline from which to measure improvement in rate of development that may result from therapeutic intervention. Occasionally plans for psychotherapy may be altered if the psychological examination clearly shows evidence of brain injury. Social workers assisting in many situations make use of varied aspects of psychological reports. Information obtained on psychological conditions frequently seems to the social worker a good base from which to start interpretation of medical and psychological findings to the parents. Findings on intellectual and emotional conditions may offer support in conferences with school authorities when arrangements for special plans or adjustments are made. When discussing a child's behavior difficulties in school, social workers may point to deviations in functioning which may create difficulties in spite of normal I.Q. findings.

Physiotherapists also rely frequently on psychological evidence: they find that it helps explain some of the difficulties they may encounter in the treatment of a child. Often psychological conditions prove to be one of the main clues to lack of cooperation of child or parent. A child's resistance, a mother's apparent laxity, a slump in rate of progress may turn out to be results of special attitudes or relationships which were most obvious in the psychological interview.

Teachers in or outside the hospital usually appreciate psychological reports which go beyond the statement of test results proper. These may help to clear their doubts or explain some vaguely noticed but puzzling deviations which intelligence ratings alone might have failed to explain. On this basis a teacher may be able to plan special concessions for some child or feel encouraged to give special attention to another severely handicapped one who, without this type of psychological appraisal, might be excluded from educational opportunities because he cannot be tested by ordinary methods.

Besides their practical value to nonpsychological colleagues, our studies seem to have varied merits for the psychologists among us.

Among the practical and immediate demands after each psychological examination is the customary discussion of the results with parents. Test findings may be used to interpret some of the family's immediate problems, such as behavior difficulties or failure in school. Often some of the everyday difficulties can be explained and distress about them can be alleviated when the parents are enabled to see them in a broader context. The psychologist can coordinate her own observations and those of the parents, can try to interpret these observations or to compare the patient's situation with a normal child's life. Usually these discussions are effective only if a parent can feel that the examiner really has come to know the child and does not judge his actions from the "tests" only. Many parents of younger children find it easier to accept opinion or advice if they have been present during the examination and can see for themselves that the child gave a true picture of his behavior and his skills.

Frequently, the psychological study involves a request to predict the future. Caution and restraint are necessary for a number of reasons: often the psychologist may be asked about mental ability and educational potentialities only. However, the question—whether, for instance, a child may be expected to finish high school—usually conceals broader issues: most parents and other interested people would like to know what kind of person a child can be expected to become, what kinds of adjustments he will be able to make, and how to help him to develop most satisfactorily. There may be some tentative answers for the question about mental potentialities. The level of maturity as it is revealed in the course of the study may reflect the rate of development up to that time; measure and quality of learning ability may show the rate and manner in which new acquisitions are apt to be made. For most initiates, these findings tend in the majority of cases to imply tacitly what may be expected in the future. However, definite statements and far-reaching predictions frequently seem premature. Except in some few isolated and clear-cut cases, less categorical pronouncements are in order. An offer to reappraise the situation after an interval of a year or so is sounder and in many distressing cases more humane. Even where predictions about mental development can be made with reasonable certainty on the basis of one examination, they alone are not the answer to the questions concerning adjustment in the future. This depends on, besides test results, many other factors which are more difficult to assess. Many of these elude all customary techniques (including projective techniques). A forecast of what a child of five years may be like at ten would have not only to take into account what he can or cannot do, can or cannot understand, feel or stand now or later, but also it would have to consider what a child's life may be then compared with now, what his parents and teachers will have wanted, thought, and felt about him in the intervening years. It would have to add hunches about what attitudes the child may develop under the conditions, stresses, and needs which he may encounter. The following example chosen from many may help to illustrate this important point.

Certain types of brain-injured children excel in verbal facility and superficial social skills, but have considerable difficulty in reasoning and learning. Frequently, they are found by many to be charming and able while they are young; they may seem embarrassingly verbose to the same people a few years later. Often their vivaciousness is encouraged by their elders earlier in life, but curbed later on. The same children may get along well with any superficial acquaintance, but not with persons whom they meet often. As a member of a family that finds social hyperresponsiveness a virtue, a child of this type may be adored all along, whereas he may seem a bore and a liability in a more demanding, intellectual environment. He may succeed well in a school that stresses learning by rote, whereas he is apt to fail in another that requires independent constructive thinking. He may be happy-go-lucky, comfortable, and proud of himself most of his life, or he may become insecure, tense, and essentially miserable as he becomes more aware of his shortcomings.

Considerations of similarly complex factors enter into advice about how to give a child—especially a handicapped one—the best opportunity for social development and education. Besides information about what he may be able to absorb, the psychological study may show to some extent how he may react under certain circumstances. Judging from his behavior, one may find that he is emotionally ready or not for school entrance, can learn alone but not in groups, can take more responsibility, be trusted away from home, etc. However, any plan proffered is doomed to failure unless it fits into the emotional, social, and economic scheme of the family, or can be combined with the child's physical limitations or the medical expectations for him. Moderate solutions that seem reasonable and acceptable to all are usually better and longer lasting than radical plans made in sudden bursts of enthusiasm or sacrifice. Among the many things we learned from Dr. Crothers' contacts with parents was to ask them what they would like to do before entering into discussions about what might be done.

The methods and findings of our psychological examinations passed many informal tests of reliability through the years. The opinions of psychologists were in most cases corroborated by those of other professional workers, were often agreed with by parents at the time of examination or later on, and were most frequently confirmed by subsequent events. Accuracy in the estimates of mental efficiency, which naturally was one of the most stringent requirements of our unorthodox methods, was many times confirmed in various ways.

Some children who were for one or another reason "untestable" by ordinary methods when young, later had more formal reappraisal.

Whether they were tested with one of the Wechsler scales, with the Stanford-Binet, or with others of the accepted test scales, by any of the psychologists at the hospital or on the outside, their test scores generally confirmed the previous findings. Their general development and their academic achievements were in many cases further proof of the reliability of our original estimates.

Some other children were physically too handicapped when young to be tested with ordinary methods. This was still the case when they were older. However, in the meantime they had given ample evidence that the early optimistic predictions of psychologists were justified. Their families and teachers now were convinced of their good comprehension and learning ability, perhaps in spite of their total or partial inability to speak. Repeat examinations in such cases also showed their steady progress in maturity of thought.

Other children—notably those recovering from severe infections or traumata—could and had responded to ordinary procedures and had seemed adequate mentally when examined with one of the test scales. At the same time they had demonstrated deviations in some areas of functioning when tested and appraised with special methods. As these children grew older, these irregularities kept interfering with their progress. Their difficulties showed that psychologists were justified in attaching prognostic importance to such earlier specific findings as lapses in attention and deficient perceptual skills.

Such cases increased confidence in the methods and in the importance of the findings. At the same time, they gave opportunity to learn from lags or failure. At the Children's Hospital it is customary to have many of the patients return frequently for reappraisal. Return visits which included psychological reevaluation were very instructive for the clinicians: reexamination showed which of the procedures that had been used previously had best predictive value for intellectual competence as well as for particular aspects of development. In consequence, as experience collected, some methods and some viewpoints were given more stress, others less. New procedures were introduced, and new overall questions asked: for instance, the opportunity to become reacquainted with children who had been seen several years earlier often allowed the psychologist to see striking changes in the emotional attitude of a child or of his parents. Often, such attitudinal changes were found basically to result from changed demands due to new conditions, as well as to the fact that all—parents and child—were growing older. Some of these considerations helped us later to form new and possibly better judgements with regard to outlook and goal. Reexaminations also taught us, in the cases of severely handicapped children especially, to pay closer attention to auditory and visual difficulties which had not been sufficiently recognized in earlier examinations by either medical or psychological advisers.

A methodological approach which is out to obtain and use clues from many sources keeps incorporating new interests and new views into its field of inquiry. This stimulating effect adds to its value, as did the gratifying enthusiasm and devotion of a selected group of students and assistants.

The idea of writing a book about our methods and experiences grew slowly. It gained momentum through a systematic follow-up project on patients suffering from cerebral palsy that was started in our group in 1951 by Dr. Crothers. With the help of various collaborators—most notably among them, Dr. Richmond S. Paine[21]—the cases of over 1,800 patients were reviewed. All these had been seen at the Children's Hospital, many as Dr. Crothers' private patients. The oldest records dated back to the 1920's. While many patients had not been seen or heard of for many years, others had been reexamined or seen for the first time within the last few years. In order to find out what had become of these patients and to ask whether it would be possible for them to return for a medical reevaluation, 1,821 letters were written. Over two thirds of these letters were answered by the patients or their families; 615 patients were reexamined—most of them at the hospital, some at home, and a group of about 90 at institutions.[22]

All information obtained in this review of cases within the years 1951–1955 was compared with findings recorded earlier in the medical records. This study afforded an unusual opportunity to appraise varied developmental data on a large number of patients who had shown deviations from normal earlier in childhood. All cases had originally been medical patients with specific complaints and specific symptoms; they returned as individuals of their own accord or that of their families. These facts gave a wide scope to the study, but also imposed limitations on the research and its methods.

[21] Bronson Crothers and Richmond S. Paine, *The Natural History of Cerebral Palsy* (Cambridge, Massachusetts: Harvard University Press, 1959). This study was jointly supported by grants from the U.S. Public Health Service and the United Cerebral Palsy Association.

[22] Of the 746 patients heard from by letter only, 445 were living at home, 118 were in institutions, and 183 had died.

One of the primary purposes of the follow-up examination was the medical study. Thanks to Dr. Crothers' personal inclinations and approach, importance was given also to social aspects, including intellectual competence, competitive status, economic situation, and emotional attitudes of patient and family.

With the few exceptions mentioned, each patient spent nearly a full day at the hospital. Each examination consisted invariably of a medical-neurological survey and an intensive interview with the patient, his parents, or both. The majority of cases also had an electroencephalogram and a psychological examination; auditory tests, orthopedic consultations, and x-rays were done when indicated. Photographs and movies were taken of a large number of patients; these were to show gait, posture, and often behavior and skill in daily activities such as eating, dressing, and playing. Parents and patient had opportunity to confer individually with various people; besides the doctors and psychologist, they talked at length with a nurse specially skilled in the problems of neurological patients.[23]

Within the framework of this study, the psychological examination was intended primarily to establish facts about a patient's intellectual competence; data concerning his emotional stability, his attitudes toward his own physical situation or his family, his emotional attachments, his social ties, and his expectations of life were to be gathered incidentally and informally rather than systematically. The psychologist's findings and judgement on these matters were integrated into the body of information that had been gathered by all other workers.

The restricted use of psychological methods within this study was dictated by many practical reasons: limitation of time and staff and the essentially medical purpose and orientation of the investigation. Also, in many of the emotionally explosive situations, restraint of psychological curiosity was imposed by a researcher's responsibility not to upset a precarious emotional equilibrium which he might be in no position to reestablish afterwards.

For the purpose of this study those methods were given preference that yielded the most quantitative data. Psychological examination was

---

[23] Miss Barbara Sikes, R.N. was for many years Dr. Crothers' competent and devoted assistant. She took a keen interest in each patient and his particular circumstances. She and Mrs. Barbara Baker, Research Assistant, were largely responsible for the organization of most practical details. Through their warmth and understanding both contributed much to the comfort of the families, the atmosphere of the visits, and the success of the study.

centered around one of the current test scales wherever feasible. With many of the older patients, the Wechsler-Bellevue Intelligence Scale was used, with others the Wechsler Intelligence Scale for Children. With children under seven years of age, the Revised Stanford-Binet Scale was used. Where physical situation, emotional status, or time did not allow the administration of the whole scale, certain areas were selected and results prorated. These tests were supplemented by varied other procedures (described elsewhere) to examine perceptual skills, learning ability, attention spans, etc.[24] With a few seriously defective patients examinations were abbreviated, and intellectual level was estimated to the best of the psychologist's ability. Also omitted was formal examination of a small number of adult patients whose academic and professional records vouched for their intellectual competence and allowed accurate enough estimate. Most of these were interviewed by psychologists. Those patients whose medical examination took place at home or at the institutions to which they had been transferred were not examined by psychologists connected with this study. In the latter cases, psychological examinations administered at the institutions were considered evidence for classification.

Results of all psychological appraisals were classified in the following groups: superior, average, borderline, defective, low-grade defective. In terms of I.Q., these categories represented the equivalents of over 110, 90–110, 70–90, 50–70, and below 50. Special difficulties in functioning, such as perceptual difficulties, attention defects, and impaired learning ability, were, if present, reported as mild, moderate, or severe, or otherwise qualified, or their nonexistence was mentioned in the report. All personality descriptions and comments on working habits, moods, emotional reactions, etc., were reported in qualitative terms. The psychological examinations were all administered by qualified clinical psychologists. The largest number of examinations was in the hands of assistants and psychological interns, whereas a small number, especially of very young patients or those with severe handicaps, was examined by myself. With a few exceptions, none of the junior psychologists had seen any of their patients before.

Rudimentary as the reported results of psychological studies seemed to the psychologists themselves, they essentially fulfilled the purpose

---

[24] In a small number of patients, examinations by the Rorschach method were done in addition. These were later discarded, as they were found to be too time-consuming and often disturbing to the patients.

TABLE 1. Intellectual competence of cerebral palsied patients, by medical classification group

Intellectual competence category	Spastic hemiplegic group		Spastic triplegic-tetraplegic group		Group with pure extrapyramidal involvement		Group with mixed extrapyramidal and pyramidal involvement	
	No.	%	No.	%	No.	%	No.	%
Superior	9	5	3	3	11	12	1	2
Average	44	24	9	10	31	33	19	32
Borderline	57	30	14	16	20	22	12	20
Defective	39	21	23	28	19	20	14	24
Low-grade defective	38	20	37	43	12	13	13	22
Total	187	100	86	100	93	100	59	100

of the medical research intended. In general they helped to corroborate and illuminate what was otherwise known about the patient through report, academic record, or unofficial appraisal.

The findings concerning intellectual competence were largely in agreement with those of other studies made on similar cases under more rigid conditions.[25] The results showed, as others have reported, that among a group of persons suffering from cerebral palsy the incidence of mental deficiency is about 50%. If special medical classifications are considered separately, one finds among the spastic groups (those with pyramidal tract lesions) a higher percentage of defective individuals. Among the spastics, there is a higher percentage of individuals with superior or average intellectual competence in the hemiplegic group than in the triplegic-tetraplegic group, though there is in both groups a higher percentage of persons with borderline abilities than in a normal population. Among patients with extrapyramidal involvement, those with "pure" extrapyramidal, rather than "mixed" extrapyramidal and pyramidal, involvement have the highest incidence of superior and average abilities of all groups and the lowest incidence of perceptual distortions. Table 1 (adapted from the Crothers and Paine study) is based on 425 of the evaluations which were done by psychologists and by them considered reliable and representative.

[25] Florence E. Schonell, *Educating Spastic Children* (New York: Philosophical Library, 1956). Using the Stanford-Binet Scale, Schonell also found no significant difference between test results obtained by rigid testing and those yielded by modified procedures or by estimated I.Q. ratings. See also Viola E. Cardwell, *Cerebral Palsy: Advances in Understanding and Care* (New York: Association for the Aid of Crippled Children, 1956), p. 341.

For the psychologists among us, the most immediate interest of the follow-up study concerned facts other than those just mentioned. In all cases where previous psychological examinations had been recorded, comparison between results and impressions then and later were a matter of course. These comparisons yielded information similar to that afforded by the ordinary reappraisals described earlier, though on a larger scale. In the present study the time elapsed between examinations often was considerably greater than in routine reappraisals. The fact that psychological examiners not familiar with the child were in charge of the re-evaluations added another element of objectivity. Also, there was usually here more medical and social information available than was customary in ordinary medical records. Some of these advantages offset the disadvantages which resulted from pressure of time and numbers as well as from the narrowed field of psychological inquiry.

The validity of earlier estimates of intellectual competence was of great interest. Many of the older patients had been first examined by Dr. Lord or one of her few collaborators. A considerable number had been examined in their early childhood by myself or my assistants. Many children had been examined repeatedly later on by various psychologists. In most of these cases, judgements had been based on the specialized, adapted procedures which had become routine in our work.

The general impression was that earlier estimates made by psychologists even on patients with severe physical handicaps stood up surprisingly well. In many instances their constancy was greater than that of some of the medical findings. They also surpassed in many cases predictions of future competence that had been made by medical men alone without the help of psychologists. The constancy of some of the psychological findings raised various interesting theoretic questions which are not to be discussed here. The practical value which comes from the proof of constancy is considerable, especially with the type of work under discussion. Comparison between early and later estimates of intellectual competence confirmed claims made frequently in our group by doctors as well as by psychologists that even with "untestable" cases a resourceful and competent psychologist can arrive at a reasonably accurate estimate of mental competence at an early age and thereby can help considerably in the management of the case. In our particular situation it also proved that the special methods which we had chosen had been adequate to meet the demands and could be improved by more experience.

Table 2, developed by Dr. Paine, attempts to show quantitatively the results of comparison between the original and later examinations. Data in this table are based on 214 cases who were reevaluated in the follow-up study and had been seen by one of the psychologists of the hospital from three to twelve years earlier. With a very few exceptions these earlier appraisals were done when the children were under six years of age. Most of the reexaminations were made at ages ranging from ten to twenty years. In the table, the cases are grouped according to medical classifications; the over-all results of the two evaluations are compared in terms of the intellectual competence category in which they place the child.[26]

Table 2 shows that of a total of 214 cases, 157 (73%) are in the same category in both examinations; 33 (15%) are in a lower category; and 24 (11%) are in a higher one. Comparison according to medical classification shows that in the hemiplegic group and the group with mixed extrapyramidal and pyramidal involvement 76% of the cases are in the same category at follow-up as they were at original examination. In the triplegic-tetraplegic group and the group with pure extrapyramidal involvement 71% of the cases are in the same category at follow-up. Of the 57 cases found to be in a different category at follow-up, 53 are in the next higher or next lower category. The greatest number of cases that are higher at follow-up than at original examination occur in the group with pure extrapyramidal involvement. The lowest number of disagreements between original and follow-up examinations occurs in the hemiplegic group and the group with mixed extrapyramidal and pyramidal involvement.

What these figures indicate may be expressed differently, as follows: in 57 cases (those in categories "average" and "superior") the psychologist could assure parents and doctors before the child was of school age that it was of normal intelligence (in 9 cases of superior intelligence). Forty of these children developed as well and 2 even better than anticipated (a total of 42 children or 72% of the 57 cases). In 107 cases the psychologist believed the child to be mentally defective at an early age. In 91 (85%) of these cases, this evaluation was proved correct by subsequent events. Of 50 children who were originally considered borderline cases (between defective and normal) 6 were better de-

---

[26] The category of "low-grade defective" had to be excluded, since differentiation between "defect" and "low-grade defect" is meaningless and unreliable in handicapped children of preschool age, except in some isolated cases.

veloped when reexamined than they had seemed before; 18 were more noticeably defective than they had appeared when younger; 26 remained in the borderline category.

It is not easy to determine for each case the extent to which the differences between original and later examinations result from the child's

TABLE 2. Comparison of early and later estimates of intellectual competence

Intellectual competence category	No. of cases in each category, original examination	No. of cases in same category at follow-up	No. of cases in different category at follow-up	
			Higher	Lower
Hemiplegic group				
Superior	4	2	0	2
Average	17	13	1	3
Borderline	19	11	1	7
Defective	27	25	2	0
	67	51 (76%)	4 (6%)	12 (18%)
Tri/tetraplegic group				
Superior	0	0	0	0
Average	6	2	1	3
Borderline	14	4	4	6
Defective	39	36	3	0
	59	42 (71%)	8 (14%)	9 (15%)
Group with pure extrapyramidal involvement				
Superior	5	5	0	0
Average	13	10	0	3
Borderline	6	5	0	1
Defective	27	16	11*	0
	51	36 (70%)	11 (22%)	4 (8%)
Group with mixed extrapyramidal and pyramidal involvement				
Superior	0	0	0	0
Average	12	8	0	4
Borderline	11	6	1	4
Defective	14	14	0	0
	37	28 (76%)	1 (3%)	8 (21%)
Total	214	157 (73%)	24 (11%)	33 (15%)

* Five of these cases suffered from kernicterus.

Note: Ratings for the last examination were based on the numerical results that had been obtained (see page 25). For the earlier estimates many of the psychological reports had to be reclassified to match the present classification. The earlier data were all derived from clinical material. At the time of the first examination the psychologist tried to help in planning management and arranging for a setting in which the child might develop to the best of his potentialities in spite of physical handicap. At that early age it was not essential to predict exactly how bright a child with average abilities might turn out to be or just how defective a seriously retarded child might become. As has been pointed out elsewhere, psychological findings were not expressed in definite quantitative terms. Therefore, the classification done years later (by the medical investigator) is in some cases based on the "intent" of the psychological report found in the medical record; it does not represent a psychologist's research-oriented rating as it would if either longitudinal studies or methodological research had been planned from the beginning.

condition or from incorrect original appraisal. In a number of cases physical deterioration went with decline in mental alertness. In some others it seemed that improved physical condition and increased opportunity for experience had bettered the mental situation also. However, study of the psychological records reveals some other significant causes of possible errors. It appears that most of the disagreements are found in cases where the first examiner tended to place more emphasis on the child's ability to use or respond to language than on other signs of comprehension. For instance, the most flagrant disagreements between original and later estimates are found in the group with pure extrapyramidal involvement—often amongst the earliest patients. Of the 11 cases in this group who were originally thought to be defective but turned out to be of borderline (6) or average (5) intelligence when examined more than ten years later, 5 had by then proved to be deaf or hard of hearing. (Medically, they belonged in the kernicterus group.) The others all had more or less serious speech delays due to dysarthria. In some other instances where the original estimates were lower than the reevaluations, children classified in other medical groups had difficulty in speaking and learned to talk late. However, errors of prediction probably due to overemphasis on the importance of speech development also occurred with children who talked early. They had earned high ratings as young children because of their verbal fluency; later this facility was not as useful to them, since at higher age levels good performance is determined more by reasoning power than by fluency of speech alone.

The follow-up study furnished other information of interest about questions that had come up but could not be answered from our previous more incidental reevaluations of former patients. We had had many opportunities to convince ourselves that some of the special areas of functioning which we were accustomed to investigate in our patients were important for appraisal. However, seeing many children whose special constellation of difficulties limited their progress in childhood, some of us frequently wondered what some of these conditions might mean in the long range view. Would, for instance, perceptual distortion and attention defects be as handicapping in later years as in early childhood? Would physical factors, such as impaired motility and resulting dependence on others that may alter development at certain stages of early childhood, have the same impact later on? How would changes of any of these conditions be reflected in social adjustment and development? Dr. Crothers' study of a large number of cases that presented innumerable variations of circumstances helped us with some of these questions. From the group of cases for which repeated previous examinations had been recorded we could get some few answers, together with new questions. It became possible to trace the development of certain psychological facts common under certain circumstances in certain groups of children with similar conditions in spite of individual variations. The data available do not lend themselves to statistical treatment, since they derive from clinical observations and are by-products rather than research findings. Neither the earlier psychological examinations nor the psychological follow-up investigations were intended for this type of research. Nevertheless, it became possible to consider comparable cases in small groups and to describe in predominantly qualitative terms their psychological situations at varied stages of their development.

Aside from this factual interest, some of the descriptions included in this book may serve to stress the continuity of certain psychological phenomena. They also may help to show in our field the merits of a broad clinical approach that is specifically oriented toward the study of each child as an individual with his own particular circumstances.

The primary intent of this book is to advocate a clinical orientation that considers simultaneously many aspects of a patient's life situation without forfeiting the advantages of obtaining quantifiable data wherever possible.

At the initial stage of book planning, we intended merely to describe certain techniques that might in complicated cases make the clinician less dependent on the few available instruments by which to appraise psychological functioning. By describing some of the techniques which had proved useful to us, we hoped to revive parts of some of the older test scales or developmental studies that are not usually included in the equipment of present-day clinical psychologists. As was mentioned before, many of these procedures can be put to good use because of the suitability of their material and the age norms they provide. We planned, in addition, to describe various ways, tested in our own experience only, in which behavior manifestations of children could be elicited and studied through methods adapted from genetic studies and partly at least based on developmental norms. Other clinical child psychologists might then feel in a position to choose from this arsenal of tests those that seemed appropriate to an individual case.

However, it soon became clear to us that probably none of the methods we planned to describe could claim any special merits except in relation to their usefulness within the style of our examinations. For this reason, we decided to show separately the details and possibilities of specific methods and the ways in which they are being used in the total examining process. Therefore, a special section has been reserved for the presentation of techniques. In this section many varied test materials are described, and suggestions are offered about how to present them and what responses to look for. For each group of procedures are given some brief discussions of developmental processes that are involved. This should help to orient the reader and to give him leads with which to evaluate an individual performance. Established norms are quoted where they are available. For some of the variations and modifications of our own invention, the tentative norms developed through our own experience only are given and so designated. There is no attempt made anywhere to discuss any statistical rationale. The aim of the presentation of techniques is not to prescribe rigid rules, but to suggest ways in which to use materials as diagnostic tools.

Our own likes and prejudices are obviously reflected in the choice of the techniques that are presented here: much emphasis is placed on nonverbal techniques, especially on those suitable for children of younger age levels. The grouping of materials is done by functional entities, such as "following, finding, retrieving," or "matching, sorting, grouping." This arrangement seemed practical even if there is naturally much overlapping, since one type of procedure may in some ways fit under one or the other heading. Why one technique has been described in one group rather than in another is subject to much argument and theoretic quibbling, which we hope to avoid by admitting how arbitrary our decisions often were. Aside from the functional groupings that form several chapters, three chapters are entitled, respectively, "Blocks," "Paper and Pencil," and "Pictures." There is no excuse for this except personal fancy based on fond memories of a former teacher who insisted that any child psychologist worth his salt should be able to evaluate a child reliably without any other equipment but paper, pencil, and a magazine. We added blocks.

Special techniques designed to investigate emotional development have been purposely omitted from this book. In our experience, most of the more common projective techniques failed to prove satisfactory with children with cerebral defects. Even where their use is technically possible, the results are often misleading and ambiguous because of the perceptual distortions that may prevail. The Rorschach method often can furnish meager findings only, which can be found with other non-projective methods as well. Interpretation of picture material as used in the TAT[27] or CAT[28] has similar defects. In this regard, further study is needed to learn more about this group of children. It would seem important, among other things, to determine whether and how children with perceptual distortions can identify with symbolized representations of people or interpret actions and events represented in pictures.

Just as descriptions of the tests would be valueless without reference to the style of our examining procedures, so enumeration of techniques would be meaningless without illustrations of their application to various clinical circumstances. Therefore, a selection has been made of some specific case situations that show most clearly how our methodological approach applies to varying physiological, psychological, and social conditions. By describing the same children at varying significant age levels, we hope to show the continuity in the method. For each child at each age level there is a detailed, running, play-by-play account of the psychological examination itself. This demonstrates the combination of interview, observation, and accumulation of measurable data that characterizes our approach. Why certain individual procedures are chosen by the examiner at certain points should—so it is hoped—become clear to the reader who follows the reasoning of the examiner, which gives unity to the examination. While each examination follows a plan that emerges from the individual situation, the reader may see a basic formula underlying the construction of most examinations. He may be interested in following in detail the description of all phases of all examinations; or he may choose to read the general descriptions and comments at various age levels only; or he may wish to concentrate on the sections headed "Stages of Development and Their Problems," which summarize impressions gained from study of children similarly impaired.

One of the aims of the presentation is to show the flexibility of the method, which allows a reasonably accurate appraisal even in so-called "untestable" cases. While the method is therefore especially suitable for children with neurological difficulties, it can provide useful

[27] H. A. Murray, *Thematic Apperception Test (and Manual)*, 3rd revision (Cambridge, Massachusetts: Harvard University Press, 1943).

[28] L. Bellak and S. S. Bellak, *Children's Apperception Test Manual* (New York: CPS, 1949). Also Raymond Holden, "The Children's Apperception Test with Cerebral Palsied Children," *Child Development*, Volume 27, Number 1, March 1956.

information on other patients with all kinds of disturbances of psychological functioning.

Of the seven cases which have been chosen as illustrations, four children are suffering from cerebral conditions dating from birth or before. They show behavior patterns and psychological difficulties characteristic of children with problems similar to theirs. Some of these may be apparent without intensive study, from descriptions and casual observations; others are brought into focus by the psychological examination. Each of these four children is described at fifteen months, at four years of age, at seven, and at twelve. Three other children described in an additional section illustrate situations resulting from injuries acquired at different ages. Each of these three children is described at several age levels following injury, at some with more detail than at others.

The form of presentation thought to be most effective necessarily points also to some of the most common problems that accompany neurological difficulties in children. It should help to convey how with advancing age some of the problems change complexion with the changing emotional climate that surrounds the child. It should also show how acquired injuries may affect development in different ways, depending on the age of the child, the attitudes of the people around him, and the type and severity of impairment. For three of the cases of cerebral palsy due to birth injury, some of the previously mentioned material from Dr. Crothers' follow-up study may help to show parallel developments in groups of children with comparable physical and mental situations.[29] For the fourth child injured from birth, material from ordinary hospital records furnishes similar though less detailed evidence.

The special physical, mental, and social conditions illustrated by the case portraits were selected not because they occur most frequently in practice, but because they show distinct differences in the constellation of psychological problems and make different demands of the examiner. The psychological situations illustrated cover only a small fraction of those which the clinician may find in pediatric neurology in general, in cerebral palsy in particular, in pediatric psychiatry, or in the education of children with cerebral defects. But the cases described

---

[29] The criteria for the selection of cases for this purpose were the following: those children were chosen who fitted the same medical classification and had within limits similar physical or mental situations. We had to restrict ourselves to a more or less limited number of cases for which we had well-documented records of several psychological examinations at significant intervals done by reliable examiners with methods relevant to those described.

here often may resemble those of other patients with similar problems in other combinations.

The children described in the case portraits are the following.

(1) Paul is a boy with a left spastic hemiplegia caused by birth injury.[30] In spite of intellectual abilities only somewhat below the normal limits, he shows psychological distortions and behavior difficulties that might easily pass unnoticed in examination with conservative test scales alone.

(2) Bobby is a severely handicapped boy with an extrapyramidal cerebral palsy and severe athetosis and dysarthria.[31] Unable to walk or to use his hands and hardly able to talk, he presents a difficult problem in testing, though he obviously has good intellectual endowment.

(3) Jimmy has a moderately severe extrapyramidal cerebral palsy with some athetosis.[32] His problems are intensified by an almost complete lack of communication caused by auditory difficulties of the kind often associated with a history of erythroblastosis fetalis with kernicterus. His irregular intellectual development, together with his behavior difficulties, present serious impediments to appraisal.

(4) John is a boy with hydrocephalus and serious motor involvement of the lower extremities.[33] Though seemingly alert, socially responsive, and talkative, he has serious intellectual limitations which are

[30] Of 469 patients reexamined and reclassified as cerebral palsied in Dr. Crothers' follow-up study, 189 (40%) were spastic hemiplegics. Of these, 58 (approximately 30%) had mental abilities on the borderline level, like Paul. In 115 of these cases (61%), motor impairment was classified as moderately severe. Of 92 children under 12 years of age, 16 (17%) were "competitive with concessions" whereas 36 (39%) were considered "noncompetitive."

[31] Of the 469 patients reexamined and reclassified as cerebral palsied in Dr. Crothers' follow-up study, 164 (35%) had extrapyramidal lesions, of which 103 (24%) were classified as non-mixed, as in Bobby's case. Of the 93 of this group who were given psychological examinations, 31 (33%) had average intellectual abilities, while 11 (12%) had above average abilities. Dysarthria and athetosis were each classified as severe in, respectively, 37% and 40% of the cases. Of 46 children under 12 years of age, 10 (28%) were considered competitive, whereas 11 (31%) were considered competitive with concessions only.

[32] Of 103 cases with pure extrapyramidal cerebral palsy seen in Dr. Crothers' follow-up study, 20 (19%) were thought to be due to neonatal erythroblastosis with kernicterus. Of 35 patients with known kernicterus, 12 (40%) had normal mental ability, like Jimmy, as against 11 (37%) with borderline ability. Hearing loss was severe in 28 (80%) and was considered questionable in 7 (20%) of these cases. Motor impairment was moderately severe in 6 (17%), as in Jimmy's case, but severe in 10 (28%) and mild in 19 (54%). See also Randolph K. Byers, Richmond S. Paine, and Bronson Crothers, "Extrapyramidal Cerebral Palsy with Hearing Loss Following Erythroblastosis," *Pediatrics* 15:248–254, March 1955.

[33] Traits similar to those illustrated by John were described as characteristic of hydrocephalic patients by Ford, by Kanner, and by other workers. See F. R. Ford, *Diseases of the Nervous System in Infancy, Childhood, and Adolescence* (Springfield, Illinois: Thomas, 1952), p. 252; Leo Kanner, *Child Psychiatry* (Springfield, Illinois: Thomas, 1948), p. 265. The frequency of paraplegia as a neurological complication

not necessarily represented in numerical test results obtained in preschool years.

(5) Ann, a normal baby at birth, had pneumococcus meningitis[34] at six months of age. She shows characteristic deviations that may occur after a serious infectious disease in infancy.

(6) Rose, having had measles encephalitis[35] at five years of age, from then on has had increasingly obvious learning difficulties which are reflected in her general behavior and which are not uncommon in children who progress normally up to the time of a serious trauma.

(7) Jack, after a head injury[36] at seven years of age, has had stormy years of unsatisfactory personality development which, though perhaps latent before, was apparently intensified by aftereffects of the accident. He demonstrates the complications that may result when an insult to the nervous system upsets a delicate equilibrium achieved between a child and his environment.

The portraits of Paul, Bobby, Jimmy, and John are to some extent "ideal type" constructions rather than actual case reports. They are based on experiences with many cases of the same kind. This

---

of congenital hydrocephaly has been discussed by Paul Yakolev, "Paraplegia in Hydrocephalus," *American Journal of Mental Deficiency* 51:561–576, April 1947.

[34] In a paper delivered at the 55th meeting of the American Pediatric Society in 1948 in Quebec we reported about periodic reexaminations and follow-up studies of 105 children who had been ill with various forms of meningitis. Evidence of severe brain damage was found in 40% of children who had had pneumococcus meningitis before the age of two years. (See John A. V. Davies, Edith Meyer, and Harriet Hyde, "Follow-Up Study of Patients Who Have Recovered from Meningitis," *American Journal of Diseases of Children* 79:958–961, March 1950, Society Transactions.) In subsequent unpublished follow-up studies of children since 1949, the incidence of severe damage was found to have diminished, although it continues to be considerably higher than in some other forms of meningitis.

[35] The consequences of measles encephalitis in children were studied in a joint investigation with Dr. Randolph K. Byers (see Edith Meyer and Randolph K. Byers, "Measles Encephalitis: A Follow-Up Study of Sixteen Patients," *AMA American Journal of Diseases of Children* 84:543–579, November 1952). It was found that in some serious cases psychological irregularities tend to outlast medical findings. The character of the psychological deviations may vary with the age of the child and also seem to depend on individual differences. Of nine children who had a protracted course of measles encephalitis, all six who were under seven years of age showed psychological deviations. With three of them, the outcome in terms of social behavior was considered good, with two bad, and with one poor.

[36] The consequences of head injuries in children are well known and have been described by various authors. Because of the many gradations in severity of injury and resulting symptoms, it is hardly possible to estimate the number of instances in which situations similar to Jack's occur. However, problems like his are familiar to many workers in child guidance clinics. See Lauretta Bender, *Psychopathology of Children with Organic Brain Disorders* (Springfield, Illinois: Thomas, 1955). Also Bronson Crothers and Elizabeth Lord, "Appraisal of Intellectual and Physical Factors after Cerebral Damage in Children," *American Journal of Psychiatry* 94:1077–1088, March 1938. Also Kurt Goldstein, *Aftereffects of Brain Injuries in War* (New York: Grune and Stratton, 1942).

method was chosen in order to bring out more clearly than any actual particular case study would do certain important points. The case portraits of Ann, Rose, and Jack are based on actual cases.

All portraits are designed to point out the chief problems of these children as we saw them and also the examining procedures that helped to identify them best. The case portraits should also show how all concerned try to cope with problems, to remedy some, and to circumvent others. How modest such efforts have to be, and how frustrating the results often are, may also be apparent through many of the presentations. Since no ready-made solution of some problems ever seems to exist, definite prescriptions will be avoided and a general attitude in the management of our patients only implied.

It has been mentioned before that the views and methods discussed here may apply to other kinds of cases as well. For instance, the large group of cerebral palsied children with tetraplegia (Tables 1 and 2) may combine various features described in the case portraits. Varied degrees of motor involvements, together with any of the psychological characteristics shown, may create similar problems and require comparable handling. Also the much-discussed group of children with brain injury but without appreciable physical defects[37] may in their combination of distorted functioning in behavior and learning call for some of the considerations discussed here.

[37] See Alfred A. Strauss and Laura E. Lehtinen, *Psychopathology and Education of the Brain-Injured Child,* Volume I (New York: Grune and Stratton, 1947); and Alfred A. Strauss and Newell C. Kephart, *Psychopathology and Education of the Brain-Injured Child,* Volume II (New York: Grune and Stratton, 1955).

Part One

CASE PORTRAITS

A—Defects Dating from Birth or Before

PAUL

Spastic Hemiplegia

Paul was born with a spastic left hemiplegia which has retarded his development and created behavior problems. His main deficiencies in mental functioning are short attention spans and inability to organize perceptual clues. These result in considerable difficulties whenever he has to understand, judge, or adapt to situations which involve complex relationships, whether intellectual, emotional, or social. He functions easily, however, when he can respond directly and immediately in relatively simple circumstances. As he gets older and life becomes more demanding, his assets and liabilities change in relative importance and appear in a different light.

His motor difficulty and his responsive attitude make him appealing as a baby. They outshine his immature and undifferentiated approach to his environment. He is still hyperresponsive at four years of age. He is easily excitable and becomes overwrought and difficult when he meets many stimuli at once; he is unable to organize them properly and becomes anxious and frightened when he does not understand. He is baffled by the demands of those around him and also by their reactions to his shortcomings. By seven years of age he has learned to respond with more equanimity to routine social requirements and has become more secure in his relationships to people. His learning difficulties are now his chief problem and a source of frustration for himself and his family. At twelve years of age his lag in social and intellectual comprehension becomes increasingly detrimental to future development. His sensitivity to pressure increases; the simple tools of adjustment which he is able to manage fit him for only a limited range of life situations.

41

Using Paul's case as an illustration, this chapter presents a description of the psychological study of a child with spastic hemiplegia and irregularity of mental functioning. This detailed account of the examination procedures at various ages illustrates how the special character of Paul's cognitive functions is revealed in his behavior as well as in his performances in various test situations. It shows how findings of the examination used as a frame of reference can help to interpret the emotional climate, attitudes, and specific problems that appear at each stage of Paul's development. The last section of the chapter describes the stages and problems of development illustrated by Paul and found, when compared with other case records, to be prevalent in children with similar difficulties. It shows also how certain responses in specific test situations seem to be characteristic for this group, how they vary with age, and how at each stage they can be understood as coherent and representative of psychological factors which determine the child's adjustment to his life situation at the time. This section also points to the questions and problems parents and doctors most commonly bring to the psychologist's attention and briefly shows how findings and interpretations of the psychological study are used as a basis for guidance.

PAUL AT FIFTEEN MONTHS

Paul is the second of two boys, the other one being seven years older. A left hemiplegia was first noticed at the age of five months when he used his right hand exclusively for reaching. In early infancy the child kicked with his right foot more than with his left. Now, at fifteen months, the left hand is always held fisted. The baby was late in sitting, but has been sitting independently since ten months of age. He still has some difficulty in pulling up to a sitting position and when he stands he does not support his weight on his left leg. He has never crept, but started to propel himself on his buttocks, using his right hand as support. Lately he has become more active than he was. He has no words, vocalizes some, has perhaps said "Mama" a few times; he does not yet have any reliable tricks. His parents find him sweet and pleasant, but much slower in development than their other boy. They are delighted that he is getting livelier now. He has more interest in toys now, though they find that he still puts most things in his mouth. He likes to be played with and to watch things in motion. He then gets excited, bounces and laughs, and even occasionally becomes a bit hysterical.

In the psychological examination he shows the following behavior.

When blocks (see Techniques: Chapter I:1[1]) are offered to him one after another, he reaches for the first block with his right hand, puts it in his mouth, reaches with the same hand for the second block, places it on the table, reaches for the third one, and puts it on the table. The Examiner[2] removes the first block from the child's mouth; he does not object, but grasps for the second block and then reaches for the next one. He does nothing else with any of the blocks, loses interest, smiles, and turns to his mother. (His behavior in this situation compares with that of normal children of approximately ten months of age.)

When a red plastic ring is offered to him and then hidden under a nearby cloth (T:V:4) he seems to like the ring, grasps it with his right hand, starts to put it in his mouth, gives it up easily when E reaches for it, smiles, follows her movements when the ring is hidden under the cloth in front of him to his right. He starts pulling at the cloth, plays with the corner of it, becomes absorbed in this activity and apparently forgets the ring. (His interest and comprehension in this situation are at approximately the ten-month level.)

He shows similar immature behavior in the next situation. When a small white pellet is placed in front of the child, he grasps the pellet awkwardly with thumb opposing fingers, drops it, does not try to retrieve it, forgets about it, and looks for another one. When a bottle is presented with another pellet beside it (T:V:8), he is very interested in the bottle. He mouths the bottle and pays no attention to the pellet. When E puts the pellet in the bottle and then empties it out, he does not seem to notice the pellet. He watches E's manipulations, gets hold of the bottle again, but shows no interest in combining the two objects. (Behavior below twelve-month level.)

Presented with the red ring with string attached (T:V:6) he reaches not for the string but directly for the ring even though it is out of his reach. Then he discovers the string, plays with its end, looks surprised when he dislodges the ring, happily manipulates it, bangs it on the table top, loses it, and looks for it. When the situation is repeated, he again reaches directly for the ring and shows no interest in the string. (Behavior at approximately ten-month level.)

When given the Wallin pegboard A (a wooden board with six round

[1] Hereinafter "Techniques" will be referred to as T, and the chapter by its number. All test materials and procedures mentioned in connection with the case portraits (Part One) are described in detail in the chapters on techniques (Part Two). Complete information concerning the sources of these materials and procedures is also given in Part Two.

[2] Hereinafter "Examiner" will be referred to as E.

holes in which fit wooden pegs, T:IV:1), he grasps the peg offered
to him, and puts it in his mouth. E points to the hole, he grasps her
pointing finger, laughs, takes the peg out of his mouth, throws it playfully, apparently expecting E to pick it up for him. E places the peg
in one hole, baby tries to remove it; at first is unsuccessful, then suddenly pulls it out, seems surprised, throws it again. Starts playing with
the board, pokes his fingers in the holes. A peg is offered to him again
and placed in the board before his eyes; another peg presented to him is
ignored. He seems to get bored and somewhat restless. (Behavior below fifteen-month level.)

Shown a picture book (*What Baby Sees,* a book with six to eight
pictures of common objects on each page, T:II:1,2), he grasps the book
in his right fist, waves it back and forth. The book opens; he pats the
pages without looking at any pictures. E points to a picture of a dog; he
starts playing with her finger again and pats the book as before. He
vocalizes some undifferentiated "da-da-da" as he has at various times
during the observation period. (Behavior at approximately ten-month
level.)

COMMENT

From this brief observation period E concludes that Paul is a pleasant,
lively baby who seems to enjoy being with people and does not discriminate between familiar ones and strangers. He is socially responsive and
is not resistant to interference by adults. He seems somewhat vague.
He does not show much interest in anything outside his immediate range
of activity. He handles all objects alike—banging them or putting them
in his mouth without discrimination. He does not stay with any
activity for long and does not seem to learn easily from what he sees.
There is no evidence to show that his actual comprehension of situations might be more mature than his one-handed performances indicate. His general behavior, his interests, and his learning ability are all
at approximately the ten- to twelve-month level.

PAUL AT FOUR YEARS

The child walks with a marked left-sided limp; he has been getting
around more or less speedily since the age of twenty-two months. He uses
his right hand predominantly; the left is held fisted most of the time,
but he uses it to steady objects. He uses his left arm to help out and to
store things. He did not talk until he was thirty months old, but accord-

ing to his parents he talks fluently now. He does not converse about past events, but instead verbalizes on subjects within the immediate situation. He is described as being very lively, getting into everything, needing a lot of supervision. He does not stay with any one activity for long, and is, on the whole, not very reliable. While he was considered even tempered and easygoing in the past, he now is easily irritated and has frequent temper tantrums. Though one can easily distract him from what he wants, he is often insistent and whiny. His parents find him rather exhausting, though lovable. They feel that most of his difficulties are due to his excessive speed and impatience. He can be sent on errands in the house, but is liable to "forget"; he is described as "destructive," breaking his toys frequently, scribbling on walls, and scattering things. He does not get along well with other children; boys his own age overwhelm and overexcite him. He plays reasonably well with younger girls, but is occasionally too rough with them. Punishment does not seem to teach him, but is being practiced with some frequency from a sense of parental duty. Toilet training is still unreliable; there are "accidents" during the daytime and regular bed-wetting at night.

The psychological examination has to determine the child's intellectual and emotional situation. His mental functioning, including verbal and perceptual comprehension, appreciation of meaning, use of language, learning ability, and reaction to stress, has to be evaluated. This may help the psychologist to explain some of Paul's difficulties, to outline expectations for future development, and to advise about educational planning.

When the child enters the examining room, his mother tries to hold on to him. When she is asked to let him go, the child darts across the room toward some toy he has spied. Mother seats herself apprehensively; E sits down too and displays the test materials. Child is immediately attracted and rather soon responds to the invitation to be seated. E suggests that mother remain in the room but be as inconspicuous as possible, thus giving E a chance to establish her relationship with the child.

Seguin Formboard (T:IV:6)

A board 16 x 10 inches, with insets to fit ten forms (circle, oval, square, lozenge, elongated hexagon, rectangle, cross, triangle, star, half-disk).

Paul immediately picks up hexagon, tries it quickly in several places without any apparent preconceived idea. Says excitedly, "Where does this go?" without addressing himself to anyone in particular and without waiting for an answer. Releases hexagon and picks up another form. Proceeds as before, repeating, "Where does this go?" E hands him the circle and points toward the correct recess. Child fits it properly and seems pleased with success, relaxing somewhat. Seems to respond to E's quiet admonitions: "Take your time; look around and see first." Success with square, oval, and rectangle. Tries star in recess of cross, gets impatient and starts to work haphazardly, as before. E points toward correct spot. Child tries, but can't fit star properly; is helped, seems reassured, places cross without help. Tries triangle in lozenge, then lozenge in hexagon, gets impatient, tries to remove the ones he had placed by picking at them with his good hand. E helps him to turn the board over and begin again. (His behavior in this situation compares with that of normal children below the three-year level.)

When the Seguin formboard is repeated, Paul's performance is similar to the foregoing. He has learned almost nothing from his previous trial; most mistakes are repeated. When the child becomes restless, E tries to shorten the procedure, and helps him place the most difficult insets to give him some feeling of completion.

MATCHING COLORS (T:VI:2)

Four boxes, 3½ x 2 x 1 inches, each of a different color (red, yellow, green, and blue) and each containing six disks to match the color of the box; the boxes open like match boxes.

E starts to display the boxes. Paul grabs them, insisting, "Let me, let me." He pulls hard at the boxes. He is impetuous and awkward and does not realize the boxes open like match boxes. He almost ruins one of them. He picks up some assorted disks that came out of the boxes, and starts to collect them in his paralyzed left hand. (He opens the left hand with the right.) He no longer pays attention to the boxes. E demonstrates how to match the disks with the boxes. Paul becomes interested in the process of pushing disks into the boxes over their tops. He pays no attention to colors. E demonstrates with three more disks. The child tries to restrain her, insisting whiningly, "Let me do it, let me do it." After having placed a red disk again, E hands another red one to the child. He places it correctly, picks up more red ones, and boxes them all. When no red disk remains, he picks up a green one and places it in the red box. E says, "It does not go there." Paul remedies his error, then places two green ones and later several yellow ones correctly;

then he puts a blue disk in the green box and adds more blue ones. From then on he fills the blue box with assorted chips. He seems to have lost interest. (Behavior approximately below three-year level.)

PICTURE VOCABULARY AND MEMORY FOR PICTURES (T:II:7,8)

Black and white pictures of common objects, presented three, four, or five at a time; the child names them as they are laid out; one is taken away while he is not looking, and he must guess which picture has disappeared.

He names each picture with emphasis and assurance, tries to grab the cards and pile them. He becomes interested in the suggestion to "play a guessing game." He does not listen much to E's directions. Upon request, he enthusiastically closes his eyes tightly; then he turns to his mother to show her his eyes closed; he now becomes absorbed in this aspect of the "game." He does not open his eyes again until E asks him specifically to "look again." E asks, "Which one did I take away?" He points first to one of the remaining pictures and says, "This one." E shakes her head. He points to the other of the pictures left on the table and tries again, "This one." E asks, "Which one is in my hand?" He turns to her, tries playfully to grab the picture from her hand; she shows it to him, he names it triumphantly. The procedure is repeated with the same pictures and renewed explanations. A different picture is taken away. He still does not understand the game. All pictures of the set are shown to him one after another. He names twelve of seventeen pictures correctly. His errors are man for arm, fork for knife, lamp for telephone, dog for horse, and cake for cowboy hat. (While his behavior and comprehension on the memory procedure are below the three-year level, by Revised Stanford-Binet standards he reaches the four-year level in the naming of pictures.[3])

PICTURE BOOK

SPONTANEOUS (T:II:1). He names objects quickly and spontaneously without errors.

DIFFERENTIAL POINTING (T:II:4). ("Show the wheels of the wagon; the tail of the lamb, etc.") He points to the correct parts.

IDENTIFICATION (T:II:5). ("Which one do we eat with?"

---

[3] Here, as in all following instances where the Revised Stanford-Binet directions are not strictly adhered to, ratings by Stanford-Binet standards are used to help estimate levels of performance rather than to give absolute measures.

"Which one goes on our feet? etc.") He points correctly for all questions, including "Which one brushes your hair?" and "Which one combs
your hair?" but not "Which one fixes your hair?" He seems to expect a
question about a new object: he points to the toothbrush. After this he
gets tired of the task. He begins to point correctly to "all animals." On
the last pages, he quickly and without discriminating points to any
picture and says each time, "This is an animal." E asks, "Is it really?"
He becomes amused and continues playfully. Asked for "all things
to eat," he starts correctly, but in high mood, and hilariously designates
many nonsensical pictures. During the last tasks child has become very
excited and gets up from his chair.

Since he seems to need some outlet, a ball is introduced; he starts
to throw it roughly at E and then at his mother. E suggests that he roll
ball from one end of the table to the other. He becomes interested and
absorbed in this new game for a short while, then loses the ball and
returns to his chair in a quieter mood. E produces blocks. Since the
child has a tendency to easily become too exuberant, and since his staying power for any one material is short, E decides against spontaneous
block play.

BLOCKBUILDING (T:I:2 AND FIGURE 1)

THREE-BLOCK BRIDGE. Paul copies straight bridge immediately
but has difficulty with bridge with oblique top; he tries to give the two
base blocks some incline, but gives up and puts them in normal position. Then he tries to top them with third block poised at an angle.
Since the base blocks are too far apart to be bridged, they get pushed
further apart by his efforts. He tries to steady them with the help of his
left hand; the gap between the base blocks continues to be too wide.
He gives up. (His performance shows comprehension comparable with
that of normal three-year-olds.)

STRAIGHT BRIDGE (REPEATED FROM MEMORY). After a new
model has been removed, Paul places two blocks now without any gap
between them; on this he piles a wobbly structure of five blocks; they
fall; he gives up.

PUTTING BLOCKS IN BOX (T:I:3)

Paul throws all the blocks pellmell into the box and then gets up.

ANIMAL PICTURES (T:II:10)

Two cards with black and white pictures of twelve different animals. The child is to match these.

E says, "Find me one just like this one." He hardly listens, briefly surveys the cards, then looks around for something else to do. E says, "Look here, this is *my* rabbit, where is yours?" He responds now, and with obvious pleasure points to the correct picture, saying, "Here is mine." To "Here is my cat, where is yours?" he again responds correctly. Then he gets carried away by the game and points haphazardly to one animal after another, saying, "That is *my* cow and that one is *my* cow." At some point, he finds "his" elephant without error, but then goes on to point to different other animals, exclaiming, "This is *my* elephant and this is *my* elephant." (Behavior well below three-and-a-half-year level.)

WALLIN PEGBOARD C (T:IV:2)

A wooden board, 13½ x 3 x ½ inches, with three round and three square holes in which fit wooden pegs.

He works very quickly, picking up whichever peg is nearest to his reach, fills the holes in succession. Places round peg in square hole, is left with a square peg for a round hole, removes a round peg from its hole to try the square one instead. Similar trials which follow indicate his lack of comprehension of form relations. When finished, each hole has been filled by trial and error method. (Behavior at two-and-a-half- to three-year level.)

When the test is repeated, he uses the same working habits and gives no forethought to where the pegs might fit. He is again left with a square peg for a round hole and wants to give up; says, "They do not fit." E says, "You made them fit before." He starts again, but does not finish; is satisfied with the fact that "they do not fit."

PAPER AND PENCIL

IMITATING DIRECTIONS (T:III:4). He imitates horizontal and vertical scribbles and properly differentiates the two directions. He does not steady his paper with his left hand; E holds the paper in place for him. (Performance at two-and-a-half-year level.)

IMITATING SIMPLE FORMS (T:III:4). For cross, he marks two separate lines that do not intersect. For square he marks a round scribble. (Performance at two-and-a-half-year level.)

DRAWING A MAN (T:III:3B). He starts with a poorly drawn circle; says, "That is a man." E says, "Draw the very best man you can do." He produces another somewhat larger circular scribble and says, "That is a man." E: "Where are his legs?" He adds two lines which are vaguely parallel but not connected with the scribble: "Here are his legs." E: "And his mouth?" He draws a horizontal line above the scribble, then goes on distributing similar marks haphazardly on his paper. (Performance at three-year level.)

COMMENT

The psychological examination confirms many of the traits described by the parents; Paul is quick, impatient, and impetuous. In his desire to be independent, he gets himself into trouble; his motor awkwardness causes small accidents such as spilling and dropping of objects. He becomes disturbed in difficult situations and either tries to avoid them or becomes stubborn and excited. In the examination he tries to change activities after failure. He is very happy when he is successful and not critical about the level of his successes. His bouts of hilariousness and excitability, though not unusual for a child of his age, have an overly tense quality.

Paul has an adequate name vocabulary, but all through the examination his spontaneous remarks are restricted to expressing immediate desires rather than ideas. His ability to comprehend meaning is limited (identification); he also is slow in understanding complex situations and is carried away by any new stimulus. He does not learn easily from new experiences. His form comprehension is shown to be poor in his first trials and does not improve easily with repetition (Wallin pegboards, Seguin formboard, drawing). His comprehension of spatial relationships is weak (block bridge) and his motor deficit often hinders him in improving this comprehension by practical experience (oblique block bridge).

He is socially responsive, but in a primitive, immature, and demanding way. He seems interested only in immediate gratification of his wishes. In relation to a social partner, he responds to approval or disapproval but he seems insensitive to the more differentiated reactions which his behavior elicits.

His performances are very irregular and range from nearly adequate in vocabulary to a poor two-and-a-half- to three-year level in areas of ideation and perception. Poor attention spans, limited learning ability, and a lack of social sensitivity, together with awareness of his own shortcomings, will cause him many frustrations and difficulties and will make his educational career stormy.

PAUL AT SEVEN YEARS

Paul, now seven years old, still walks with a limp and uses his left hand very little. He has become more efficient in the use of his left arm. He uses it to carry objects by holding them pressed against his body with his upper arm. According to his parents, his behavior has improved when compared with three years ago. He obeys better and can be trusted. He stays with the same activity for longer periods; he still prefers rather simple toys, repeats the same games with them, and does not seem inventive or constructive in his games. He has adjusted better to the household routine, occasionally likes to help his mother in the house; he likes to put things away for her. He becomes disturbed and difficult because of changes or irregularities in routine. Paul is at his best during the day when he is alone with his mother. He gets more tense in the afternoon when his brother and neighbors return from school. Though he looks forward to seeing them, he usually ends up in tears very soon because he pesters his brother and is left behind by children of his own age. He has not had any formal schooling. His mother has taught him some letters and numbers, but finds it difficult. He seems to remember one day; forgets the next. While he cannot read, he surprises his family with his sure recognition of brand packages and labels on phonograph records. His family has accepted the fact that Paul has to be handled with more indulgence than other children, that excitement and confusion must be avoided, that often decisions have to be made for him, and that he does not respond well to reasoning. While the home situation at this time does not present many problems, the parents wonder what should be done with regard to schooling. They realize that such concessions as he gets at home cannot easily be duplicated.

When invited by E into the examining room, Paul readily leaves his mother behind. He hardly listens to the explanation that she will wait for him in the waiting room. He seems to be more subdued and more docile than he was a few years ago. While he inspects the room with his eyes, he no longer darts toward what attracts him, but seats himself soon. He seems apprehensive and slightly awed.

SEGUIN FORMBOARD (T:IV:6)

He starts spontaneously to place the insets and has no difficulty except for a brief trial of lozenge in hexagon, which he corrects. He states emphatically and repeatedly, "That is easy for me." He obviously is becoming more at ease as time goes on.

FIVE-FIGURE FORMBOARD (T:IV:7)

A wooden board with five recesses (square, oval, round, hexagon, cross) and eleven wooden insets to fit into the recesses, two for each except three for cross.

When the board is presented to him, he says without inspecting it, "That is easy for me, too. Do you have a harder one?" E: "This is a little harder. I'll help you if you can't do it; you try first." Child says, "You do not need to help me; that is easy." Picks up the half-oval. "Where does this one go? Do not help me; where does it go?" Tries it haphazardly in various places. E points to the correct hole. Child makes placement and spontaneously adds the other half. Continues correctly with round form, then various trials and errors with cross. E removes wrong cross piece. Paul pays very little attention to this help and makes same placement, but corrects spontaneously; briefly confuses segments of square and those of hexagon. E points to one of the segments of the square. Child tries to fit it into the recess with its points against the sides. E helps by turning it properly. Paul completes square. Hexagon presents great difficulties, and he becomes unhappy and impatient. E helps. When the five-figure formboard is repeated, Paul places all forms except hexagon, which presents same difficulties.

MARE AND FOAL PICTURE BOARD (T:IV:13)

The colored picture board shows a mare and a foal in a field with two sheep and three chickens; seven pieces are cut out, to be fitted in the recesses. Cut out pieces are head of mare, head of foal, lamb, chicken, front legs of mare, front leg of foal, piece of meadow.

Paul does not seem to look at the picture at all but treats insets solely as form pieces, as was proper in preceding tests. Several trials and errors; longitudinal pieces are tried in longitudinal recesses. If they do not fit, he tries to hammer them in with his fist. Finally places all pieces correctly, except the two pieces showing heads of horses. (Performance at approximately four-year level.)

HOW MANY. (Horses, houses, chickens, etc.) Counts with emphasis: one, two horses; one, two, three chickens. Seems to enjoy this activity and does not find it beneath his dignity; obviously he enjoys the praise he receives.

Picture Vocabulary and Memory for Pictures (T:II:7,8)

THREE PICTURES. (Coat, block, car.) He names them immediately. Car picture is removed while he is not looking. E: "Which one did I take away?" Paul: "The car."

FOUR PICTURES. (Hat, knife, airplane, ball.) He names them all. Hat is removed. E: "Which one did I take away?" Paul: "The car." E: "That was before. Which one is gone this time?" Paul: "The airplane." E: "No, that is right there. Which one is no longer there?" Paul: "I do not know; I do not want to play this any more." E: "Try once more." Same four pictures presented again in different order. Ball is removed. E: "Which one is removed?" Paul: "The ball."

FIVE PICTURES. (Cane, horse, flag, key, cowboy hat.) Horse is removed. E asks which is gone; Paul says the ball, and that he does not want to play this any more.

With more pictures to remember, the task becomes more difficult, and he forgets the principle of the game, though he understood in the first trial and in the repetition of the second. All pictures are named correctly. (While his behavior and comprehension on the memory procedure are at approximately a four-year level, he passes without difficulty in the naming of pictures, which by Revised Stanford-Binet standards is normal for children from five years of age on.)

E: "Let us look at some more pictures." She tries to turn to the Birthday Party picture (see below), but Paul declares, "I do not want to look at pictures. Don't you have more games?" He gets up. E: "Let us look at a few pictures that are funny. You tell me what is funny about them." Paul: "I do not want to look at pictures." E puts her arm around him; he cuddles briefly and gives an unwilling look at the picture and then becomes interested.

Picture Absurdities (T:IX:11)

MAN IN TREE. (A man sitting on a tree sawing off the limb on which he is sitting.) Paul: "The boy is cutting the tree down." E: "What is funny?" Paul: "He will get an awful spanking." E: "Why?" Paul: "He might hurt himself; he might fall down." E: "And then?" Paul: "He will get an awful spanking." E: "What is funny about the picture?" Paul: "I do not know—because he got spanked."

MAN ON SCALES. (A man on scales with books in his arms.)

Paul: "He is looking at the clock." E: "What is funny about the picture?" Paul: "The clock is not going, and he does not even know it."

CAT AND MICE. (Mice playing around a cat, climbing on her back and eating her food.) Paul: "The cat is playing with the mice." E: "What is funny about it?" Paul: "They are having fun; the mice are all over the place; they are drinking the cat's milk. She does not even say anything." (By Revised Stanford-Binet standards, Paul fails on seven-year level.)

PICTURE DESCRIPTION (T:II:6)

GRANDMOTHER'S STORY. (Children listening to a woman telling a story while kettle is steaming and food is boiling over on the stove.) Paul: "That is a boy and a girl and a mother. She is telling stories." E: "Anything else?" Paul: "Smoke." E: "What about it?" Paul: "The kettle is boiling over." E: "And?" Paul: "I do not know anything more." E: "And the mother?" Paul: "She is telling them a story, about Little Red Riding Hood." E: "And the children?" Paul: "They want to go out playing, they do not like stories. . . . I do not want to look at pictures any more." E: "Let us look at one more only, and I'll give you something easy to guess."

BIRTHDAY PARTY. (Children dressed up for a party with presents in their hands ringing the doorbell at a house; a birthday cake is seen in the window.) Paul: "A boy and a girl; they want to go in." E: "Why?" Paul: "They want to see their mother." E points toward window in the picture. Paul: "It is a window and a cake; it is somebody's birthday." E: "And the children?" Paul: "They want to get in to see their mother." E: "Whose birthday is it?" Paul: "Somebody's." E: "Guess whose it is." Paul: "I do not know." E: "I think it is a child. How old is it?" Paul: "I do not know." E: "Look at the cake." Paul: "It is a birthday cake." E: "Count the candles." Paul: "Four." E: "Count again." Paul: "Five. Five candles." E: "How old is the child going to be?" Paul: "I do not know." (By Revised Stanford-Binet standards, Paul just about scores on six-year level.)

Paul's responses to the picture absurdities and the picture description tests are revealing in several respects. He obviously talks easily and fluently; his reasoning processes, however, are still quite primitive. He perceives many details of a situation, but does not combine them in a coordinated system (Birthday Party). His sense of humor is simple and realistic. His ideas follow each other in a chain without reference to the starting point (Man in Tree). From the emotional point of view, tension and insecurity seem to show in his need to see his mother and in his fear of imminent realistic punishment or ridicule ("he does not even know it."), and his resistance to more formal teaching situations (Grandmother's Story, and his attitude about pictures in general).

E produces boxes with blocks. They seem to reassure Paul. He sits down again.

BLOCKS (T:I:2,4)

Twelve red and twelve green one-inch blocks.

SIX-CUBE PYRAMID. (Red.) Imitates correctly.

OBLIQUE BRIDGE. Is clumsy; his left hand is no help; he tries to keep base blocks in position while placing top block at the proper angle. Succeeds.

SIX-CUBE STEPS. Arranges three blocks horizontally with four blocks vertically at one end; omits middle step. E shows him block by block how to proceed; he learns and later repeats correctly.

SIX-CUBE PYRAMID. (Red base, green top.) His structure is correct, but no attention is paid to the arrangement of colors. E: "Make it just like mine, the red ones below." He imitates correctly, but says: "I do not want to play with blocks any more."

SERIAL PATTERNS (T:I:5). He is to alternate one red, one green, one red, etc. He understands immediately and likes the task. He is then to alternate two green, one red, two green, one red, etc. Correct until all green blocks are used up, then continues all red, saying, "Look how *long* I am making mine." E: "Is it still all the same way we started—two green, one red?" No response and no checking.

COUNTING (T:I:7). Paul counts twelve blocks correctly.

ISOLATING SMALL QUANTITIES FROM LARGER ONES (T:I:8). E says, "Give me seven blocks . . . (four blocks . . . nine blocks)." Paul counts correctly, makes a mistake with nine, but corrects. Does not enjoy himself, seems to become tense; gets up.

GOLDSTEIN-SCHEERER STICK TEST (T:VII:6 AND FIGURE 12)

Plastic sticks in four different sizes.

Starts spontaneously to arrange the sticks "log cabin" style, piled on top of each other. Asks, "Do you have more? Do you have large ones?" E produces a design that resembles a house (10). Paul imitates with different irregular sizes, poor angles, continues adding sticks on, no recognizable shape. Paul: "See what I am making?" It is a car—it looks like a fence. Paul: "See my fence." E: "Let us make little things." Paul: "Let me make it."

REPRODUCING FROM MEMORY. (Various simple figures made of three to five sticks.) Reproduces various forms with gross mistakes in size and orientation. The pitchfork form is reproduced like a star. Presented with a reversed E, he names it spontaneously and seems delighted to recognize it. Does not identify an F; copies it by adorning one long stick with four teeth.

SORTING AND COUNTING STICKS. Understands, carefully lines up sticks of one kind and starts counting. E: "How many tiny ones have we got?" Answers correctly. He likes the task. E: "How many tall ones, etc.?" Counts correctly, but does not want to continue.

COMPARING CONCRETE QUANTITIES (T:I:9)

E shows Paul a square made of four sticks. E: "You make the same." When he has finished, she asks, "How many sticks have *you* got?" Paul counts his sticks. E: "How many have I?" He counts again. It is not obvious to him that two configurations made of identical sticks in identical shape and size must contain an identical number of sticks.

OPPOSITE ANALOGIES (T:IX:5)

E: "Let us play a game. I start it, and you finish it. I say: 'A father is a man, a mother is a. . . .' " Paul: "Girl." E: "A brother is a boy, a sister is a. . . ." Paul: "Girl." E: "In daytime it is light; at night it is. . . ." Paul: "Dark." E: "The sun shines during the day; the moon. . . ." Paul: "In the day." E: "The rabbit's ears are long; the rat's ears are. . . ." Paul: "Long." E: "The dog has hair; the bird has. . . ." Paul: "Wings." E: "The snail is slow; the rabbit. . . ." Paul: "Is a rabbit." (By Revised Stanford-Binet standards, Paul passes on four-year level and fails on six- and seven-year levels.)

PICTURE COMPLETION (T:IX:12)

A card with five incomplete (mutilated) pictures. Missing are leg of table, sleeve of coat, tail of cat, mouth in face, wing of bird.

Paul makes only one error in naming the missing part. About the bird, he says, "His feet are missing." (By Revised Stanford-Binet standards, Paul passes on five-year level.)

Pictorial Identification (T:II:9)

A card with pictures of objects which the child is to identify by pointing in response to questions such as "Show me the one that can fly, can swim in the water, etc."

Paul points to all pictures correctly. (By Revised Stanford-Binet standards, he passes on four-year level.)

IDENTIFICATION IN REVERSE. E: "Now you make me guess. Ask me another one." Paul: "I do not know." Then repeats as he was asked before, "Show me the one that can fly." E: "Ask me something new, something I did not ask you." Paul: "Where is the apple?" E: "But you better not tell me which one you mean—it is too easy that way. Just talk about it, and see whether I can get which one you mean." Paul: "Which one is the apple on the tree?" And later, "Which is the bird that makes peep peep?"

Animal Pictures (T:II:10,11)

Paul matches pictures correctly. Names nine out of twelve correctly. Mistakes: reindeer for horse, camel for tiger, bear for pig. (Performance at approximately five-year level.)

E: "Which one gives milk? (Which one gives Easter eggs?)" Paul answers correctly. E: "Which one gives bacon, cheese, nuts?" Paul: "I do not know." (Performance at approximately five-year level.)

Conventional Manikin (T:IV:10)

A human figure made of wood, to be assembled from six separate parts (head, body, two arms, two legs).

Paul reverses each arm and leg, fits pieces carelessly. (Performance at four-and-a-half- to five-year level.)

Paper and Pencil (T:III:1)

Paul: "I do not like to make pictures."

Copying Forms (T:III:5 and Figure 2)

CROSS. Correct, but very big and sloppy.

SQUARE. Correct; his stroke is poorly coordinated, and angles are not closed firmly.

DIAGONAL CROSS. He lifts his left arm and gives the paper some incline, but then proceeds to draw the cross parallel to the sides of the paper, which results in same design as first cross.

TRIANGLE. Lines do not meet in angle. Paul says, "I can't do it. . . . I can make an A." Produces a large A which covers the page. Later says, "I know how to make my number." Produces P (for Paul), which consists of vertical stroke and an arc which do not join properly.

RECOGNIZING LETTERS (T:XI:8)

Letters are drawn successively by E; child is to name them. He knows a B and an E. To P he says, "That is my number." To T and later to W, "I do not know that one. I do not want to do this any more."

MEMORY FOR FORMS OR DESIGNS (T:III:5 AND FIGURE 2)

BRITISH FLAG. Paul draws a rectangle with enclosed unorganized lines. When asked to copy same design, he draws a rectangle with a cross inside.

MEMORY FOR DESIGNS (T:VII:1 AND FIGURE 4)

A card showing the design is exposed for ten seconds and is to be reproduced from memory. The card has two figures (1) a square with another square enclosed so that its points touch the sides of the first, and (2) two vertical lines of different lengths and connected at the bottom by a horizontal bar; each is topped by a small square, and both squares point in the same direction.

Paul ignores the first figure; produces for the second two shapeless, roundish lines (representing the squares) connected by a wobbly horizontal line. E: "What else would you like to draw?" Paul: "I can't draw. . . . I can make a house." He scribbles very quickly a vaguely circular marking with three vertical strokes, saying, "Here are the windows." "A roof" for two lines meeting at an angle. Later adds a "door" protruding below the bottom line of the "house," then adds "smoke" beside the roof, but not connected to it. "I do not want to make pictures any more."

COMMENT

In the psychological examination Paul seems to be less active and hectic than he was three years ago. He still is resistant to demands and likes to be independent, but now expresses this in words rather than in actions. He is sensitive to his shortcomings, knows in which areas they will show most, and is apprehensive of tasks which he cannot fulfill. He has apparently been exposed to educational efforts and is rather set against these. He continues to show verbal facility, but his actual name vocabulary is limited (animal pictures). He expresses facts rather than thoughts. He comprehends simple, immediate, verbal connections (opposite analogies, pictorial identification), but not underlying thought processes (pictorial identification in reverse). His reasoning processes lack coherence and fail to integrate all given facts (picture absurdities and picture description). He has acquired information and academic skills (numbers and letters) which would place him on approximately kindergarten level. His most important liabilities are perceptuo-motor difficulties. His form comprehension is primitive (formboards). He appreciates details rather than integrated wholes (Goldstein-Scheerer sticks, forms). His own visuo-motor productions (drawings) are very poor, not only because of poor motor coordination but because of inadequate comprehension of spatial relationships.

Except for these areas of special difficulty, Paul functions on a borderline level. Though improved, his short attention spans continue as one of his many liabilities. His tendency to respond to isolated stimuli in an immediate and uncontrolled fashion is reflected in his personal social adjustments and accounts for labile reactions to the outside world. When he tries to avoid failure, he resorts to primitive attitudes. His apparent resistance to adults masks a desire for affection and acceptance. He seems sensitive and easily guided if not met head-on.

In view of these findings, Paul should start slowly only on academic schooling. He would do rather poorly in academic competition and needs concessions to protect him as much as possible from frustration.

PAUL AT TWELVE YEARS

Paul is still rather small and undeveloped for his age. He walks with a marked limp; his left arm and hand are stiff. He seems wiry, nervous, and tense, and has abrupt and awkward angular movements. He looks anxious and harassed.

For the past three years he has been in a special class. He likes school and the teacher, but does not get along well with the other children. They like to tease him and to egg him on. Frequent emotional outbursts result. When he is irritated, he "loses his head," and is apt to hurt children. The neighbors therefore are somewhat uneasy about him. Nevertheless, he moves around freely in the neighborhood, runs errands for his mother, and no longer loses either his way or his change. He can recognize some printed signs on streets and busses, but does not read enough for information or pleasure. According to his teacher, he reads at approximately second-grade level.

His family finds him more competent than his school grades indicate. He knows his father's tools and tries to help in simple carpentering. In spite of his stiff arm, he has found effective methods of manipulations in situations that interest him; he is very proud when praised for such skills. He does not have any one favorite activity and never stays long with anything he does. He likes to accumulate sundry objects, which he picks up when and where they appeal to him. His father tried to start him on more systematic projects, such as stamp or postcard collections, but after some initial enthusiasm Paul was not interested enough to continue. On the whole, his family is more worried about his emotional instability than about his limited capacities. They feel that he could take care of himself if he could be more self-controlled and even tempered. His mother finds him gentle and sensitive at heart, and easy to handle if not met head-on. She describes him as generous and ready to share. There have been various instances of petty stealing, all of them caused by his desire to do favors for his family or for an occasional friend at school.

Since last seen in E's office, at age seven, the child has had various psychological examinations at different places. The most recent one was an unfortunate experience with a school psychometrist who was to find out whether Paul was ready for transfer to the normal grades. This examination was done in a hurry and resulted in frustration all around. His parents were unwilling to accept as correct a Stanford-Binet I.Q. of 55 and were appalled at the recommendation for institutionalization. Paul was much disturbed by the event. According to his mother, he has since then become sensitized against "testing." Because of both mother's and child's apprehension, E decides to proceed in two sessions. The first one will be designed to set everybody at ease by getting acquainted.

Paul comes with E with his head hanging, a picture of suppressed apprehension and unwillingness. He is closed up and unresponsive.

E suggests, "I thought you might like a puzzle," and produces one without waiting for an answer.

FIVE-FIGURE FORMBOARD (T:IV:7)

Paul looks at it unsmilingly, starts very quickly, saying that this is "easy." He proceeds correctly and speedily except for some brief hesitation and trial with the hexagon.

CASUIST FORMBOARD (T:IV:8)

A wooden board with four recesses (three circles of varying sizes and one oblongated oval). There are twelve insets to fit into the recesses, three to each of the two larger circles, two to the smaller circle, and four to the oval.

Again he starts very quickly in a somewhat aggressive manner; apparently he wants to show that he is competent and would like to get through as quickly as possible. He has some difficulty with the oval; at first he accepts help reluctantly, but he seems relieved and less tense when he finds that he may obtain assistance from E.

REY NONVERBAL LEARNING TEST (T:VIII:1 AND FIGURE 16)

Four wooden boards, each with nine pegs arranged in rows of three. On each board all pegs but one are loose. Child is to find fastened peg on each board and remember its position.

Paul does not listen well to instructions and wants to start hastily before they are completed. While his search procedure is systematic on the first board, it becomes less so on the next. In spite of instructions and E's repeated reminder that "there is a different one on each board," he first tries with each new board the peg which proved to be correct on the previous board. Whenever his trials finally lead him to the correct peg, he exclaims with some triumph and challenge, "Here it is!" The next round shows considerable unevenness in approach. While there seems to be hardly any learning and comprehension in the first three rounds, he adjusts better in the next ones; soon it can be noticed that he has learned the positions of the pegs but has difficulty remembering their proper sequence on the four boards. When upset about his inability to succeed, he becomes indiscriminate in his choice of pegs, and seems to forget all his previous experiences with them. Success alternates with failure. On several occasions he spills boards and pegs while transferring the boards from one pile to the other. He handles them too quickly and carelessly and does not take into account how loosely the pegs are attached. After fifteen rounds the test is interrupted—no reliable learning has taken place. (Performance at zero percentile for his age.)

Since Paul now seems bored and discouraged, a very simple situation is introduced to lift his flagging spirit.

MEMORY FOR PICTURES (T:II:8)

THREE PICTURES. Success on first trial.

FOUR PICTURES. Success on second trial.

FIVE PICTURES. Success on first trial.

The irregularity of this performance seems at least partly caused by his tension, which is still apparent.

DRAWING

E: "Would you like to make a picture?" He looks dubious. E: "How about a lady who is walking in the rain?"

LADY WALKING IN THE RAIN (T:III:2). He seems to be relieved as soon as a specific theme is suggested. He starts quickly and rather sloppily. He tries a figure in profile, but adds legs and feet in front view; one of the legs has double lines, the other single ones; feet are shapeless and only loosely attached to the legs. Paul: "She needs a dress and a pocketbook." He sketches a dress which covers the figure but does not avoid transparency. Adds, "She has flowers on her dress." Very carefully he draws small flowers on the dress. They are arranged in rows. He gets tired of this tedious activity while finishing the second row; he gives up. He spends some care on a hat with a feather and finally forgets the pocketbook he had intended to do. He declares his picture finished and seems pleased with it. The figure has no arms or hands. E: "Remember what we were going to draw?" Paul: "A lady." E: "What about her?" Paul: "It is raining; she needs an umbrella and rain." He draws an umbrella which does not cover the head; adds one arm to hold the umbrella; carefully outlines spokes and adds a tassel at the handle; no rain. (Performance at zero percentile before E's suggestions.)

MEMORY FOR DESIGNS

ELLIS VISUAL DESIGNS TEST (T:VII:2 AND FIGURE 5). Each of a series of ten designs is presented to the child for five seconds. He is then to reproduce it from memory.

He does very poorly; he distorts the forms, overaccentuates the angles, and reverses some of the designs (3, 4). He regularizes shapes which are meant to be uneven (4, 5), etc. His strokes lack direction and coordination. E tries to determine which of his errors are due to lack of motor control and which, on the other hand, are due to a lack of comprehension of spatial relationships. E: "Are they the way you want them?" Paul: "No, it is no good." E: "What is wrong on this (4)?" Paul: "This (the dip) should be in the middle." These questions and answers confirm that not only his production but his intentions also contain many errors of form comprehension. Task is interrupted after design 7. (Score: three points, well below zero percentile for his age.)

    BENTON VISUAL RETENTION TEST (T:VII:4 AND FIGURE 8). A series of seven design cards, five of them with three forms arranged in specific sequence, size, and spatial position. The basic shapes are simple (circle, squares, triangles); some have slight modifications only. The cards are presented to the child for ten seconds and the designs are then to be reproduced from memory.

    Paul: "That is easy." He does not look long enough when presented with first and second design; after a start on the third design, he asks to have it shown again because he "did not see it all." Gets impatient and a little whiny when this is refused. (Score: two points, well below average.)

    Paul: "I do not want to draw any more." E: "Could you write your name on your drawings so I know who made them?"

WRITING (T:III:2 AND XI:9)

Writes his name rather quickly and sloppily. E: "Will you write it as fast as you can? It does not need to be good." Paul complies with pleasure. The product is similar to the first one. E: "Now write it slowly and as well as you can." Paul starts with a very careful and flourished P; then continues in his previous, quick, careless way. Refuses to write his address and declares that he does not know how to write anything else. He sounds a bit irritated and on the verge of becoming resistant and negativistic.

WOOD PICTURE COMPLETION TEST (T:IX:13)

A series of colored pictures mounted on plywood, showing a succession of activities illustrating a schoolgirl's day. Each picture has an inch-square cutout; 60 one-inch pieces go with the set. These include the correct solutions and a collection of extra pieces intended as incorrect solutions or planned alternates. The child must choose which piece to insert in each picture.

    Paul seems glad to get a "game." He begins by fitting blank insets in three of the pictures which he chooses at random. E suggests he look the pictures over and try to find "things" which would fit. Paul next places a purple squirrel beside a purple shadow, a rope next to other ropes, a cat next to a reading child, and a dog following a walking child. He removes two of his first blank placements and replaces them by more appropriate, though not correct, choices (an empty basket in the hands of a child leaving a store; a piece of clothing much larger than other garments on the same line). He has now gained courage to make some choice instead of using blanks which do not commit him to any decision. After he has finished, E questions him about some of his choices. He confirms that he chose some insets because their color corresponded (purple squirrel to purple shadow), or because they showed the same thing (rope to rope), or because of other one-to-one relationships (child with dog or cat). Obviously, he has not considered all relationships involved in each picture, and particularly has not taken notice of the fact that the pictures present a continuous story. (Score: forty-five points, well below zero decile for his age and near fifth decile for ages seven-and-a-half to eight-and-a-half years.)

The session is interrupted here. It seems to have fulfilled its purpose since it ended on a pleasant enough note, and the child got accustomed to E. With hardly any questions to answer and with "things to do," the testing situation seemed on the whole less menacing to him than he had expected. E has gained an initial impression and can form her first hypothesis.

COMMENT

Paul still seems to be the same insecure and sensitive child of years before. Obviously he has experienced many failures and has become increasingly aware of his difficulties.

With his aggressive and resistant attitude he tries to ward off criticism which he has come to expect. He has become more subtle than he was in avoiding difficult situations (word writing). When he is not able to do so, he becomes upset and easily goes to pieces. Then he is apt to lose previous gains (Rey nonverbal learning test) and to become childish and insistent in his attitude and in his demands (drawing from memory). His reasoning is, in general, impulsive and shortsighted; in trying to solve a problem, he pursues first clues without checking or appraising the whole of the situation (Wood picture completion test). He gets easily involved in details and forgets his goal (lady walking in the rain). His performance improves when the adult supports him with kindly and systematic suggestions (drawings, Wood picture completion test). Paul is hindered in learning and reasoning by his obvious difficulties in perceptual organization (memory for design tests, formboards,

Rey nonverbal learning test), even in situations in which he is reasonably comfortable emotionally. He seems to function on a borderline level.

This first impression tallies well with previous examinations and is confirmed by his parents' reports. However, it is necessary for E to verify this initial appraisal in a second session. It would seem a good plan next time to give Paul a more formal examination with a standardized scale. This will, perhaps, clarify some of the confusion about his I.Q. and, therefore, will be useful in contact with school authorities.

When he arrives for his second visit, Paul starts immediately to take the lead in the situation. He allows no time for greetings or conversation between E and his mother, but hurries silently ahead of E into the testing room. He goes to get the formboards himself, since he knows them from his previous visit. Sitting down, and still without words, he points toward E's chair, inviting her to be seated, too. He seems comfortable and pleased when all is again as it was before. He completes the formboards more speedily than the first time, but he has brief hesitations with some of the difficult pieces. E: "What else would you like to do?" Paul: "I do not want to make pictures!" E: "How would you like to play with pictures that are all made?"

PICTURE ARRANGEMENT (T:IV:14 AND IX:10)

A series of pictures which, when placed in the right order, tell a story. The pictures are presented to the child in disarranged order, and he is asked to put them together in the right order. The three introductory series are not sequences of events, but single pictures cut in pieces.

DOG. (In three parts.) Paul says, "That is easy"; he completes the picture quickly and correctly. (Two points.)

MOTHER. (A mother playing with her child with an electric train.) At once he puts together the two pieces of the traintrack (O and Y); briefly tries to place the figure of the mother (T) at the wrong end of the track (OYT), then corrects spontaneously (TOY). (Two points.)

TRAIN. (An engine in two parts, I and R; a tender, O; a lorry with coal, N.) First fails to put the two engine parts together, places IORN; notices his error when the wheels do not fit together; then corrects (IRON). (Two points.)

SCALES. (A man with a suitcase looking at scales, A; the man is standing on the scales, his suitcase beside him, B; man walking away suitcase in hand, C; presented in order ACB.) E: "This time

you have to put them together so that they will tell a story." Paul:
"They do not fit." He is ready to give up. E repeats directions. He tries
to fit the floor lines on the picture. Seems discouraged. E suggests that
it is one story about the same man. He understands the suggestion and
completes the arrangement without errors (ABC). (No credit.) E: "Why
did he put the suitcase down?" Paul: "It is too heavy." E: "How do you
mean that?" Paul: "He would weigh too much." Though his first reply
is ambiguous, his second explanation shows his comprehension of the
situation.

FIRE. (A boy warned by his mother not to play with matches,
F; matchbox and curtains are on fire, I; the fire engine speeds along,
R; fireman at the burning house, and the boy crying, E; presented
in order REIF.) Paul looks at the pictures and arranges them correctly
in twelve seconds (FIRE). (Five points.) E: "Tell me about it." Paul:
"She gives him a match, he plays, he starts a fire, he is running, the
policemen come, they put out the fire, he is crying." E: "Why?" Paul:
"He is scared."

BURGLAR. (A burglar opens a window from outside, T; climbs
in, H; opens drawers, gets money and jewelry, U; a policeman arrests
him when he climbs out of the window, G; presented in order HGTU.)
Paul arranges pictures correctly in fourteen seconds (THUG). (Five
points.) E questions him about story. Paul: "He climbs in the window,
he climbs in the window, he finds something, the cop gets him."
E: "What does he say?" Paul: "He should not climb." E: "And then?"
Paul: "The cop will go and tell his mother." E: "And?" Paul: "She will
give him a spanking and send him to bed." E: "What is he going to say?"
Paul: "He will cry." E: "Why?" Paul: "Because he got a spanking."

FARMER. (A farmer sowing corn, Q; the corn is growing, a
scarecrow in the field, R; the corn is ripe, S; a truck driving the corn
to market, T; presented in order STRQ.) Paul arranges the cards with
some errors, QRTS. He starts to explain: "He is sowing his corn, Q;
the corn is growing, R; he drives to town, T; then he tastes it, S—No,
that is wrong." He exchanges T and S. Correct QRST. (Four points.)

PICNIC. (A dog following a man with a picnic basket, E; he
approaches and tries to get the chicken, the man and woman do not
notice him, F; the dog eats the chicken, G; they unpack their basket
and find the chicken gone, H; presented in order HEGF.) Paul arranges
the cards with errors, FEGH. (No credit.) He explains, "The dog likes

the turkey, F; he follows them, E; he eats it, G; they are surprised he took their dinner, they are mad, H."

SLEEPER. (A man in bed shuts off his alarm clock, P; goes back to sleep, E; he eats breakfast, his wife tells him that he is late, R; he runs to work, C; he goes to sleep at his desk, Y; presented in order RPYEC.) Paul arranges cards in order EPRCY, which is correct except for reversal of first two pictures. (No credit.) He explains: "He is asleep, E; the alarm clock rings, P; he has breakfast, R; he runs, C; here he is asleep again, Y." Procedure interrupted here. (Total WISC score: twenty points.)[4]

Paul's performance in the picture arrangement test shows characteristic peculiarities. The first three pictures are put together by fitting lines rather than by examining picture content. This principle is at first carried over into Scales. Remnants can still be observed when, in the following series, after making his choices, he tries carefully to fit the edges of the cards also. For him, many of the pictures seem to have gross differentiations only; he overlooks the finer points (Burglar, Sleeper). Furthermore, his verbal explanations reveal distortions in perception, reasoning, and social comprehension. In Fire, the mother's outstretched, scolding arm becomes for Paul an arm that offers the match to the child. Paul uses no independent judgement to test this unlikely hypothesis. He confuses the functions of policemen and firemen; to him both are figures of remote authority, whereas the mother continues to represent direct authority and is the person to whom the child is fully responsible. She in turn is at the root of the child's actions (she is indirectly causing the fire). In Burglar, the mother administers punishment while the policeman scolds only for climbing into the window, not for stealing. Whether or not Paul's own personal experiences with petty stealing lead him to repress the idea of theft altogether remains a matter of conjecture.

When Paul's performance on the picture arrangement test is evaluated according to standard WISC procedure, these distortions of comprehension do not affect his scores on Fire and Burglar, since he was able to place the cards in correct sequence. However, on Picnic and Sleeper

---

[4] Here, as in all following instances where the WISC (or Wechsler-Bellevue) directions are not strictly adhered to, ratings by Wechsler standards are used to help estimate levels of performance rather than to give absolute measures.

his scores are affected by his failure to perceive and coordinate details, even though he understands the main themes well enough.

Picture Completion (T:IX:12)

A series of twenty picture cards in black and white. In each picture a part is missing and is to be identified by the child.

Paul gives correct responses for the first seven pictures: comb—tooth, table—leg, fox—ear, girl—mouth, cat—whiskers, door—hinge, hand—fingernail. (Seven points.) On the next pictures, his responses are as follows: To card with a spade missing, "I do not know; I do not play cards." (No credit.) To scissors with a screw missing, "The paper is missing." (No credit.) To coat with buttonholes missing, answers "Button." (No credit.) To fish with dorsal fin missing, answers "The wing on the other side." (No credit.) To screw with slot missing, answers "The line there." (One point.) To fly with antennae missing, answers "Nothing missing." (No credit.) To rooster with spur missing, answers "Nothing missing—the little thing here." (One point.) To profile with eyebrow missing, answers "Nothing missing." (No credit.) To thermometer with mercury missing, answers "Nothing missing." (No credit.) From here on, Paul casts only a brief glance at the picture and repeats automatically, "Nothing missing."

His failure on card and coat involve lack of proper number concepts or poor form comprehension. Successes on screw and rooster show his occasional awareness and interest in small lines or details; his repeated "nothing missing" seems to show his defeatism as well as rigidity of response when he has to face problems. (Total WISC score: nine points.)

Block Designs (T:VII:8)

A set of one-inch blocks, each with one white, one blue, one yellow, one red, one red/white, and one yellow/blue side; a set of cards printed in color, each showing a design that can be made by assembling four (nine) of the block surfaces. The child is to arrange four (nine) blocks according to the model card. The WISC designs are all in red and white.

CARD A. Succeeds on first trial. (Two points.)

CARD B. Succeeds on first trial. (Two points.)

CARD C. Inverses triangles. (No credit.)

CARD I. Succeeds (in thirty-five seconds) after making some trials and errors. (Four points.)

CARD II. Uses three all-red and one all-white side instead of red/white sides; he is not satisfied, becomes restless, and starts turning the blocks; he discovers the blue sides and starts to arrange a square made of four blue sides; he reaches for the rest of the blocks and starts to add more blue ones. "I do not want to do these any more. I'll show you what I can do with those. Don't take all those away. I'll need them all." (Total WISC score: eight points.)

Paul seems to have reached his peak in block designs, but in order to check this without antagonizing him at this stage, E falls in with Paul's new interest in block sides of colors other than red or white. He becomes interested in a "new" task.

BLOCK DESIGNS (T:VII:7 AND FIGURE 13)

Same colored blocks as above. The Kohs designs are made up of all colors (blue, yellow, red, white, blue/yellow, red/white).

CARD I. Immediately arranges two blue blocks next to each other, corrects and tries having corners meet. He adds red blocks into the free spaces, all blocks touching in the center in a diamond effect with spaces in between. Paul is not satisfied, but now keeps on trying and succeeds.

CARD II. Arranges two red ones as base, one yellow above and one blue on top; is dissatisfied, turns blocks idly; then for the first time seems to become aware of the yellow/blue sides; looks for a second one, and succeeds in arranging correctly.

CARD III. Starts with a blue base and solid yellow top row. Not satisfied, he changes one yellow into blue. E demonstrates and undoes her model. Paul is to try again. He now uses correct blocks, but places triangles parallel and not converging. E arranges four blocks for him as a model to copy. Paul now succeeds by copying block by block. Card III is presented to him again. He rearranges as he did before, with triangles in wrong position. Paul now gets restless and seems a bit moody; brushes all blocks aside, and wants to quit. E persuades him to try one more and promises to help.

CARD IV. He uses correct blocks, but cannot arrange them correctly. Once he seems to have the proper solution, but he does not recognize it as correct and destroys it while trying further. E demonstrates; test is interrupted. (Performance at approximately seven-year level.)

Paul apparently takes no notice of the similarity between the Kohs and the WISC designs; he does not transfer what he has learned from one design to another, or from a demonstration to a repeat production. His success in the second Kohs design (Card II) seems accidental; the yellow/blue blocks happened to get into the correct position, but he is incapable of duplicating this arrangement later.

Obviously Paul is now ready for a complete change in situation. E suggests "we do things in our head now." Herewith she introduces:

OPPOSITE ANALOGIES (T:IX:5)

Paul succeeds on the easy ones, then—E: "The rabbit's ears are long, the rat's ears are. . . . " Paul: "Short." E: "The dog has hair, the bird has. . . . " Paul: "Wings—no, feathers." E: "Snow is white, coal is. . . . " Paul: "Hot." E: "Wolves are wild, dogs are. . . . " Paul: "Nice." E questions this answer. Paul says, "Very tame." (By Revised Stanford-Binet standards, Paul passes on eight-year level.) During this task, Paul regains some assurance; he seems pleased and bursts out with his answers.

OPPOSITE ANALOGIES (T:IX:5)

E: "Lemons are sour, but sugar is. . . . " Paul: "Sweet." E: "Boys grow up to be men, and girls to be. . . . " Paul: "Mothers." E: "A knife and a piece of glass both. . . . " Paul: "Cut." (Note: the second WISC item, "You walk with your legs and throw with your. . . .'" is omitted because of Paul's own physical handicap.)

SIMILARITIES BETWEEN TWO THINGS (T:IX:2)

A series of word pairs are read to the child one after another, with the request that he state in what way the subjects are alike.

E: "Plum—peach." Paul: "You eat them." (One point.) E: "Cat—mouse." Paul: "Have a tail." (One point.) E: "Beer—wine." Paul: "You drink them." (One point.) E: "Piano—violin." Paul: "They play." (One point.) E: "Paper—coal." Paul: "I do not know. You can write on paper. I do not know about coal; it is black." E: "What is it used for?" Paul: "Some people burn it when they have no oil." E: "How about paper?" Paul: "It can burn, too. They both burn." (No credit.) E: "Pound—yard." Paul: "You can pound things." (No credit.) E: "Scissors—copper pan." Paul: "You cut with scissors. I do not know what you do with a copper pan." (No credit.) E: "Mountain—lake." Paul: "I do not know." E: "Salt—water." Paul: "Salt water tastes awful." E: "In what way are salt and water alike?" Paul: "I do not know." (No credit.) His first four answers show his preference for practical functional solutions. From the "paper—coal" question on, he arrives at a correct answer only after some of E's suggestions.

Total WISC score on Similarities: seven to eight points.

COMPREHENSION TEST (T:X:3)

A series of questions testing general comprehension.

E: "What is the thing to do when you cut your finger?" Paul: "You put a band-aid on. You wash it good first." (Two points.) E: "What is the thing to do if you lose one of your friend's balls?" Paul: "You give it back; you got to find it or you have to buy him a new one." (Two points.) E: "What would you do if you were sent to buy a loaf of bread and the grocer said he did not have any more?" Paul: "Go and tell my mother." (One point.) E: "What is the thing to do if a fellow much smaller than yourself starts to fight with you?" Paul: "You do not fight, you tell his mother." (One point.) E: "Why is it better to build a house of brick than of wood?" Paul: "It is better, it does not burn as fast." (One point.) E: "Why are criminals locked up?" Paul: "They do bad things like stealing and robbing and they have to go to prison." (One point.) E: "Why should women and children be saved first in a shipwreck?" Paul: "They can't swim." (No credit.) E: "Why is it generally better to pay bills by check than by cash?" Paul: "I do not know. You write checks. It is like money, but it does not cost anything." E: "Why?" Paul: "Because it is just paper." (No credit.) E: "Why is it generally better to give money to an organized charity than to a beggar in the street?" Paul: "He may not need it so much; Red Cross takes care of soldiers and everything." (No credit.) (Note: omitted is item 5, "What should you do if you see a train approaching a broken track?" and also the last four items of the series.) (Total score: eight to nine points.)

Again Paul's answers are interesting beyond the actual score; he shows evidence of meager verbal comprehension. His interest and reasoning power is limited to the sphere of his immediate personal experiences. One senses a certain rigid and slightly moralistic quality and lip-service to admonitions from adults, especially from his mother.

FACTUAL INFORMATION (T:XI:10)

A series of questions testing general information.

E: "From what animal do we get milk?" Paul: "Cow." E: "What

must you do to make water boil?" Paul: "Put it on the stove." E: "In what kind of store do we buy sugar?" Paul: "The A & P." (Score including WISC questions 1–3 omitted: six points.) E continues on the same theme. E: "Where do you buy your bread?" Paul: "I buy it in the store at our corner." E: "What do you pay?" Paul: "I do not know." E: "What does it cost, a loaf of bread?" Paul: "I do not know; you have to ask my mother. I take the money she gives me." E: "How much does she give you?" Paul: "Sometimes she gives me a dollar, and I have to bring back the change, and not buy anything else." E: "What is change?" Paul: "Dimes and nickels and pennies." E: "How many pennies make a nickel?" Paul: "Five." (One point.) E: "How many pennies in a dime?" Paul: "Ten." To "How many nickels in a dime," Paul answers, "Five—no, two"; to "quarters in a dollar," he says, "I think four." To "nickels in a dollar," he responds, "I do not know." E: "What can you buy with a nickel?" Paul: "An ice cream cone—a small one. I am not buying any candy any more. I am saving my pennies for a bike. I know how to ride a bike. My mother is afraid. But she says I can have one if I save all my pennies." E: "When did you start to save?" Paul: "Yesterday." E: "How much money do you have to have for it?" Paul: "I do not know. An awful lot." E: "How much?" Paul: "Perhaps ten dollars." E: "You think you can save enough to get all this?" Paul: "I do not know. I got already sixty-two cents." E: "How much more do you need to get one dollar?" Paul: "I do not know. Have you got any other games?" E: "Let us first do a few more of these questions—all right?"

E: "How many days in a week?" Paul: "Seven." (One point.) To "what are they," he answers correctly. E: "Who discovered America?" Paul: "George Washington; he was the father of the country." (No credit.) E: "How many things make a dozen?" Paul: "Twelve." (One point.) E: "What are the seasons of the year?" Paul: "Summer, fall, autumn, winter, spring." (One point.) E: "What is the color of rubies?" Paul: "I do not know." E: "Do you know what rubies are?" Paul: "No." E: "They are a precious stone." Paul: "Stones are sort of gray." (No credit.) E: "Where does the sun set?" Paul: "East—no, west. When the sun is in the south it is the middle of the day." E: "Where does it set?" Paul: "East." (No credit.) E: "What does the stomach do?" Paul: "I do not know; it helps us keep the food, that is where the food goes; it has to go through the stomach." E: "What does the stomach do?" Paul: "I do not know; it holds food." (No credit or ?) E: "Why does oil float on the water?" Paul: "I do not know; it floats. . . . " (No credit.) E: "Who wrote *Romeo and Juliet?*" Paul: "I do not know." E: "Did you ever hear those names?" Paul: "No." (No credit.) E: "What is celebrated on the Fourth of July?" Paul: "I do not know; they have firecrackers; they are very noisy." E: "Why firecrackers?" Paul: "They have a nice time; my mother says when I get older I can have fire-crackers; they are dangerous. . . . " (No credit.)

Paul seems to get very tired of answering questions. He has reached his limits. (Total WISC score: ten to eleven points.)

DRAWING A BICYCLE (T:IX:14)

Child is to draw a picture of a bicycle and explain how it works.

E: "About this bike. Tell me more about it. Can you show me on a paper what it will look like? It does not need to be a good picture. Just so it has all it needs." Paul draws very fast two somewhat elliptical wheels, two pedals between them, a handlebar attached with crude strokes to a front wheel. He looks at the drawing dubiously, discards the pencil, and declares: "I can't make a bike. It is too hard." E: "How does the bike go?" Paul: "You have to push the pedals and that makes the wheels go." E: "How?" Paul: "I do not know. There is the chain." He adds a chain which goes from the center of the rear wheel to the center of the front wheel. "It turns. You can get hurt when you put your fingers in." E: "What about the pedals?" Paul: "They turn the wheels." E: "And the chain?" Paul: "It turns the wheel." E: "What makes the bicycle go?" Paul: "The wheels and the pedals and the chain." E: "How do the wheels turn?" Paul: "When you pedal." E: "Sometimes you do not pedal and the wheels turn. Why?" Paul: "I do not know." E: "You want to show me on your picture how the bicycle goes?" Paul: "The pedals make the wheels go and the chain turns. Do you have more games? I do not like making pictures."

Paul knows the various parts of a bicycle well enough, but has rudi-mentary notions of the relations between the parts; he knows that the pedals act on the wheels and that the chain does, too; he also knows that the chain moves when the pedals are in action; but he cannot co-ordinate these actions clearly enough in his mind to be able to express them either in words or in his sketch.

E suggests, "Let us do some more puzzles." Paul looks dubious.

OBJECT ASSEMBLY (T:IV:11,12)

A series of separate figures cut in five to seven parts, to be assembled by the child.

MANIKIN. Paul looks at the pieces with some suspicion at

first, then immediately says, "That is easy—it is a boy"; he arranges the pieces correctly, but gets one leg longer than the other; he leaves it this way, obviously not sure of it, then keeps fingering the leg pieces without finding another solution; then suddenly readjusts and interchanges the leg pieces correctly. (Four points.)

HORSE. Paul assembles the horse roughly first, obviously recognizes the head and the rear part, and soon the front leg; spends a good deal of time trying the small end pieces of the legs, inverts them; he is left with the middle piece, for which he does not find any spot; he leaves it aside, saying, "It does not fit"; looks at the legs and rearranges them correctly and spontaneously. E interrupts at ninety seconds. (Four points.)

AUTOMOBILE. E asks, "Do you think you know what this is going to be?" He handles the pieces idly for a moment, then discovers a wheel, puts the wheel together, and says, "It is a car." Assembles both wheels, but cannot do anything more with the pieces, keeps inverting pieces and gets very obviously annoyed and discouraged. E interrupts task at about ninety seconds. (Approximately two points.)

FACE. Since it becomes clear soon that Paul cannot make anything of the individual pieces, E suggests that this is supposed to be a face. Paul still seems unhappy and at a loss. By pointing to the largest piece, E suggests that this is "one of his eyes and his ear, etc." He finds the other eye piece, puts it next to the midline, removes it, finds that two of the headpieces fit, later assembles them to the face part and attaches the eye. Wants to give up. E interrupts task. (Even if E's suggestions were allowed for scoring, Paul would earn only one point in credit.) (Total score: ten points.)

E says, "You know nickels and dimes very well. Let us do some more things with numbers." Paul: "I am no good at numbers; I hate numbers." E: "What I mean is really very easy. You can say your numbers; you know how to count, of course." Paul: "You mean one, two, three—that is easy."

COUNTING (T:XI:2)

He counts quickly up to thirty. E interrupts him with, "Can you count backwards from twenty down?" He proceeds slowly but correctly. E: "Now I am going to say numbers, and you say them just the way I say them."

REPEATING DIGITS (T:VIII:5,6)

DIGITS FORWARD. He has no trouble with three, four, and five digits forward. With six digits he stumbles on seven, five, four, nine, three, one and five, two, eight, seven, four, six; but he succeeds with two, four, six, eight, ten, twelve which seems to sound familiar to him.

DIGITS BACKWARD. Three digits, correct. To seven, five, two, eight he repeats eight, two, seven, five; to four, one, nine, six, he says "nine, six . . . no, six, nine, four, one." He gets annoyed and restless. He dislikes working with numbers and does not seem to notice that he is wrong. Obviously, he would like to quit. E says, "Let us do one more. How about five, four, three, two?" Paul: "Three, two, four, five." Set to say numbers backward, he fails to recognize the familiar series and therefore continues to make mistakes even with this simple sequence of numbers. With equivalent digit series, his total WISC score would be eight points.

Since time is running short, E decides to try some arithmetic despite the fact that Paul does not seem to be in a good mood for it. It may perhaps show interesting sidelights on the way Paul is able to function under stress. E: "Could you do just a few very simple arithmetic problems? You do not have to do this—it is not like school—but I would like very much to have you try. We will start with very easy ones, and you may stop when you want to—just as they do on the quiz programs on TV. Try this one."

ARITHMETIC PROBLEMS (T:XI:5)

A series of arithmetic reasoning problems which increase in difficulty.

E: "If I cut an apple in half, how many pieces will I have?" Paul: "Two—that is easy." E: "John had four pennies and his mother gave him two more. How many pennies did he have altogether?" Paul: "Six." (Score: including WISC problems 1 to 3 omitted, five points.) E: "James had eight marbles, and he bought six more. How many marbles did he have altogether?" Paul moves his fingers and furtively glances at them. He is counting the solution out on his fingers. "Fourteen." E: "Very good. Do you want to try one more? A boy had twelve newspapers and sold five. How many did he have left?" As before, Paul uses his fingers, adds up by them, and comes up with an answer, "Sixteen." E: "Try again. What did you do?" Paul: "I added twelve and five." E: "I'll read it again." E now emphasizes the words "have left," but makes no other suggestions. Paul: "Is that subtraction? Isn't it?" He uses his fingers again and comes up with the correct solution, "Seven." (Overtime and suggestion account for his earning no credit for this belated solution.) E: "Now let us see this one. At seven cents each, what will three cigars cost?" Paul: "Ten." E: "Why?" Paul: "Seven and three is ten." E: "It is multiplication." Paul: "I have not had sevens—I can't do these things." E: "Have you had threes?" Paul: "Yes." E: "Now let us say, 'At three cents each, what will seven cigars cost?' " Paul: "Seven threes . . . one three is three, two threes is six, three threes is nine, four threes is twelve, five threes is thirteen, no, is fifteen, six threes is eighteen, seven threes is . . . twenty-one, eight threes is . . . twenty-four , . . " E: "What were you trying to find?" Paul: "Seven threes is twenty-one." E interrupts task. (Total WISC score: six points.)

Paul runs into difficulty as soon as he has to choose operations himself. He has some of the simple arithmetic facts at his disposal; he knows additions within ten, and by using his fingers is able to add small numbers beyond ten. He knows some multiplication tables by rote; he has to repeat the whole series and cannot muster multiplication facts out of context.

The second session, devoted predominantly to the WISC material, interspersed with some other relevant tests, went along rather satisfactorily. Its emotional climate was variable, but remained reasonably serene. E remained intent on avoiding frustration and negativistic attitudes. The sequence of the tasks was arranged accordingly. At the beginning, the various picture tasks continued the game atmosphere of the previous session and this was carried over into the block designs. After this, Paul seemed ready for more verbal situations. E tried to make these as attractive as possible by starting them with simple tasks (analogies). During the information questions, conversation relieved apprehension which might have been aroused by questions on school learning. Paul had the opportunity to show some everyday competence not necessarily tapped by the WISC questions. Later, when disagreeable subjects (arithmetic) were introduced, they were preceded by easy tasks with numbers (counting).

COMMENT

Throughout the testing situation, it was felt that Paul's achievements represented as nearly as possible his optimum level of intelligence. Without the careful manipulations described above, this would probably not have been the case.

In terms of numerical test results, he has on the performance scale an I.Q. of approximately 69, on the verbal scale approximately 75, and on the full scale approximately 70.

Perhaps more important than these numerical results are the somewhat less tangible facts which emerge from the psychological interview and which are summarized below.

At twelve Paul still requires concessions which a normal child has usually outgrown before this age. Paul has not yet learned how to control his fears and negativistic attitudes. He does not yet know how to accept failure as part of life, but becomes upset and unruly when faced with a difficult situation.

The examination has shown disabilities which account for his slow progress in intellectual matters and which are equally responsible for his immature attitudes in situations demanding flexible adjustments. Many situations are threatening and stressful for him because he comprehends only superficially and in simple terms. As he did in some of the tests (picture arrangements, bicycle), he reacts too impulsively to his first immediate perceptions and is unable to make comparisons or predictions on the basis of previous experiences. He is slow to learn from experience, but learns best in the secure emotional climate of familiar situations.

His immature, tense, and often apprehensive attitude, his slow and frequently erratic adjustments, added to his physical appearance and motor handicap, are bound to make an unfavorable first impression on the casual outsider. This, in turn, contributes to making Paul even more self-conscious and insecure than other adolescent boys with whom he shares many characteristic traits.

To those who are close to him and understand him, Paul is a gentle, sensitive, and essentially emotionally uncomplicated person. He is quick to perceive friendly and encouraging attitudes and responds to them readily. He is, in general, not unduly suspicious of adults and accepts and depends on their authority. When he is on guard, it is mostly against displaying his own shortcomings because he is interested in establishing pleasant relationships with others. He is rather childlike and direct in his confidences and egocentric statements.

It seems important to gear future plans so that Paul can develop his favorable personality traits more and more. He will have to have success and satisfactions. With his reasoning and learning ability still only on an eight- to nine-year level, and his academic achievements not beyond second- or third-grade level, it is to be assumed that Paul will not go much further or become happier in school. He may consolidate some gains in certain academic subjects, but he is unlikely to reach an intellectual level at which techniques become tools for higher learning. Though he still has to continue in school, he needs a supplement of other activities. For Paul, other goals and aspirations must take the place of the conventional ones. It does not seem too early to develop in him interest and possibly skill in practical matters (carpentering, painting, cooking). Some simple but real achievements in this direction might enhance his self-respect and make him more acceptable to others. He will probably always remain a person who must depend on the good will and friendship of a few. He will have to be protected from social situations which are too complicated for him to handle.

He will continue to be amenable and comfortable enough as long as he can live in a sympathetic environment. His family is willing and, at least at present, able to give him the protection he needs without resorting to public resources.

STAGES OF DEVELOPMENT AND THEIR PROBLEMS

Paul's psychological development through the years follows a pattern found to be prevalent in children with brain injury resulting in hemiplegia and irregularity of mental functioning. Such patterns, identifiable in some form at each age level, are determined largely by the child's physiological development and partly by his life experiences. Some aspects of the pattern are specific for similarly handicapped children; others are common to most children because they are inherent in the process of growing up in a similar culture with similar educational and emotional standards.

At fifteen months Paul is retarded in his motor development; he is limited in his ability to get around and to use his hands. His contact with the world of objects remains superficial. He is attracted by objects in his direct view or reach. He shows little initiative and enterprise because most stimuli remain undifferentiated and unspecific for him and leave no prolonged imprint. He has a few simple patterns of reaction to stimuli of varied sorts. His undifferentiated and scantily adapted responses make him socially a friendly, unperturbed baby who smiles at everybody and everything. His invariably good-natured attitude masks a lack of discrimination of the finer shadings and moods which cause a normal baby of this age frequently to be shy and oversensitive to new impressions. Paul's shortcomings, however, are at present no serious hindrance to him; in many ways they are an asset. He is still fully able to live up to the demands of his life situation. He creates friendly, warm, and indulgent feelings in those around him, and can be easily loved, comforted, and entertained. Although his parents are rightly worried about the lag in his motor development and especially about his stiff hand, they are unaware of his serious limitations in comprehension. They have not yet fully visualized the impact of his handicaps on his future development.

At four years of age Paul's motor impairment still makes him clumsy and insecure when moving around. He still is more involved in experimenting with his own body movements and precarious equilibrium than in investigating objects. While other children at his age examine and try to comprehend their surroundings, Paul still has no well-defined notions about qualities and properties of objects. Among many others are his perceptuo-visual and sensory difficulties, which delay his ability for fine discrimination. He has a set of poorly organized responses which are more primitive than those of other children at his age. The normal child's visual, auditory, and social perceptions are embedded in organized structures which are responded to as wholes. But Paul reacts quickly and immediately to successive isolated stimuli which lack coherence and, therefore, elicit only unrelated, disconnected responses.

In the language field, Paul was late in talking. Now he quickly establishes auditory connections. He repeats properly what he hears and associates certain word sequences with certain sounds, objects, and situations. The speed of these responses masks their superficial nature as well as their lack of selection and discrimination. Superficially, these learned phrases do credit to his "good memory," but actually they are automatic registrations which lack the plasticity and flexibility of intelligently learned material.

At this age, undifferentiated directness still characterizes his social responses. The friendly baby who returned the smiles of those around him has developed into the child who, aware of his social environment, reacts impetuously to attitudes of approval or disapproval, to pressures or freedom. However, he is unable to see these attitudes against their background; he does not understand their causes and conditions and has difficulty in discriminating which of the various personalities in his surroundings display them, and when.

Paul no longer fits as smoothly into the demands of his life situation as he did in earlier years. He seems awkward physically and socially. He encounters many situations which are too complex for his means of adaptation. Content and comfortable under simple conditions, he becomes erratic, hyperactive, and disturbed when he meets a confusing multitude of stimuli. He causes disapproval, resents it, and gets more of the same. His parents recognize the vicious circle but do not know how to get out of it. They try to equip him better for the world by applying more pressure. They become exasperated with him and with themselves. Uneasy emotional attitudes are the result of an increasing awareness that there will be much cause for worry about Paul as time goes on. They are now beginning to realize that the educational concessions which he will require will set him and them apart from the usual course of a normal child's life.

At seven Paul has learned better control of his own body. He still reacts intensely to the immediate stimuli which he encounters. Now he is hyperactive mentally rather than physically. He has poor mental staying power and short attention spans. At this age his lag in form discrimination interferes with the production and comprehension of forms and symbols more than with the manipulation of objects. His ability to make quick associations helps him to remember simple, everyday routines and experiences. But at this age a retentive memory for auditory clues and series no longer suffices for adequate achievements in the language field. An undifferentiated vocabulary and failure to comprehend underlying meanings become hindrances to communication and understanding. His tendency to respond to isolated details now interferes with orderly reasoning processes. He has developed more differentiated social behavior patterns, but still is unable to respond adequately to social demands. He is still pleasant and amiable as long as he is comfortable. He now reacts to subtler social pressures than he did before. This makes him appear suggestible in many instances and defensive in others. He still is more than normally dependent on the emotional and social protection of his family. His parents themselves have become more secure. They are ready to defend him in difficult situations and they receive some immediate satisfaction from his response to their wiser and more indulgent management.

At twelve Paul, like other children of his age, has had more opportunity for experiences of living. He has shown skill in acquiring simple common-sense information. His ability to make quick associations, together with his attraction to details, help him remember facts which may remain unnoticed by others who try to understand broader connections. He can activate these facts readily because they have not been absorbed into more elaborate structures of thought. By the same token, he continues to have much difficulty in reasoning and in learning. His social sensitivity has continued to increase; he is more vulnerable to failure and criticism, but is still quick to sense friendliness and sympathy. His life situation has become more complex. He can fit it in some ways but not in others. This variability is perplexing to many people and creates around him conflicting attitudes and demands. His family knows him best and makes life easiest for him. He is less rebellious at home than is common for children his age. At this age level the simplicity of his reactions can be an asset as long as no unexpected situations require judgement and flexibility. His parents direct their concern almost entirely toward a future in which they may no longer be able to protect him fully.

Analysis of case records of children with spastic hemiplegia indicates that the pattern of development illustrated by Paul is in some ways repeated in many cases of this group.[5]

Between the ages of fifteen and thirty months, most of the babies studied are described as placid, content, responsive and alert. Only a very few are irritable and easily upset, and this disposition is, in these few rare cases, usually explained by confusing home situations or physical conditions. Though most of these babies are noted for their social assets and some for their imitative skills, all are slow in developing language. In the test situation all except a very few have some difficulty in form discrimination or orientation. These defects show mostly in tests such as pegboards, formboards, and blocks (T:IV:1–5 and I:1,2). These babies have difficulty in distinguishing between directions of strokes when scribbling (T:III:4) and are usually poor in understanding the relationships of objects and containers (T:IV:3 and V:8). They

[5] This discussion is based on the study of case records of 26 children with hemiplegia involving arm and leg (right, 17; left, 9). Of these children, 8 had two psychological examinations, 11 had three, 5 had four, and 2 had more than four. (Total number of examinations was 80.)

Interval between first and last examinations was more than three years in 3 cases, more than five years in 8 cases, more than eight years in 8 cases, more than twelve years in 7 cases.

Mental ability at last examination was above normal in 2 cases (8%), normal in 6 cases (23%), borderline in 11 cases (42%), below borderline in 7 cases (27%).

Motor impairment was severe in 6 cases (23%), moderate in 13 cases (50%), mild in 7 cases (27%).

All these children walked independently before the age of four.

frequently persist in undifferentiated banging and throwing of objects. Since these babies have only limited use of one hand, their difficulty in discrimination can easily pass for motor awkwardness alone.

The evaluating psychologist must note that future intellectual competence usually is more accurately judged by a child's adaptive skills than by his social responses. Psychological appraisal at this early age can frequently help to steer the family's expectations. The psychologist can emphasize the personality assets of the child, can point out how to develop them further, and can prepare an indulgent atmosphere for the time when intellectual liabilities may become more noticeable.

In their preschool years many of these children are still described as alert, responsive, and friendly. Many accept strangers without shyness or concern. Responding immediately to friendly attitudes, they appear sunny and chatty. All react badly to pressure and frequently become hectic or confused, like Paul. By four-and-a-half years of age, all except a very few have learned to talk. Verbal ability varies from fluent to poorly enunciated. Skill in producing automatisms such as nursery rhymes, number series, ABC, songs, or adult phrases is common (T:XI: 1,2). Verbal fluency contrasts in many cases with difficulties in verbal comprehension.

In the test situation these children may win high vocabulary scores on picture vocabulary (T:II:7) or picture description (T:II:6) tests, but they have difficulty in understanding questions. The younger children may fail in picture book questions or in conversation about things "that are not there." Those four to five years old may be able to identify pictures (T:II:9) by direct verbal-visual association, but may fail when identification in reverse tests their comprehension of the underlying process. Their fluent conversation, usually limited to immediate associations, may, to the unwary observer, appear to be meaningful conversation. Many of these children find it very difficult to sustain attention to any one task; others find it impossible to attend to a variety of stimuli at once. They may become distracted by new stimuli or remain excessively aloof from them. This can be observed in various of the above-mentioned test situations, as well as in memory for pictures (T:II:8).

Perceptuo-motor ability is more or less significantly low in all these children. In some it is defective *per se;* in others it is low only in comparison with verbal and social skills. At preschool age levels perceptuo-motor difficulties show in the tests involving pegboards

(T:IV:1,2,4), formboards (T:IV:5,6,13), blockbuilding (T:I:2), and drawing (T:III). Imitation of strokes (T:III:4), copying of designs (T:III:5,6), free drawing, or subject drawing (T:III:1–3) may reveal these disabilities. Primitive perceptions are apparent in varied test items. There may be relatively minor oversimplifications and confusions of direction in matching tests (T:VI:4,6,7), stick designs (T:VII: 6), and the like. There may, in older preschool children, be severe distortions in drawings and inadequate preposterous trials in fitting insets into formboards and such. Diagnostically significant for the whole group, as for Paul, is the discrepancy between verbal-social and visuomotor skills. Equally important is the discrepancy between automatic associative verbal ability and verbal comprehension. True learning ability is, in most cases, lacking, in spite of good auditory memory.

The behavior difficulties not uncommon at this age are, in many cases, explained by the child's other problems. Children described as quiet and responsive in earliest years frequently become hyperresponsive, erratic, and quickly upset when they meet the greater demands of their preschool years.

The psychological examination at this age level can clarify the situation and enable the adviser to give guidance and help in educational planning. The rate of the child's mental development is most adequately determined by appraisal of reasoning and verbal comprehension. Level and character of motor skills and quality of perceptuo-motor functioning furnish important clues by which to predict how well the child will later get along in school. At this age level it can be especially deceiving to judge competence by verbal fluency alone. In many cases it is well to prepare early for a possible delay in school entrance in order to avoid disappointment and undue pressure. When such advice is put off until school age is reached, it is often not easy to dissuade parents and even teachers from having the child "try to get something out of school, anyway." However, the undesirable result of such trials often persists throughout his school career. Too much pressure to keep up will harass him; too much leniency, however, will lower his own level of aspiration. In both instances the gap between the handicapped child and his normal contemporaries is widened instead of bridged, and the child's self-image is the more distorted. Development of personality assets can often, in the preschool and kindergarten years, be furthered by the child's close daily contacts in his home and neighborhood, which give him and his family more success, more satisfactions, and more opportunities to learn than a school situation into which he does not fit. With physio-therapeutic sessions mandatory in many cases, the child often has as much of his time scheduled as is good for him. But categoric advice in one or the other direction must here—as always—be avoided. Imagination and foresight must decide under which circumstances each child will find the most harmonious and relaxing climate in which to grow up.

Many case records describe children *between six and ten* as cooperative, friendly, and eager to please. Some seem hyperresponsive, others defensive and tense. In contact with a stranger, such as the psychologist, their mood is often determined by the expectations which they bring to the testing situation. The more mature children are often the most apprehensive ones. The simpler, immature, and verbose children are apt to trust their ability to please by social grace and verbal skill. Unfortunate experiences in school or elsewhere have made some more wary than others.

Their performances may vary. Those children who in earlier years showed ability to repeat automatically learned series such as nursery rhymes, still frequently are found to have a good immediate auditory memory, which enables them to repeat digits (T:VIII:5) and sentences (T:VIII:7) and perform other rote tasks (T:XI:1–3). Many have acquired verbal auditory associations which help them to succeed in opposite analogies (T:IX:5). Vocabulary scores often continue to be high, especially in picture vocabulary (T:II:7 and XII:1) and in concrete ranges of oral vocabulary tests (T:XII:2). Reasoning is frequently uneven; children with less mental impairment succeed, with the help of previously acquired experiences, in identifying differences (T:IX:1) or similarities (T:IX:2), which are tasks that can, when a certain level of maturity is reached, be solved in one quick, intuitive process. However, many children fail when the task becomes more complex, and it becomes necessary to keep in mind various parts of the problem simultaneously, as in identifying both similarities and differences (T:IX:3). In the same way, picture arrangements (T:IX:10) and verbal absurdities (T:IX:6) are solved by some children with the help of intuitive grasp, but cannot be handled when the series becomes more complex and the factors which have to be considered are too numerous. Many children of this group, however, show by their trials and errors in these tasks that they have rather adequate common sense and social experiences. Like Paul, they can also succeed often in comprehension (T:X:3) or information

(T:XI:10) on the lower levels because they are alert to social clues and social details.

Difficulties in reorganization of material are usually outstanding in many areas. Digits in reverse (T:VIII:6) are, in the majority of cases, less well solved than digits forward (T:VIII:5). Formboard tasks (T:IV:6–9) are done more slowly and usually with a great many trials and errors as soon as fine form discrimination or size discrimination is requested. Block designs (T:VII:7,8) are, at this age, usually done poorly. Scores on object assembly tests (T:IV:11,12,14) are often, though not regularly, depressed. Difficulties in organization are, in this test, most evident when the original directions are altered so that the object to be assembled is not named to the child. Drawings (T:III: 1–3), memory for designs (T:VII:1,2,4), and copying designs (T:III:5 and VII:3,5) are, in the majority of cases, the most significantly failed items. Regardless of the degree of motor skill or impairment, most children in this group show in these tests characteristically distorted or retarded performances. One may find either oversimplification or overemphasis on detail in various areas of functioning. Global primitive solutions or exaggeration of details in drawings or in other form matters are equaled by similar undifferentiated solutions or overstressed individual factors in other tasks. Important features may be ignored, less significant ones singled out, and main themes ignored in reasoning tasks such as picture arrangements (T:IX:10), Wood picture completion test (T:IX:13), or verbal absurdities (T:IX:6).

Various types of attention difficulties remain common among these children, especially in tasks which involve a prolonged and organized process. Learning tasks (T:VIII:1–3) frequently rate significantly below other performances. This may, in some cases, be due to the child's inability to stick to one line of thought and to keep focused on one set of facts. In other cases, one finds the opposite kind of attention difficulty; the child may fail to pay attention to all necessary aspects of the situation but persist doggedly in one track of thought only.

In academic areas the achievements of this group are uneven. Reading difficulties are very common owing to various causes, among them the disability in form discrimination and orientation. Spelling occasionally comes easily to a child who apparently learns the sequence of letters like other automatic series. Frequently, this accompanies inability to write or print the spelled word because the child does not know his letters. Some children at this age, thanks again to their association memory, have learned to recognize certain street signs, headlines, etc., as a skill which can pass for reading. Such performances may be as impressive to the casual observer as was the child's ability to recognize brand packages and victrola record labels in his preschool years. Arithmetic is significantly deficient except in a few children in the younger grades.

The characteristic pattern seen in Paul and other children with similar difficulties can also be found at this age, with some variations, in those hemiplegic children who have higher mental abilities. Verbal-social skills are often developed more highly in them; some children, given social and educational opportunities, develop elaborate vocabularies which make them appear precocious. For others, interest in everyday events develops a stock of readily produced information about current events which is not often found to the same degree in normal children of their age. Immediate memory prevails; prolonged learning presents more difficulty. At this age level many reasoning problems like picture arrangements can be solved by intuitive grasp of simple relationships (T:IX:10). The task is more difficult, however, if background experience is lacking and need for elaborations and construction is more urgent. Difficulty in organizing new material is, in this superior group, most apparent in block designs (T:VII:7,8), memory for designs (T:VII:1,2,4,5), and other similar tasks. In school these children often read avidly but slowly. In arithmetic, they love computation but hate problems.

(Such characteristic patterns of functioning are apt to be blurred in children with low mentalities. Poor visuo-motor ability and serious attention and learning difficulties may, or may not, accompany verbal fluency. If they do, performances in vocabulary tests (T:XII) are often low because there is not enough differentiation of meanings of words. The automatic series which have been acquired by these children are based on the simplest associations only.)

At this age level the test characteristics of the hemiplegic group may be summarized as follows: relatively high performance in verbal tasks such as vocabulary, common sense questions, and everyday information; irregular performance in reasoning, with best achievements in tasks which can be solved quickly and intuitively, but poorest performances in those that require coordination of multiple factors; more or less serious difficulty in learning and attention tests; and generally low performances in most perceptuo-motor tasks.

In the psychological examination mental efficiency is appraised by careful distinction between those achievements obtained with the help of verbal associations and auditory memory and those based on adequately coordinated reasoning processes. At this age mental progress depends on ability to adjust to and comprehend new situations swiftly and to learn from them. Good immediate auditory memory is no longer sufficient, since with progressing age the child meets increasingly complex situations. Adequate structuring and logical objective reasoning processes become more and more important for him. Again it is the appraisal of the child's reasoning level that yields the best single clue to his mental level. Investigation of his learning ability and study of his perceptuo-motor functioning help best to predict his academic and educational progress. Behavior and attitude of the child must be of great concern to the examiner. They help to determine how well the child will be able to make the best use of his endowment in the new social experiences which lie ahead of him.

Psychological examination leads to reappraisal of school and home situations. Depending on the school's reports, parents may have varying degrees of insight into the child's mental situation; pressures for academic achievement and better behavior can occasionally be significantly modified when test results are well interpreted to the parents. Some complaints about behavior may appear to them in a different light when these can be explained by constitutional difficulties rather than by educational failure. In some families, however, the emphasis on accomplishment is so great that any substandard measure is difficult to accept. The psychological examination often helps in taking stock, in remedying school attitudes, and in giving new focus to the family. At this age level it becomes increasingly important to provide the child with opportunity for success, regardless of how modest or insignificant it may seem. Some children can use their good memory for repeating songs, poems, or prayers; others can use their friendliness to become popular in a circle of adults in the neighborhood. Any kind of success makes both the child and his parents happier and paves the way for smoother progress.

In the years between eleven and sixteen these children, in general, display more signs of self-consciousness. Many previously carefree and cooperative children now are less confident of their own abilities. On the surface they are still friendly. They may seem to like to meet new people, but frequently are anxious to set the tone of the examination and to avoid sensitive or demanding subjects. The record notes bear descriptions such as "overtly friendly, but guarded," "puts on a good show," "acts nonchalant," "senses failure," "works hard," "is eager to please." The chattiness which was displayed by many of the children at an earlier age is no longer as prominent. Some children may still be conversational about their own affairs, but rather closemouthed during the examination. Their social awareness has obviously taught them through the years that they no longer can rely on their verbal fluency alone when they want to please adults. In some children the previously noted ability to make quick associations now may show up in verbal tasks such as vocabulary and abstract words (T:XII:2). An unfamiliar word on the list sounds similar to and reminds them of another familiar word which they are apt to define instead. Part of a statement in a comprehension question (T:X:3) or verbal absurdity (T:IX:6) may remind them successfully of a recent event. The same ability for superficial quick connecting still allows them to show their interest in everyday events (T:X:2) as it did before. However, scores in comprehension (T:X:3) and information (T:XI:10) may be uneven where current events questions require, at this age level, more solid background information and underlying reasoning. Some children's former interest in and preoccupation with details develops at older age levels into anxious meticulousness. They often are slower now than they were previously to start out on an unfamiliar task; they may ask for more directions and additional information. Others again throw themselves upon a detail of their own choosing, as they did before, but their attitude appears more desperate and less carefree or secure than it was before. Many of them now become flustered and embarrassed, and seem to expect failure and ridicule. They refer more frequently, directly or indirectly, to their own physical or mental shortcomings. The characteristics of functioning described at earlier levels are still prominent. Performances in reasoning tasks become more irregular. Discrepancy between rather good solutions in tasks which can be solved in one quick glance, such as some similarities (T:IX:2), verbal absurdities (T:IX:6), and others which demand more complex reasoning, such as arithmetic, are more in evidence. Most of the children discussed here continue to have serious problems in perceptuo-motor functioning. This is evidenced by low scores in memory for various designs (T:VII: 1,2,4,5), copying of complex figures as in the Bender visual motor Gestalt test (T:VII:3) and the Rey-Osterrieth complex figure test (T:VII:5), and, in general, in block designs (T:VII:7,8). Occasionally some of these children attain high scores in block designs or in some memory for design test, which at first glance seem surprising. Here again study of the process rather than of the end result shows that the solution was obtained by the cumbersome adding of detail to detail favored by some of the brighter, more meticulous children.

Learning ability continues poor among these children. Learning tests (T:VIII:1–3) show low scores. Some children acquire through rote memory many varied bits of information which add up to a good stock of learned items and enhance their performances in tasks such as information (T:XI:10), current events (T:X:2,3), and vocabulary (T:XII:2). Judged *per se,* these scores do not necessarily bear witness to the labor which was involved when the child went through the process of learning the facts. The larger number of children in the group are slow where comprehension must precede learning. Valuable additional insight in the quality of learning ability can be obtained when the time and effort spent on a child's academic education are compared with the achievements. Most children in this group lag behind their normal grades or have a hard struggle to keep up. Reading skills continue uneven in this group. Those who know how to read fluently often fail in subjects which emphasize reading comprehension rather than reading skills (history, social science). Arithmetic is commonly poor in children who have passed the age at which memorized arithmetic facts and simple mechanical computation alone can bring success. Usually they have difficulty in choosing the proper operation or in keeping an operational plan in mind. Occasionally, however, some arithmetic problem is solved by intuitive grasp of a number combination.

At this age an estimate of mental ability is arrived at by the careful study of reasoning ability, perceptuo-motor functioning, and learning ability. It is often deceiving to rely, as one might in certain adult cases, on a comparison between total verbal scores and total performance scores in order to identify mental disabilities due to brain injury.[6] Also it is not only unreliable to consider single items such as block designs or object assembly tests (WISC or Wechsler-Bellevue) as foolproof tools

---

[6] David Wechsler, *The Measurement of Adult Intelligence* (Baltimore: Williams and Wilkins, 1944), pp. 148ff. In the revised 1958 edition, published after this manuscript was completed, Wechsler discusses in detail some of the complex problems involved also in the diagnosis of brain injury in adults. See *The Measurement and Appraisal of Adult Intelligence* (Baltimore: Williams and Wilkins, 1958), Chapter 13. Also Donald O. Hebb, "The Effect of Early and Late Brain Injury upon Test Scores, and the Nature of Normal Adult Intelligence," *Proceedings of the American Philosophical Society* 85:275–292, February 1942.

for diagnosing organic difficulties, but also dangerous to judge the degree of such involvement by the value of these individual scores. At this age the total verbal score and the total performance score may be more nearly equal than they were in earlier years, when performance scores were usually well below verbal scores. Verbal tasks such as similarities and vocabulary may now demand more active and constructive reasoning than they did at younger age levels. Performance tests (picture arrangement, picture completion) now contain more elements of social and visual experience, and therefore for some children are easier now than they were in earlier years. The above described piecemeal solutions in block designs (T:VII:7,8) also may add to the numerical score of the performance scale. Often the psychologist's concern centers around the patient's behavior and social attitudes even if at this period the parents are often more interested in educational and academic advice only and dismiss personality problems as normal for the age.

Children with an over-all rating of just normal or better often present a more acute problem than those who are more impaired mentally. In spite of their physical handicaps, they may have been able to stay more or less in competition with their contemporaries up to this time. But now, with the work becoming harder, some are subject to additional educational pressure. Others are resentful when those around them seem defeatist and no longer seem to believe in them. They then drive themselves hard in order to show how capable they are. The result, in both cases, is much tension and discontent, which are heightened by the problems of adolescence. Less able children, like Paul, are at this age usually somewhat more protected from academic pressures. Educational and professional standards have been relaxed earlier for them. Occupational problems become more acute.

The psychological examination should help to clarify expectations and to arrange for the happiest solution for the years immediately following. For some children, the psychologist tries to diminish pressure, but also tries to avoid undermining the confidence others may have in the children. For others one may wish for more opportunities and experiences. This happens especially when failures in school have so marked the child that those around him no longer think that he may become more able, successful, and independent in any field, no matter how modest. Occasionally, some planning for other activities relieves tension and monotony for parents and child.

Extrapyramidal Lesion, Athetosis Dysarthria

Bobby was born with an extrapyramidal lesion which has resulted in severe athetosis and dysarthria. His intellect is potentially intact; he has adequate reasoning ability. His chief problems are his physical helplessness and his inability to express himself by speech or motion. These deficiencies profoundly influence his development and distort his relationships with people, objects, and ideas. His over-all situation does not change much through the years. However, the problems which concern his adjustment take varying forms as he grows older. As a baby he appears remote and unresponsive because of his inability to move and his difficulty in expressing emotions. However, his family recognizes his growing awareness and comprehension. At age four he is still completely dependent physically and lacks social and emotional experiences outside his immediate family; his experiences are restricted to what he sees, hears, and observes. He understands language, but is unable to use it effectively for communication. His limited opportunities for exploring and using what he knows keep him somewhat aloof and remote. At seven, having gained a minimum degree of independence, he can develop closer relationships with people and things. Since he now communicates through language in spite of his severe speech difficulty, he gains satisfaction through his intellectual competence, which is now becoming obvious to all. At age twelve his receptive intelligence is still his best asset. His slow and cumbersome speech continues to make communication difficult and to hinder learning through exchange of ideas. This factor, added to other consequences of his physical impairment, causes him to become more lonesome and remote as he grows older.

Using Bobby's case as illustration, this chapter presents a description of repeated psychological evaluations of a child with severe athetosis and dysarthria. This detailed account of the study procedure shows how Bobby's adequate comprehension and reasoning ability are, in spite of his physical difficulties, revealed through his responses to various test situations, and how at each period of his childhood they, together with other information, are interpreted by the psychologist in terms of personal social adjustment. The last section describes how the specific psychological trends and difficulties illustrated by Bobby at each stage of his development are in some ways common in similarly disabled children, as was found by comparison with other case records. It also points out briefly how the psychologist identifies some of the problem areas and tries to solve a few of the questions that arise.

BOBBY AT FIFTEEN MONTHS

Bobby's development has been extremely slow from the start. At five and six months of age, his mother noticed that his fists were still tightly clenched and that he did not grasp anything. He has never been able to hold up his head. He still does not sit, but flops over in jackknife fashion when placed in a sitting position. He usually lies on his back, his head turned to one side. He uses his hands hardly at all, but does somewhat better with his left than with his right. He is unable to roll over; therefore, someone in his family gets up several times each night to turn him over. He is difficult to feed; he does not chew, often does not swallow, and regurgitates. He still lives on a semiliquid diet. He is fed five or six times a day because his mother finds that he becomes less tired and eats better when fed small amounts frequently. She knows that the baby not only recognizes his bottle but also distinguishes between milk and orange juice in it. He is said to have been "trained" for several months; when he is wet or soiled he cries until his mother comes to pick him up. She can distinguish sounds meaning hunger or discomfort from those expressing pleasure.

When brought to the psychologist, Bobby is placed in the examining crib; he lies there rather quietly with his legs outstretched stiffly and crossed slightly. His face seems expressionless, but his eyes show life and some apprehension. He follows his mother with his eyes as long as she stays in sight; when she inadvertently goes beyond his field of vision, he looks more perturbed and agitates his arms and head in jerky, uncoordinated movements. He relaxes when his mother talks to him. A red ring is moved in front of him, first slowly sideways, and later quickly (T:V:1,2). His arms become agitated; again the left seems to move more than the right. He is unable to approach the ring effectively with either hand but follows it with his eyes without turning his head. A screen is set up; the ring is moved slowly toward the screen, then is made to disappear behind it and come out the other end (T:V:7). At first Bobby keeps looking at the spot where the ring disappeared from his sight. However, after the procedure has been repeated twice, Bobby has learned that he can expect to see the ring again at the other end of the screen. As soon as it disappears, he shifts his gaze to the other side. (Normal babies learn to react this way when they are about twelve to fourteen months of age.)

Bobby also shows his comprehension in the next situation (T:V:4). A set of jingle bells is shown him; then placed under a nearby cloth. He keeps staring at the spot and seems pleased when E uncovers them again for him. This is repeated several times. After this the bells are moved to a spot farther away and hidden under a cloth there. It seems clear enough that this time Bobby expects to have them uncovered there. His interest in the situation is very obvious. (His mother comments that Bobby "just loves" to watch people playing with things for him.)

Presented with a picture book (T:II:1–3), Bobby's eyes move from one color spot to the next. He becomes somewhat agitated when his mother asks him, "Where is the doggy?" and fixates on the correct page. When it has been turned, his mother asks him the same question. The child looks about the page without finding a point to fixate. He seems to search for the previous page at the proper side of the book. He later smiles at the dog when the page is turned back for him. All through these situations the child hardly vocalizes, though he produces a few undifferentiated gutteral sounds.

When placed in a sitting position on his mother's lap with his head supported by her, he is presented with a pellet and bottle (T:V:8). At first he notices the bottle alone; later he becomes aware of the pellet which is being dropped out of the bottle. He pursues it visually and smiles when the performance is repeated for him. E opens his fisted right hand and puts a block in it. Bobby loses the block and seems startled to see it dropping on the table. When the same experiment is repeated with the left hand, his hand seems to open somewhat more easily. He holds on longer and better, taps the table top with the block clenched between palm and thumb; when the block falls out of his hand, he agitates his hand as if wanting to retrieve it, but does not succeed. In the sitting position, the experiment of the ring disappearing behind the screen does not succeed again. Bobby seems to tire quickly. With his poor head control, he cannot follow an object as well when he is sitting as when he is lying on his back. He sees only what is immediately in front of him and appears oblivious to what goes on just outside his visual field. When put on the floor, he stares at a shelf which happens to be in front of him; he remains motionless and bewildered; he starts to cry but stops when his mother talks to him.

COMMENT

The observation period has shown that this baby is more observant and alert than he appears at first glance. He is aware of being in a strange place and is ill at ease in new surroundings. However, he has only limited means of expressing his discomfort.

There is evidence that his perceptions and his comprehension of objects and motions are nearly adequate for his age (ring disappearing behind screen, bells hidden by cloth). He also seems to comprehend some language (picture book). He fails to notice very small objects at first. Obviously he has had little experience with any objects, especially very small ones. Lack of effective manipulation, locomotion, lip movements, and sound production must seriously limit the scope of his interests and activity. For the time being it seems reasonable to assume that most of Bobby's retardation is due to motor impairment rather than to a lack of intellectual endowment. Already at this early age his personality development is being affected by his physical limitations. He is unable to develop patterns of independence and initiative which enable the normal baby to deal more and more effectively with his environment. Whether his potentialities can develop enough to be effective despite these difficulties remains to be seen.

BOBBY AT FOUR YEARS

Bobby's progress has been very slow; he still does not walk at all. He can, with support, maintain himself in a sitting position for a short while, but he has a tendency to slide backwards and out of his chair. He can do very little with his hands, but uses the left somewhat more than the right. Both hands have jerky, uncontrolled movements. He cannot stand independently, but for short periods can lean propped upright against a wall or a chair. According to his mother, his ability to stand has not improved much in the past two years. At home he sits in a specially constructed chair. Various walkers have been tried at different times during the past years but were found to be unsatisfactory. At present he can push a three-wheel "Taylor Tot," but needs help to guide it in the right direction. His parents continue to carry him about since there is no way in which he can get around independently. The family, though distressed about his poor motor development, takes pleasure and pride in more and more obvious signs of mental competence (T:X:1). They understand his speech, which is hardly intelligible to outsiders. They claim that Bobby talks in sentences, understands everything, and can express his views. They find that he closely follows his mother's activities around the house. He knows routines and is always well aware of any change. He knows where things are kept and when they are needed, and notices what or who is missing. He likes to watch television and identifies commercials and props of several shows. He has definite favorites in foods and recognizes those which he does not like, even in disguise (eggs in milk, for example). He never wets, but becomes unhappy and restless if not attended to promptly. He is described as a good and thoughtful child who is sensitive to the moods of his family. His mother, a lively, tense, insistent person, has centered her life around Bobby's care. She spends a great deal of time with him and admits that she somewhat neglects the rest of the family. She never goes out with her husband; he accepts this as apparently unavoidable. Bobby's seven-year-old sister is an independent, somewhat tempestuous little girl. In her relationship with her brother, she vacillates between self-effacing adoration and occasional stinging abuse. For the latter she is usually severely reprimanded. Both mother and father smile when Bobby, fully aware of such scenes, enjoys his sister's disgrace and repentance as much as his own role as wronged hero.

Bobby's parents request a psychological evaluation at this time in order to assist them in educational planning. They also hope it will convince doubtful relatives and friends that Bobby has great assets and help stop the flow of free advice on how to run their difficult life more efficiently and with less "sacrifice."

Bobby enters the office of E on his father's arm. He seems passive and vaguely smiling, while his mother is tense and managing. Since none of the available seating facilities seem to her suited to Bobby's purposes, E proposes that his mother hold Bobby in her lap. The mother seats herself near the table, but Bobby, turned halfway toward her, leans backward in her arms. He mumbles to her, but either ignores or does not notice E. The mother's hands are joined around the child's waist and are therefore a barrier between table and child.

BLOCKS (T:I:1,4)

When E produces two boxes and two sets of blocks (one red and one green), Bobby's mother looks at them apprehensively and explains that Bobby "cannot do anything with these because he cannot use his hands!" E has to ask her to turn Bobby and to hold him so that he may at least see the blocks and have as free a range of action as possible. Bobby, who has remained passive and quiet until this point and is now nearer to the table with his head drooping a little, becomes aware of the blocks. Uncoordinated general activity increases; he starts thrashing about. With the palm of his left hand he gets a hold on a green block, but involuntarily sideswipes several others which fall onto the floor. Startled by this, Bobby loses the block he held precariously.

SORTING COLORS (T:I:6 AND VI:1)

E places the boxes wide apart, holds up a green block, then slowly places it in one of the boxes; she picks up a red one and places it in the other box; picks up a green one and places it in the box with the first green one. When she picks up a red one again, she watches Bobby trying to strain in the direction of the first red block. E places a red block in Bobby's left hand. He makes attempts toward the box with the other red blocks but drops the block near the box, not into it. His excited movements sweep a few blocks from the table again. When Bobby's father, trying to be helpful, picks them up again, E stops him with a sign and retrieves the blocks herself. She tries to make the parents observers who do not actively participate in the situation and hopes that this may facilitate direct contact between herself and Bobby.

Bobby grasps another green block and strains toward the green box. E tilts it somewhat to make aiming easier for him. He is pleased when he drops the block into the box and angles for another one. E helps him take hold of it again; he tries for the correct box once more, but drops the block on the floor. It is now obvious that Bobby intends to sort the blocks by color and that he has noticed that the situation calls for this even before E has made any suggestion to that effect.

In order to avoid undue strain on Bobby so early in the examination, E decides to test his continuous interest and comprehension of the task by suggesting sorting by proxy. E: "You tell me where to put it." She holds up each block and watches to see toward which box he strains. For six consecutive trials Bobby indicates correctly where the blocks should go. His immediate comprehension and unhesitating choices show that this task is easy for Bobby. (His performance is comparable to that of normal children of three- to three- and-a-half years.)

Bobby's interest and eagerness increase his involuntary motor activity. His mother, who herself is more at ease now, admonishes him to relax. His father, volunteering to hold him, sits on a small stool in front of the table with the child held between his knees. This new position gives Bobby more freedom of action and at the same time his excessive flailing motions subside somewhat. More and more he accepts the idea that he can show what he wants done and need not handle all materials on his own. The two next procedures are done by proxy.

SERIAL PATTERNS (T:I:5)

The red and green blocks are to be arranged in a pattern: one red, one green, one red, one green. The child must choose which color is to come next. For Bobby the blocks stay in their respective boxes, which are placed far apart to avoid ambiguity.

Bobby makes the correct choice for the next five blocks. Obviously he has understood the principle of the pattern as well as do normal three-and-a-half-year-old children.

DECROLY MATCHING GAME (T:VI:4)

A matching game with sixteen small pictures representing common objects which are to be matched with identical pictures on large cards.

Bobby correctly chooses places for the first five pictures (apple, star, square, train, pear). Then he makes his first error by putting the triangle on the sailboat. His mother gasps, "Now, Bobby!" E signals to her to resist admonishing Bobby. He continues to choose correctly with the exception of the flag which is placed on the umbrella and the pitcher placed on the watering can. Flag and umbrella have a superficial resemblance, as do pitcher and watering can, triangle and sailboat. (Performance at least at four-and-a-half-year level.)

IDENTIFICATION BY GROUP CONCEPT (T:VI:4 AND II:5,9)

E: "Which ones can we eat?" Bobby looks around, fixates on the apple and makes an attempt at naming it slowly and indistinctly. Then he finds the square and mumbles something which his mother interprets as "cooky." E: "Which ones are up in the sky?" He looks at the disk and says "moon," then at the flag and utters some sounds which are interpreted as "parade." Bobby overlooks the star. His mother volunteers: "I guess he has not seen any stars. Bobby is not a night owl." Bobby mumbles to his father who interprets proudly that Bobby asked to go to see "Uncle Jack." Bobby observed a parade from Uncle Jack's window about four weeks ago.

E decides to explore the area of language comprehension and reasoning further and to continue on the same line by producing:

PICTURE BOOK (T:II:1,5)

E says: "Let us look at the book and find all the animals in it." She turns the pages slowly. Bobby indicates correctly the horse, lamb, dog, rabbit, and elephant. He omits the duck. Bobby knows how to choose pictures which are relevant to a concept and is able to disregard others. He comprehends the questions and groups objects by practical concepts which are derived from his immediate experience. When he designates the flag as belonging in the sky, E remembers that this is not an uncommon solution for immobile, handicapped children who spend much time looking up toward things above them.

IDENTIFICATION BY USE. E: "Which one writes?" Bobby indicates pencil. E: "Which one do we sit on?" Bobby indicates chair. E: "Which one tells us what time it is?" Bobby shows clock. (His comprehension of this type of question is at approximately the four-year level.)

E wishes to confirm her impression of his good comprehension by additional test procedures, but decides to continue to use the picture book. Black and white card material (T:II:9), ordinarily used with normal children, has more pictures to a page than a picture book. Since Bobby must indicate his responses largely through his poorly directed motions, this may lead to ambiguity.

IDENTIFYING ANIMALS BY NAME. E says, "Let us see more of these animals you found; where is the lamb?" E turns the page. Agitated, Bobby points toward the horse. E: "Where is the elephant,

. . . the dog?" Both correct. E: "Where is the horse?" Bobby chooses the lamb. His first error between horse and lamb is confirmed. E: "Where is the chicken, . . . the duck?" He does not find either. His name vocabulary may not be as good as his other performances. But in order to be definite about this, one would need more proof.

Now Bobby shows increasing signs of fatigue. He thrashes around more and drools profusely. His mother tries to wipe his mouth; he seems annoyed at this and tries to ward her off.

Seguin Formboard (T:IV:6)

As an introduction to the task, E places the round inset and the cross. Bobby is looking on. E, holding up the oval inset, asks where it goes. Bobby tries to point correctly for it and the square. When E holds a triangle, Bobby indicates the place for the lozenge. He is correct in showing the proper place for the rectangle; for lozenge, however, he indicates the elongated hexagon. E places the star to avoid fatigue.

When the Seguin formboard is repeated, E removes lozenge, hexagon, triangle, and oval. She holds up hexagon; Bobby shows oval but corrects his error. She holds up lozenge; Bobby responds correctly.

It seems that Bobby is able to recognize immediately the similarity of the simpler forms. He has hesitations about the more difficult ones (hexagon, lozenge) and seems predominantly guided by some outstanding form characteristic (pointedness, etc.). His are not unusual first choices for children of his age; however, normal children can soon correct their errors through trial and error methods which are impossible for Bobby because of his motor impairment.

Picture Completion (T:IX:12)

E asks what is missing in pictures. To table with leg missing, Bobby answers "plates." To coat with sleeve missing, he answers "man." To cat with tail missing, he answers "a cat." Examination interrupted.

Comment

The examination was restricted to a small number of items. The child's disability precluded the use of many materials. While more tests could have been introduced, they probably would not have added enough information to justify more fatigue for the child and possible increasing apprehension for the parents. All through the examination E was much aware of both these dangers. Since the psychological examination was designed to profit parents as well as child, much attention had to be paid to the parents' feelings toward it. The mother's almost hostile attitude gradually disappeared when E showed signs of appreciating Bobby's competence. However, she remained ready to explain and defend. Therefore, E tried to rely on techniques which were likely to introduce a minimum of frustration for all concerned.

The examination, sketchy as it may have seemed, on the whole has fulfilled its purpose and has thrown light on several of the most important aspects of Bobby's situation.

The extreme degree of his disability necessarily keeps him fully dependent on his mother and father at an age when most children have gained a certain amount of freedom. Bobby still needs them to support his body, to help him move, to feed him, and to interpret his wants. For his mother, this has resulted in an intense and exaggerated feeling of responsibility and prolongation of earliest protective tendencies. She has unconsciously set a wall between the child and the world. (During the observation period this could be seen in her objection to all available seating arrangements in which he would have been independent of her and in the way in which she at first held him shielded from the table.)

Bobby, in turn, is influenced by such apprehension. During the examination he kept himself passive and aloof at first. However, he is not centered exclusively on his mother. He had no objection to switching over to his father; after a while he communicated only occasionally with either one of them. He showed initiative and curiosity when presented with test material; he was intent on dealing with it without help. He resented being interrupted to have his mouth wiped. In contact with a new situation, he was more interested in the objects themselves than in E. He did not try to communicate with her for some time. Gradually, however, he adopted the method of showing her, instead of attempting to do things on his own in his inefficient way. Considering that he is neither accustomed to social exchange with strangers or to independent exploration of entertainment material, he adapted surprisingly well to the new situation.

The test performances, meager as they may seem, show that in many areas Bobby's comprehension and reasoning ability are within normal limits (Decroly matching game, picture identification). His errors in form matching, his insecurity in differentiating animal names, and possibly his unadapted responses in the incomplete pictures, seem to show that his development is about normal for his age, but not superior as his family likes to claim.

For the moment, it may be only academic, not practical, to question whether Bobby's lack of experience has held him back mentally from what he was "meant" to be or whether he has developed as much mental power as his potential endowment permits. The more important evidence which results from this examination is that at age four, Bobby, though seriously handicapped physically, shows promise of normal mental abilities; within his limitations he seems to be ready for more experience and more independence than he has had so far. In a day nursery school for handicapped children, he might become interested in learning some locomotion within his means; he may gain more balance by activities on the floor and may learn to roll over and thereby get from place to place under his own steam. He would also learn to live in a group with others who have similar difficulties and similar rights, and so would grow socially and emotionally. Bobby himself may have some conflicts in his adjustment to a new group since his mother will find it hard to relinquish any part of his care to others. The child at first may be torn between loyalty to his mother and pleasure in the new experience. But with both parents most enthusiastic about the plan, the experiment seems worth trying.

BOBBY AT SEVEN YEARS

Bobby, now seven, continues to be a severely handicapped child. He still cannot stand independently and does not walk. He cannot sit without being supported. He cannot creep; occasionally he drags along a few inches on his abdomen, but usually he gets around the floor by rolling. There are still many involuntary movements which involve his head and his hands, which he still uses very poorly. As before, he can grasp somewhat better with his left than with his right hand. His speech is laborious and very slow; those who take time to listen to him carefully can understand him reasonably well. He talks much more than he did and likes to use long sentences.

Three times a week for the past three years he has attended a nursery school for children with cerebral palsy. There he has been encouraged to roll on the floor and to try to get things for himself when he wants them. His joy in being more independent has been recognized by his parents. His father built an apparatus which enables him to turn the pages of a book. His mother has been gratified by the success of her effort to teach him how to read. Both parents are proud of him and his accomplishments. They are inclined to have standards for him which are too high. Their endless imaginative ideas about how to improve his situation have offered these enterprising people an outlet for their frustration and has given them prestige among other parents at the school which Bobby attends.

Bobby is examined on one of his regular mornings in school. In order to avoid the strain of changing to a different position, he comes directly from the playroom seated in his special chair. Even so, his involuntary chaotic movements are momentarily increased by his excitement about the unusual event. He is in a cheerful mood; he seems accustomed to friendly contact with adults. He gives the impression of an older person who, because of an infirmity, has to be tactfully helped by others; intuitively one treats him in a matter-of-fact manner and avoids appearing overly patronizing.

The following considerations guide E while she plans the course of the examination which is to help in preparing some educational program for Bobby.

The examination must be short since the child is known to tire quickly. However, it should bring out a picture of Bobby's abilities, special difficulties, working habits, and personality characteristics. While E will soon find out how much or how little Bobby can do motorwise, at first she will avoid tasks which involve much manipulation. His efforts to accomplish them would strain him unnecessarily and leave him too exhausted for further testing. Also, he might feel soon that her demands are all beyond him anyway. He knows condescending and "kind" adults all too well; he may readily assume that E would happily accept almost anything he might produce. Such a low level of aspiration would result in less than his best achievements. Though manipulative tasks are undesirable, the use of verbal material also has its limitations at this stage of the examination. Each of his verbal responses will take a great deal of time because of the child's serious speech impairment. Therefore, E has to choose only the most relevant questions and pick those which do not call for lengthy or complex answers. Bobby is difficult to understand for those who do not know him well; until E gets used to him, it will be necessary to postpone verbal tests which might leave her in doubt about what he has said.

Since verbalization and manipulation are limited, the child will have to communicate by pointing and gesturing in some tasks. Test material must be set up in spatial arrangements and sequences which preclude errors of interpretation. Each task involving new test material also means new motor and visual adjustments for Bobby. Therefore, it will be easier for the child and the observer to limit the number of changes and make the most of each material. E will have to be on the alert for the child's moods and emotional reactions in the testing situation—even more than she would with a normal child. Signs of frustration may be more difficult to appreciate, since Bobby's means of expression are so limited. In this sensitive child, responses may be seriously influenced by some slight upset. All along Bobby must be assured that E is neither shocked nor baffled by him and that she understands him without difficulty. She begins by introducing blocks.

SERIAL PATTERNS (T:I:4,5)

E: "We want to arrange the blocks one red, one green, one red, one green." E arranges four of them, saying, "You tell me which to take. I'll do it, and you tell me which." Bobby indicates four consecutive blocks correctly; he tries to strain toward them himself and approaches them with his left hand.

E now explains that blocks are to be arranged two green, one red, two green, one red, etc.: "You tell me which and I will do it for you." Bobby does not hesitate; he indicates correctly the next six blocks to be placed. E: "Which ones will be left over?" He predicts correctly by indicating the red blocks. E: "Why?" Bobby: "Use—more—greens." In spite of E's instructions, Bobby consistently follows an impulse to try to get hold of the blocks in order to arrange them himself. He upsets the blocks which are in front of him and tries without success to rescue them. He becomes embarrassed, and therefore even more chaotic in his movements. He kicks E accidentally and looks apologetic. The next material is presented to him; he continues to strain toward whatever is presented to him in order to get hold of it.

PICTURE ARRANGEMENT (T:IX:10)

SCALES. E: "It is all one story about the same man, but the pictures are mixed up. Tell me how to put them so it all makes one story about the same man. Which one comes first?" Bobby describes the first picture: "Going to work" (C). He looks at the next: "Is at work" (A). Next: "On the scales" (B). He reads the pictures off like the pages of a book. E puts series in correct order, ABC, says: "Now tell me the story." Bobby: (to A) "Is at work"; (to B) "Weighing himself"; (to C) "Coming home with his bag." E: "Why did he put his bag down here?" Bobby: "Too heavy, weighs too much." E: "But he did not put it down here (C or A). It was not too heavy for him there?" Bobby: "On the scales—too heavy."

FIGHT. E repeats directions: "These cards are all mixed up; if we put them right they will make a sensible story; you tell me how to put them." As before, Bobby reads off the pictures in the order they have been presented to him: "They fight" (B); "they fight" (A); "this is the last, he got hurt" (C).

FIRE. E: "How does the story go?" This time Bobby starts to describe the first picture on his right first, then picks out the one to his far left. His order is not the correct one, but is no longer the order in which the cards were presented to him: "Here he is playing" (F); "the fire engine comes" (R); "he is running from the house" (I); "and here he is scared, he cries" (E). Obviously he has some general idea for both pictures series, but it is not clear if he knows it is the boy who causes the fire. E: "How did the fire come about?" Bobby: "I do not know." E: "Look at the pictures some more." He does; then, as if he has discovered a new factor, he says joyfully: "He had matches" (F). E: "Let us put that one (F) first; which one next?" Bobby: "The curtain burns, he runs away" (I); "the firemen come" (R).

PICNIC. Bobby again describes the cards at random: "Going out" (F); "coming back" (E); "lost his hat" (H); "eats the chicken" (G). Again there is a question whether or not he understood the interrelationships between the events. E arranges the pictures in correct order, says, "Tell me the story now." Bobby: "He follows them" (E); "likes chicken" (F and G); "they go home—it is gone—they are surprised" (H).

BURGLAR. Bobby: "He is stealing money" (U); "the cop gets him" (G). E: "Which one comes first?" (U or G) Bobby indicates correctly (U) and adds, "He has to open the window" (T and H).

FARMER. Bobby starts describing the middle picture (T), then continues with the first to the left: "A wagon loaded" (T); "he likes corn" (S). . . . He seems to become very uncertain. He is tired, drools and thrashes around more than before. E interrupts task.

Bobby's interpretations are partially correct, even though they do not give him credit in formal WISC scores. He has some general comprehension of the pictured situations. He does not indicate causal relationships and pays little attention to details unless he is especially asked to do so. In Bobby such a tendency to rather primitive perceptual comprehension may be enforced by his unnatural motor situation. His jerky eye and head movements hinder him in scanning the complete width of the visual field at once and make it difficult for him to compare and integrate the various features he notices. As next test item E chooses:

PICTURE COMPLETION (T:IX:12)

Bobby responds as follows: to comb, teeth (correct); to table, drawer instead of leg; to fox, ears (correct); to girl, comb instead of mouth (when E asks "How do you mean that?" he repeats, "comb"); to cat, whiskers (correct); to door, lock (instead of hinge); to hand, nail (correct); to card, first says, "nothing," later starts to count the number of spades, says, "One is missing"; when E asks where it should be, it is physically impossible for Bobby to indicate clearly the correct spot (the picture is too small and his movements too chaotic); to scissors, paper (instead of screw); to coat, man (instead of buttonholes).

E now introduces the folder of Stanford-Binet material.

PICTURE COMPLETION (T:IX:12)

To table, Bobby answers leg (correct); to coat, man (instead of sleeve); to cat, nothing; to face, comb (instead of mouth); to bird, wing (correct). E points toward the hindquarters of the cat, asks, "The cat has no . . . ?" Bobby: "Tail." E points toward the missing mouth: "The face has no . . . ?" Bobby: "Comb—mouth." Bobby looks embarrassed. It dawns on E that in both pictures of faces the child must have meant to say mouth, but confused mouth and comb, probably because of the comb which had teeth missing!

ANIMAL PICTURES (T:II:11)

IDENTIFICATION. E: "Which one says 'meow?' " Bobby: "Cat." E: "Which one eats cheese?" Bobby: "Mouse." He gives these answers without looking at the pictures. Obviously, he repeats from memory what he knows. E: "Look at the picture and tell me which one of them eats nuts." Bobby: "The bear; (triumphantly) the elephant. I saw an elephant in the zoo; my uncle took me to the zoo." E: "What did you see?" Bobby: "Bears, elephants, and monkeys, they were . . . funny." E: "Did your uncle come and take you to the zoo?" Bobby: "The whole day." E: "You stayed the whole day at the zoo?" Bobby: "No, not lunch." E: "You had lunch outside?" Bobby nods excitedly, pleased that E understands. E: "Did you have it in a restaurant?" Bobby: "My uncle, he lives near Franklin Park next to the zoo. I spent the day." E: "When was that? In summer?" Bobby: "No—a Saturday. I spent the day; to get away from the house—it is a change." He says this wistfully, smiling; his manner indicates that he repeats what he has heard grown-ups say. E: "If you have been to the zoo, you know a lot about animals?" Bobby: "I got books, too." E: "Which one can climb trees?" Bobby: "The cat." E: "And another one too?" Bobby: "Squirrel; I saw a squirrel—here—in school." He volunteers: "The camel—goes without water." E: "Could you say the names of all these animals here?" E points to one picture after another, and Bobby names them slowly and with deliberation. Clearly he has a different name for each and is correct in all except one name. (Performance at six-year level.)

PICTORIAL IDENTIFICATION (T:II:9)

E: "Which one swims in the water?" Bobby: "Fish." E: "Which one do we read?" Bobby: "Book." E: "Which one gives us milk?" Bobby: "Cow." E: "Which one shines in the sky at night?" Bobby: "Moon."

IDENTIFICATION IN REVERSE. Bobby: "Which one is in the kitchen?" E: "You meant the stove, not the fish?" Bobby: "Which one is in the tree?" E: "Is it the apple?" Bobby: "No." E: "The bird?" Bobby: "No." E: "The nest?" Bobby: "Yes." E: "They are all in the tree, you know." Bobby: "What do you take when it is raining?" E: "It can only be an umbrella!"

PICTURE ABSURDITIES (T:IX:11)

MAN IN TREE. Bobby says, "He will fall; he is on the limb. He is sawing."

MAN ON SCALES. "His books are too heavy. It puts on too much weight." E: "What should he do?" Bobby: "Put it down."

CAT AND MICE. Bobby: "A lion; they are on his back." "Who are 'they'?" Bobby: "Mouses." E: "Why is it funny?" Bobby: "They are on his back." E: "Who is 'he'?" Bobby: "The lion." E: "Is he really a lion?" Bobby: "A cat—the cat looks like a tiger." (By Revised Stanford-Binet standards, Bobby passes on seven-year level.)

Bobby's flailing movements have increased during the last situations. However, he declares that he is not tired and that he is used to sitting and "working" for an hour at least. He still is full of good will and enthusiasm. E moves slowly and stalls before introducing the next situation in order to give him some time to relax.

Bobby seems to have adequate reasoning ability. In his responses to picture absurdities, for instance, and also to picture arrangements, his comprehension is within normal range for his age level. He is able to revise or to sharpen up his primitive original solutions as soon as he finds new clues, and therein shows a certain amount of healthy flexibility in his reasoning processes (identification in reverse, picture arrangements). On the proper occasion he activates material which he has learned before (information about animals, counting spades). His rather immature performances in some tasks are noteworthy for the primitive tendencies they reveal; his concern is less with structural detail than with function of pictured objects (picture completion); his picture arrangements are correct in the gross lines, but not in detail. His verbal concepts reveal some rather primitive fusions (teeth-mouth-comb and lion-cat-tiger); but when it comes to simple labeling of individual items, he seems to have an adequate name vocabulary (animal names). Reasoning ability is tested further in:

SIMILARITIES BETWEEN TWO THINGS (T:IX:2)

E asks in what way certain things are alike. E: "Bread—meat." Bobby: "You eat." E: "Window—door." Bobby: "They are both down." He makes a vertical motion. E: "How do you mean?" Bobby: "The window is down—this way—and the door is down too." E: "Can you think of anything else they are the same in?" Bobby: "They open." E: "Mosquito—sparrow." Bobby: "A bird—they are both in the tree." E: "Anything else?" Bobby: "They fly." (By Revised Stanford-Binet standards, Bobby passes on eight-year level.)

SIMILARITIES AND DIFFERENCES (T:IX:3)

E asks in what way certain objects are alike and in what way different. E: "Lemon—banana." Bobby: "A lemon is round and has a tail; a banana is down. You have to peel it." E: "What way are they the same?" Bobby: "They both have tails." E: "Pen—pencil." Bobby: "Both write; the pen is longer." E: "Shoe—glove." Bobby: "Shoe on your feet; glove on your hand." E: "How are they the same?" Bobby: "Glove has fingers; the shoe has toes in it; the glove has fingers in it." (By Revised Stanford-Binet standards, Bobby fails on nine-year level.)

Opposite Analogies (T:IX:5)

Bobby answers all correctly until: E: "The dog has hair; the bird has
. . . . " Bobby: "Wings." E: "The rabbit's ears are long; the rat's ears
are. . . . " Bobby: "I do not know." E: "Wolves are wild; dogs are. . . . "
Bobby: "Friendly." (By Revised Stanford-Binet standards, Bobby passes
on six-year level but fails on eight-year level.)

Repeating Digits (T:VIII:5,6)

DIGITS FORWARD. For three and four digits forward, Bobby
gets tense and tries to pronounce the numbers very correctly. He obviously has the impression that this task is a speech exercise. He is intent
on producing the sounds correctly. For five digits; three, five, nine, two,
eight repeated as three, five, nine, two; seven, one, six, two, three repeated as seven, one, six, two. E: "You do not need to say them extra
well; just try to think of all the numbers I say and repeat them." He
then repeats four digits correctly.

DIGITS BACKWARD. For three digits backward he repeats three,
one, five as three, one, five. For two digits, he answers "three" to two,
one; "five" to three, two. For Bobby, numbers seem to mean either
just words or arithmetic facts. He shows fair knowledge of these even
though in the test proper he fails on the seven-year level.

Recognition of Forms (T:VII:9 and Figure 15)

A large card with a series of different designs. The subject is shown
small cards, each of which has a design identical to one on the large
card, and then identifies the same design on the large card from memory
or by direct comparison.

Bobby chooses four out of five designs correctly. One design in the
shape of a reversed E is named as such and placed more quickly than
the others. Bobby has difficulty in pointing accurately. He aims at one
design and is apt to land on another one. E has to watch him closely. His
facial expression and her query reveal whether or not he is satisfied
with his choice.

Block Designs (T:VII:7 and Figures 13 and 14)

He handles the blocks and studies them; he is unable to turn them at will;
he upsets them; he drops them and becomes agitated. E says, "You
tell me how to put them," using proxy method.

CARD I. E picks two blocks, red sides up, says, "Tell me how

I shall put them for you." Bobby: "Put them together, I guess." E puts two red blocks side by side, asks "And the blue one?" Bobby: "Next to the red, I guess." E gives him a choice of position of the blue block below or beside the red one. Bobby: "Beside, I guess." He seems very insecure and vague. E repeats explanations, then places one blue next to two red blocks; asks "Where shall I put the other blue one?" Bobby: "Next to the yellow one." Suddenly it becomes clear to E that Bobby judges the blocks by their sides as well as by their tops. He has gradually slipped into a reclining position and thus sees the blocks from a different perspective. From here on E arranges the blocks in a box which she tilts to Bobby's angle of vision. She repeats explanations.

CARD II. E places two yellow/blue sides parallel (incorrect) and asks Bobby, "Is that all right?" Bobby: "They have to be the other way." To save time and more frustrating explanations, E arranges the two blocks correctly, though she is uncertain whether this is what "the other way" meant for Bobby. E: "What now?" Bobby: "Yellow." E: "Where to?" Bobby: "Under them." E places as directed, asks, "And then?" Bobby: "A red one under that one." The result is a T-shaped arrangement.

MULTIPLE CHOICE. E shows above model (design 3b of Figure 14) with correct model (1), asking, "Which one is like the card?" (II). Bobby correctly chooses (1). E shows model with blue/yellow reversed (2) and correct model (1) and again asks which one is similar. Again Bobby chooses correctly and explains, pointing to (2) "It's upside down."

COUNTING BLOCKS (T:I:7)

E places all sixteen blocks in one box, one by one; asks Bobby to count. He counts correctly from one through eleven, then "thirteen, fourteen, sixteen, seventeen, nineteen." Told to count them again, he does as before; again thirteen, fourteen, then seventeen, eighteen. He is obviously not yet secure in his number series after thirteen, fourteen.

COMPARING CONCRETE QUANTITIES (T:I:9)

E arranges two squares of four blocks each, asks, "How many are in this one?" He counts correctly, "Four." E: "How many are in the other one?" He gets ready to count again. E: "Can you tell without counting?" He seems startled for a moment, then says emphatically, "Four— it is the same."

MATCHING OBJECTS AND PRINTED WORDS (T:VI:11 AND XI:8)

E prints the words dog, chair, car, then holds up a small toy dog, asks, "Could you find the word that goes with it?" Bobby seems delighted and chooses correctly, later also chooses correctly for car and chair. E prints cup, car, cat, chair, and Bobby chooses correctly for cup, but hesitates between the words car and cat when trying to place cat.

He seems to be very proud of his reading ability; but it is obvious that he is getting tired. The session is ended.

COMMENT

Bobby's examination at age seven shows that within his severe limitations the child has obvious assets and some liabilities. He has made a reasonably good adjustment to his life situation; obviously he likes contact with strangers. His essentially adequate reasoning ability, confirmed in the second part of the examination (similarities, similarities and differences), helps him to comprehend the restricted experiences which come his way. He is capable of learning from his experiences. His judgement is frequently based on somewhat insufficient evidence gathered through his superficial acquaintance with a subject. This tendency, partly explained by his age and limited activities, in Bobby is probably reinforced by his motor handicap which, in visual tasks for example, hinders him from absorbing immediately all those factors involved in a problem (pictures). He also has difficulty in structuring his perceptions (block designs). However, the questions remain as yet unsolved whether these are due to the same perceptuo-motor disturbances which are found in other types of brain-injured children or whether his difficulties are of a different nature. In Bobby's case his good performance in recognizing designs and words and his immediate understanding of the reversed blocks in the model in block design would indicate more peripheral and experiential motor rather than central distortions. Some minor errors in spatial orientation (looking at pictures from right to left, using blocks sideways) may be directly related to his motor disability. Since it is impossible for him to move about like a normal person, Bobby can neither manipulate objects freely nor get around them. Therefore, his perceptions are not organized in a normal way. A similar lack of free exchange with his environment seems to be the cause of peculiar difficulties in another area. In spite of his severe speech impairment, Bobby uses a rather elaborate vocabulary and good sentence construction. Occasionally, he has some unchildlike, precocious phrases. There are, however, various verbal expressions which reveal physiognomic or primitive syncretic qualities usually abandoned by children of Bobby's age and mental level. In conversation rather than when trying to find a correct name, Bobby's language contains remnants of a "personal" language which has not yet been entirely destroyed by verbal practice and exchange ("down" used to indicate the shape of window and door, "tail" for stems of fruit, "comb" for teeth and mouth). Bobby, at age four, showed in other areas unusual persistence of such primitive criteria.

Since then he has come a long way; his course has justified the prediction made at that time. However, though competent and able to learn, Bobby shows enough variations from normal in his mental functioning to warrant a cautiously planned educational program. In his early days it was necessary to defend him from those who thought he was mentally defective. Now, at seven, he is more likely to need protection from those overly optimistic persons who tend to dismiss any deviations from normal development as "merely motor" or "sheer lack of experience." No matter which explanation is preferred, the fact remains that Bobby's development is stunted by irreparable circumstances. Wise concessions to his difficulties must be made in order to avoid disappointment for himself, his parents, and all others dealing with him.

BOBBY AT TWELVE YEARS

Bobby, now twelve, has become a frail-looking, thin boy with angular features. He still is unable to walk independently, but can take a few steps when held by one hand. He has marked tremor in his hands and head. While the left hand has more athetoid movements than the right, it has more strength and is used more. Still, he cannot hold a spoon or pencil with either hand. He feeds himself solids and can drink with the help of a straw. A wheelchair allows him to get around. His speech is slow and labored, but understandable. Bobby's mother died rather suddenly when he was nine years old. Shortly after his mother's death, Bobby spent a few weeks in an institution for severely crippled children. His father was reluctant to do this, but was persuaded by his relatives who thought that Bobby could not be taken care of at home without his mother. Bobby himself liked the idea and looked forward to going to school. Soon, however, he hated life in the institution; he was disturbed by the proximity of other handicapped children, many of them mentally retarded. He missed his family and his teacher and was bored with the uniformity of his surroundings. His father gladly took him home again and moved into a suburban community. Since then a quiet relative has kept house. His father has taken on most of Bobby's physical care. A home teacher comes to Bobby two hours a week and considers that he is technically in the fifth grade. However, Bobby has never been able to do any writing; he has a typewriter and with great difficulty can peck out a few words; this is so laborious for him that it is of no use in his lessons. He spends a great deal of time reading; he goes to the local library by himself in his wheelchair and consults with the librarian. In the community he has many friends, especially among adults. He has been asked to join the local Boy Scout group. He enjoys these contacts and seems contented enough to all concerned. His father encourages all his independent activities and is proud of his accomplishments; he seems to get much satisfaction either directly from or through the child. He enjoys the attention which he and his unusual family receive from neighbors and acquaintances. Bobby's sister, now fifteen, seemed more upset and uprooted by her mother's death than her brother. Later she managed to adjust reasonably well. She is now getting honor grades in the local high school and has become interested in various social activities; she has joined a rhythmic dancing group for girls and is very serious about her art; she has not yet decided whether to become a teacher of physical education or a nurse. When questioned, she declares emphatically that her brother's condition has nothing whatsoever to do with either one of these projects.

For Bobby, the question of schooling arises again. He, his family, and friends think that he may now be ready for more education. Application is being made to a nearby state school for crippled children; Bobby would live in school, but would be close to his home. The school accepts only children with normal intelligence; the state law requires a psychological examination with numerical test results in terms of I.Q. and a statement from the psychologist. The school authorities rigidly adhere to this rule, especially in the case of a child with cerebral palsy. In their experience they have too often found that children who were reported "bright" proved to be unable to learn. They hope that an I.Q. test will eliminate at least the most flagrantly unsuitable cases.

Bobby enters the examining room in a wheelchair. He is full of curiosity. He knows that the examination is a necessary formality, but that he has nothing to worry about. He has declared his confidence and has half-jokingly expressed the hope that E knows enough about him and will be prepared to do the writing for him. He is obviously tense and excited; his athetoid movements are very prominent; his head shakes wildly. He is slow in producing his first words. He holds on to his shoulder in an effort to control the movements of his left arm. A table top placed over his lap for the examination has to be discarded because it interferes with the flailing motions of his arms and legs.

E tries to decide quickly how to start. The most suitable test would be one which can be easily understood and which does not involve complicated postural adjustments or manipulations. It should also be reasonably short and well-structured, have a limited number of possible solutions, and not require much speech or social exchange. It should help to get Bobby oriented and relaxed while allowing E to again become accustomed to Bobby's physique, motions, and speech. If she becomes at ease quickly, so will Bobby.

Picture Completion (T:IX:12)

Comb: Bobby looks intently at the picture with much head-shaking; then, smiling with relief, says, "teeth." To show that she easily understands him, E repeats, "The teeth, of course, the teeth of the comb are missing." To table, Bobby responds more quickly than before, "leg." E repeats as before. He answers correctly to fox, girl, door, hand, card. To scissors, Bobby says, "Not the same—it is too round." He answers correctly to coat, fish, screw, fly, rooster. To profile with eyebrow missing, he says, "Nothing there, nothing I can see." To thermometer with mercury missing he says, "Nothing there." To hat with hatband missing he says, "Noth . . . the line that goes around the hat." To umbrella with spokes missing, he says, "Nothing missing" and repeats "Nothing missing" for cow with cleft in hoof missing and house with shadow missing. (WISC raw score: fourteen; scaled score: twelve.)

This test situation furnishes for E a first rough gauge with which to judge the level of Bobby's competence. She can now design a plan for the examination, which will be centered around Stanford-Binet items. Bobby was not disturbed by his inability to find missing parts in some of the pictures, but seemed convinced that he was correct. His first errors concerned a manual instrument (scissors) and a body-image (profile).

This first task helped to reassure Bobby, who has become more relaxed. The next item has some similarity to the previous task. Though entirely verbal, it also has short, well-defined items, does not demand many words, and is well structured.

OPPOSITE ANALOGIES (T:IX:5)

Bobby responds correctly to all questions. (By Revised Stanford-Binet standards, he passes on eight-year level.)

SIMILARITIES AND DIFFERENCES (T:IX:3)

E: "Banana—lemon." Bobby: "Same, because they are fruit; lemon you use the juice, banana you peel and eat." E: "Shoe—glove." Bobby: "Both are things to wear, but the glove goes on your hand, shoe on your foot." From the outset, Bobby has the directing idea in mind; he tries first to find a similarity, then a difference. The maturity of his approach and the high quality of his responses in both items lead E to omit any other questions of the same test, in order to save time and strain. (By Revised Stanford-Binet standards, Bobby passes on nine-year level.)

SIMILARITIES AMONG THREE THINGS (T:IX:4)

E asks in what way three objects are alike. E: "Snake—cow—sparrow." Bobby: "All are animals." E: "Rose—potato—tree." Bobby: "All have roots." E: "Wool—cotton—leather." Bobby: "All fabrics." He knows the answers immediately, but spends much effort verbalizing them. (By Revised Stanford-Binet standards, Bobby passes on eleven-year level.)

SIMILARITIES BETWEEN TWO THINGS (T:IX:2)

E: "Egg—seed." Bobby: "Both become something; both still very small, not the real thing." E: "Farming—manufacturing." Bobby: "Both important for the country." E: "How do you mean?" Bobby: "For the people. It is how they work—on a farm or in a factory—or some have shops of their own." E: "Melting—burning." Bobby: "When it is very hot—things melt like butter—when there is not enough water to put it out." Obviously Bobby sees a relationship between both words of each pair; he furnishes pertinent observations, but he does not succeed in giving precise enough answers, except for the first pair. (One plus. By Revised Stanford-Binet standards, Bobby fails on the Superior Adult I level.)

Since Bobby seems to enjoy activities with words, the examination is continued with:

ABSTRACT VOCABULARY (T:XII:2)

E: "Pity." Bobby: "Feel sorry for that person." E: "Curiosity." Bobby: "Very curious, you look into everything . . . I am!" E: "Grief." Bobby: "It is sad—almost." E: "Surprise." Bobby: "They did not know about it." (All plus. By Revised Stanford-Binet standards, he passes on twelve-year level.)

E: "Connection." Bobby: "Joined together." E: "Compare." Bobby: "See who is better." E: "Conquer." Bobby: "Defeat somebody." E: "Obedience." Bobby: "Do what is good for you." E: "Revenge." Bobby: "Get even." (Four plus. By Revised Stanford-Binet standards, he passes on thirteen-year level.)

E: "Generosity." Bobby: "Very kind—always friendly." E: "Independent." Bobby: "Helpful—does not bother anybody to do it for him." E: "Envy." Bobby: "Jealous—he got something." E: "Authority." Bobby: "He is interested—he likes to talk about it." E: "Justice." Bobby: "Law and order." (Three plus. By Revised Stanford-Binet standards, he passes on fourteen-year level but fails on Average Adult level.)

These performances show Bobby's knowledge of words and ability to comprehend language; in spite of his technical speech difficulty, Bobby uses a rather large and expressive vocabulary. Many of his definitions are based on personal experiences and reveal a somewhat narrow point of view. There are traces of egocentricity and moral righteousness (obedience, independence, authority) which are less common in normal boys of his age. The following test is designed to relieve the strain of verbal effort and allow an appraisal of form comprehension with nonmanual material:

ELLIS VISUAL DESIGNS TEST (T:VII:2 AND FIGURE 5)

RECOGNITION. Of five cards to choose from, the subject picks out the one that is similar to the design on the key card; the other four choice cards are variations of imperfect reproductions of the same design.

Bobby chooses correctly except for reversals in the third and the sixth designs.

BLOCK COUNTING

A card with pictures of piles of cubes arranged in two rows; the blocks are to be counted.[1]

---

[1] Lewis M. Terman and Maud A. Merrill, *Measuring Intelligence* (Boston: Houghton Mifflin, 1937), pp. 163, 376.

Bobby counts correctly for groups of three, five, and six blocks, respectively. He fails with the other designs. The task is difficult and nerve-wracking for him. It seems that the constant motions of his head prevent him from fixating on the designs long enough to count satisfactorily. It is difficult to ascertain whether this is the only cause of failure. (By Revised Stanford-Binet standards, Bobby fails on ten-year level.)

PICTURE DESCRIPTION (T:II:6)

MESSENGER BOY. (A messenger boy with a broken bicycle is waving for help to a passing automobile.) Bobby: "He broke his bike; he wants the car to pick him up. Looks like a policeman or a newsboy." E: "Why does he want to be picked up?" Bobby: "His bike broke." (By Revised Stanford-Binet standards, Bobby fails on twelve-year level.)

PICTURE ABSURDITIES (T:IX:11)

WINDY DAY. (A house with trees and clothes hanging on a line; the smoke, clothes, and trees are blowing in different directions.) Bobby: "It is stormy, the clothes are waving in the wind. There is smoke, the trees are tipping over." E: "Which way are they going?" Bobby tries to indicate the direction. E: "Which way is the smoke going?" Bobby points in opposite direction. E: "Is there anything wrong about them?" Bobby: "They should all go one way." (By Revised Stanford-Binet standards, Bobby fails on twelve-year level.)

In this picture, Bobby comes to the correct answer only after E's leading questions. For the first one, however, he lacks necessary background experience; though he sees policemen and newsboys on bikes, he is unlikely to meet messenger boys in a suburban neighborhood of today. Bobby does not observe well enough small details such as the telegram in the boy's hand.

Throughout the last tasks Bobby has not seemed certain of himself. His squirming and head-shaking has increased. He talks with more difficulty. He again seems to become more secure when presented with printed words.

DISSECTED SENTENCES (T:XI:6)

Three different sets of jumbled words, each set forming a sentence when read in the proper order.

He reads the words slowly to himself, then produces each of the first two sentences correctly. (By Stanford-Binet standards, Bobby passes on thirteen-year level.)

RECALL OF FACTS (T:VIII:4)

A story printed on a card is read to the subject who is asked to follow on his copy. The procedure is designed to test memory for facts.

DISTINGUISHED FRENCH ACROBAT. Bobby follows the lines of his copy and listens attentively, then answers all seven questions without hesitation. He does not need to think about his answers, but reproduces them as if he was reciting from a book, eager and intent on saying his words accurately. (By Revised Stanford-Binet standards, he passes on thirteen-year level.)

REASONING PROBLEM: THE BURGLARY (T:IX:8)

Bobby answers correctly, "Nobody was home between four and five." (By Revised Stanford-Binet standards, he passes on fourteen-year level.)

VERBAL ABSURDITIES (T:IX:6)

E: "A father wrote: 'If you do not get this letter, send me a telegram.' " Bobby: "He could not know—he did not get it." E: "A soldier complained that every man was out of step except himself." Bobby: "He was the one that did not walk right." E: "A kind-hearted man taking a heavy bag to town on his horse sat on his horse and lifted the bag to his own shoulder to make the load easier for the horse." Bobby: "It was too heavy anyway—it still was the same." E: "A man said to his friend: 'Hope you live to eat the chickens that scratch sand on your grave.' " Bobby: "He was dead—he could not eat." (By Revised Stanford-Binet standards, Bobby passes on eleven-year level.)

E: "Many more women than men get married." Bobby: "There must be the same." E: "A man wished to dig a hole to bury some rubbish; he could not decide what to do with the dirt from the hole; a friend suggested he dig a hole large enough to hold the dirt too." Bobby: "He would have still more dirt."

FACTUAL INFORMATION (T:XI:10)

Only a few items are chosen. To "Who discovered America?" "Who wrote *Romeo and Juliet?*" and "What is celebrated on the Fourth of July?" Bobby gives correct answers. E: "Where is Chile?" Bobby is correct. E: "What is the capital of Greece?" Bobby correct. E: "What other capitals do you know?" Bobby: "Rome, Italy; Paris, France;" (smiles) "Boston, Massachusetts; Hartford, Connecticut." E: "What is the capital of New York State?" Bobby: "Not New York—Albany." E: "Where is Algiers?" Bobby: "In Africa—the northern part." E: "How do you know all these things?" Bobby: "I have a globe; I study it." E: "Why does oil float on water?" Bobby: "I do not know why." E: "What is the color of rubies?" Bobby: "Like diamonds, white." His stock of information seems rich in some areas but spotty in others.

REASONING PROBLEM: ORIENTATION (T:IX:7)

A set of questions testing orientation in space by compass directions.
E: "Which direction would you face so your right hand would be toward the north?" Bobby: "West." E: "Suppose you are going East, then turn to your right, which direction would you face?" Bobby: "South." E: "Going South, turning left, turning right." Bobby: "North." E: "Going North, turning right, turning right, turning left." Bobby: "South." E: "Going West, turning left." Bobby: "South." (No credit.) He succeeds in questions which require only one imaginary turn in space (first, second, last), but is unable to think of several successive shifts in directions. Last question was added to verify this hypothesis.

REPEATING DIGITS (T:VIII:5,6)

DIGITS FORWARD. Bobby succeeds in repeating six digits forward. (By Revised Stanford-Binet standards, he passes on ten-year level.) He fails in eight digits forward. (By Revised Stanford-Binet standards, he fails on Superior Adult II level.)

DIGITS BACKWARD. Bobby succeeds in four digits backward (passes on nine-year level). He fails in five digits in reverse (fails on twelve-year level.)

The session has lasted 75 minutes. Bobby seems tired and much less enthusiastic than he was at the beginning. No more items can be added. The standard scale has been abbreviated wherever feasible. If Bobby succeeded in a task E assumed that he also would have passed the same type of task on an easier level. For instance, under recall of facts, School Concert (ten-year level) was omitted after Bobby earned credit on Distinguished French Acrobat (thirteen-year level). When Bobby repeated a digit series correctly, no other series of the same length was given. The sequence of the tasks reduced postural changes and readjustments to a minimum (card material items followed each other, as did verbal items).

COMMENT

Bobby's numerical rating on the Revised Stanford-Binet Scale varies according to the method of scoring used. If one gives him credit for all items he passed but considers as failed all items he was not given because he was believed unable to do them within the required time limits, Bobby's mental age is twelve years six months, which is equivalent to an I.Q. of 103. This method of scoring seems arbitrary. For example, Bobby probably could have named twelve animals (ten-year level) if the time limit set for this task was ignored. He could have thought of the same number of animals within the one-minute time limit, but it would have been impossible for him to say them in that length of time. Tasks such as memory for designs (T:VII:1) involve both motor skill and form recognition. One might think that, except for technical difficulties of reproduction, Bobby would have succeeded with all designs. However, his less-than-perfect performance on the adapted Ellis visual designs test (T:VII:2) suggests that he might also have had some difficulty with Stanford-Binet material on the twelve-year level, but probably not on the nine-year level.

In Bobby's case these are the obvious difficulties of using any test scale elaborated on a normal population. Still, it has shown its usefulness here as a screening tool. Since Bobby is able, in spite of his infirmity, to respond verbally, he has revealed his normal reasoning ability. He has shown how he would compare with a normal population. With an I.Q. of 100 or over, he will be accepted at the state school for crippled children. However, the numerical rating alone does not describe this child adequately. A short qualitative analysis of his performance in the test situation shows the features described below.

One of Bobby's assets is a good ability in the language field. In spite of his labored speech, he has a good vocabulary and good comprehension of speech. He also has a good memory for facts. He is able to reflect on situations which have been described to him in words. He has some difficulty in appraising pictorial situations (picture description, block counting). He does not do very well on problems involving spatial orientation and movement in space, whether they are presented visually or only verbally (Ellis visual designs test; picture absurdities—Windy

Day; reasoning problem—orientation). He has good attention spans, but gets exhausted easily. He is pleasant, cooperative, and eager to make a good impression. The present picture corresponds well with that of Bobby at age seven. His language, rich even then, has become more socialized through practice with words, whether heard or read. Some difficulties in spatial perception, such as reversals, were noted then as well as today. These may be related to his abnormal body mechanics, his lack of head control, and his inability to move effectively in space. Or they may be related to minor pyramidal injuries. He has acquired some precocious mannerisms which make him, on the whole, more popular with grown-ups than with children, with whom he has never been able to compete on equal terms. His new associations in an institution will widen his experiences, but also will open more and more the nearly insoluble question of his future.

STAGES OF DEVELOPMENT AND THEIR PROBLEMS

Bobby's psychological development through the years follows a pattern found to be characteristic for children who are severely handicapped physically but whose mental abilities are essentially normal.

At fifteen months he is still almost completely helpless. At an age when other children have started to discover their world, Bobby, because of his motor handicap, has had no chance to respond with actions to incoming stimuli. However, he obviously sees and hears. Within his limited means he has learned to understand some aspects of his environment. He knows the people around him and can differentiate their varying means of expression. He understands some language clues; he knows that objects move, and how. He reacts with fear and apprehension to some things and with pleasure to others. He is learning that certain of his responses produce certain actions from those around him. In a modest way he is in communication with others. His parents get satisfaction from understanding and responding to his most minute signs. They woo him for a smile on his immobile face. Stunned by the severity of his physical impairment, they are happy about evidence of mental awareness. In an emotional but determined way, they derive some pleasure from taking excellent care of his unusual physical needs. For the time being, he fills an important though unexpected role in the life of his parents.

At four years of age Bobby is still essentially helpless, unable either to move effectively or to talk unambiguously. He recognizes various people in his environment. He also knows objects around him by their movements, sounds, shapes, and other properties, but has not been able to touch, handle, or get around them effectively. He has learned to differentiate some major spatial areas. He has also learned to associate certain names with certain people and objects. Many of the names he knows have been acquired from picture books and hearsay rather than from direct contact. Aside from names, he has learned other language uses. He has heard meaningful associations of words, but has not yet been able to manipulate and experiment with words and sounds as other children do at his age and earlier. He has found means to communicate with his immediate family, but has not had opportunity to try them with others. His restricted life has offered him very little opportunity for experimentation—whether verbal, adaptive, or social. Unlike other children his age, he has hardly any occasion to use his judgement and make decisions. Since he needs intermediaries for all his activities, those around him are accustomed to act for him. Given a chance, he enjoys being mentally or physically active, but in such unusual situations he gets excited and overwrought.

To his parents, who are still overwhelmed by his physical disability, he remains a helpless baby who needs protection which they alone are able to provide. In spite of their distress, they still derive satisfaction from their painstaking care. Their main concern is far more with his lack of physical power than with his inability to attain independence. They themselves are delighted and entertained that he seems intelligent to them. They try to convince others of it, but as yet they do not know how they can help him to use his mind.

At seven years of age Bobby has changed considerably. Though still helpless, he talks more and has acquired some independent locomotion which has increased his physical contacts. Compared with a normal child's, these experiences have been extremely limited, but they have helped him broaden his interest in, and knowledge of, the world around him. As an onlooker, he has become more curious about wider spatial areas. He has learned to observe more actions of people and objects. Thanks to his good reasoning ability, he has learned to draw conclusions from them. His point of view has, because of his physical limitations, remained more restricted and egocentric than is normal for his age. Since listening is easy and satisfying for him, he has improved considerably in the language field. He has been attentive to what is said around him and has learned word combinations and sentence construction. He seems to enjoy passive contact with language more than normal children do at his age. In spite of the fact that he cannot repeat, practice, and manipulate his verbal acquisitions as normal children can, he understands the structure and meaning of language better than do some other types of brain-injured children who talk freely. However, his own limited experiences occasionally deprive him of well-defined mental concepts. This lack of precision is apparent in some of his spontaneous expressions, but since the latter usually appear in smooth and elaborate sentence constructions and are produced with great effort and poor enunciation, these indefinite or incorrect wordings are easily overlooked by the uncritical listener. For most people who learn to understand Bobby at all, he is impressively facile with language, except for his severe dysarthria. With his widened social experiences, Bobby has found new friends and admirers outside his family. He has learned to interact with them in varying roles and in varying social situations, as normal children begin to do at younger ages. He is more mature with some and less with others. In most of his social contacts he shows a somewhat demanding attitude though this is partially disguised by his overt cheerfulness. Proud of himself and eager to surprise his listener by his skills, he occasionally lacks the sensitivity to judge when his slow speech and uncontrolled movements become embarrassing and harassing to others. He is absorbed in trying what he can do and seems less concerned with what he cannot do.

Because his specific physical, mental, and social situation is unique, even in a group of children with cerebral palsy, Bobby has remained more self-centered than is normal for his age, in spite of his increased social contacts.

Bobby still has the full approval and support of his parents. An intricate system of communication has developed between them and him. Father and mother are going through a relatively serene emotional stage; they have gradually overcome the first shock and are adjusting to the slowness of Bobby's physical progress. With his learning ability no longer a subject of dispute, they now devote their efforts to developing his intellectual assets. They are inclined to magnify them for their own compensation. But with their high hopes and expectations, they frequently forget to allow for fatigue and expense in effort. In comparison with his own earlier days or with normal children of his age, Bobby is under considerable pressure.

At twelve years of age Bobby, somewhat more mobile than before, is still essentially helpless. He still talks very poorly. He has become more conscious of his physical limitations. He has more foresight in judging what he can and cannot do: he has found that, on the physical level, effort does not always pay and that he can avoid embarrassment and chaotic movements by staying clear of certain difficult situations. This restraint together with that imposed by his limited range of motion make him now appear more mature than is normal for a child of his age. Within his restricted and routinized life he has found new satisfactions in his mental resources. Thanks to the interest in language which he displayed earlier, he now obtains new information through reading and listening. He still memorizes easily. Internalized language and acquired factual material allow him now to discover mentally new combinations and bits of truth at an age at which normal children also learn from symbols as often as from actual experiences. His increased knowledge and mental activity help him to entertain himself better alone now and make others appreciate him. But, unlike normal children his age, he has not much opportunity to use his ideas constructively. He still has only very limited means of communication and expression. He cannot write; his speech is so slow and cumbersome as to practically preclude any casual discussion or exchange of thoughts. His knowledge, therefore, remains somewhat stale and unselective. Occasionally his ideas seem rigid, biased, and egocentric at an age when normal children show a surprising ability to shift their opinions and interests with any new fad, friend, or teacher that comes their way.

Bobby has become physically less appealing than he was when younger. He is painful to watch and to listen to. In many adults and most children he causes pity, awe, or guilt feelings. While he has many casual acquaintances, he has no real friends and no true companionship. Probably to protect himself emotionally, Bobby has now a slightly remote, somewhat standoffish and cool attitude which is often masked by his superficial friendliness. He tries to influence people by being factual rather than by being emotionally responsive. As in earlier years, he tends to ignore or to remain somewhat insensitive to the subtler emotions of others.

His relationships with his immediate family have become more objective, in spite of his immediate physical dependence. While other children his age become gradually freed from their most intimate family bonds in order to establish new attachments, Bobby seems to remain emotionally uninvolved and lonesome. For normal children of his age such an emotional stage may be a transitory one which will be quickly succeeded by new opportunities and circumstances. With his limited chance for experiences, the hope for any radical emotional or social change for Bobby seems meager.

New developments and the passage of time have gradually transformed parental attitudes. Having finally accepted the fact that Bobby, in spite of his mental potentialities, will not be able to take care of himself, his father now believes that a permanent plan for his protection is essential. While he, with his wife, was anxious in earlier years to develop Bobby's assets for successful and gainful use, he now can relax pressure. Confident in Bobby's personality and intelligence, he trusts him to become popular with new people. His relations with Bobby, however, are more stereotyped and less dynamic than those of father and son at that age under normal circumstances.

Analysis of case records of children who are equally seriously damaged by an extrapyramidal palsy indicates that the trends and stages of development illustrated by Bobby are in many ways representative for this group.[2] However, the combination of symptoms and the severity of disability vary particularly widely among children in this group.

For example, among the similarly injured children whose case records were studied, there are some who have never walked independently and whose speech impairment is as great as Bobby's. Others walk better but talk as poorly; others talk more easily but cannot walk, or differ from Bobby in ability to use their hands or control their heads. Some have had convulsions at one time or another. When Bobby was very young his doctors considered his disability to be of purely extrapyramidal origin; however, later neurological examinations revealed some minor signs of pyramidal involvement. The group whose records were studied

[2] This discussion is based on the study of case records of 27 children with extrapyramidal palsy. Of these, 6 cases were classified as pure extrapyramidal palsy; 10 showed mild pyramidal signs; and 11 were classified as mixed pyramidal and extrapyramidal palsy.

Ten of these children had two psychological evaluations, 7 had three, 5 had four, and 5 had more than four. (Total number of examinations was 86.)

Interval between first and last examinations was more than two years in 1 case, more than three years in 3 cases, more than five years in 8 cases, more than eight years in 6 cases, more than twelve years in 9 cases.

Mental ability at last examination was above normal in 4 cases (14%), normal in 10 cases (37%), borderline in 12 cases (44%), below borderline in 1 case (5%).

Dysarthria was severe in 4 cases (14%), moderately severe in 9 cases (33%), mild in 7 cases (25%), nonexistent in 7 cases (25%).

General motor impairment was severe in 8 cases (30%), moderately severe in 11 cases (40%), mild in 6 cases (22%), nonexistent in 2 cases (8%).

Six of these children were unable to walk independently.

includes some children whose disabilities are of purely extrapyramidal origin; others who, like Bobby, show minor signs of pyramidal involvement; and still others whose disabilities are of mixed extrapyramidal and pyramidal origin.

The presence of these variations, in addition to the individual circumstances that always differentiate each case from others with similar handicaps, permits at best the description of some common developmental and psychological trends that distinguish this group.

The most obvious problems of the babies *between fifteen and thirty months* are, in general, overwhelmingly physical. Failure to grasp, to kick, to turn, and to acquire balance while sitting or later while standing, are the most prominent symptoms noted in the records. Feeding difficulties are common. Psychological examinations are rarely requested before the child is fifteen to eighteen months old, and even then not frequently. Psychological considerations are postponed altogether in many cases. Often parents do not question mental development until the child's failure to speak begins to worry them. Many of these babies are described by their parents as alert and responsive, or as passive but observant. Later, in spite of their failure to talk, many are said to "understand." They like picture books and stories. Some more sceptical parents worry mostly about the baby's inability to hold on to anything. Some parents believe this is due to lack of comprehension and interest; others think it is caused by the child's inability to move. Pediatricians' attitudes range from pessimism to a "wait and see" policy. They may restrain themselves from making any predictions, but may also feel that the child's motor inability precludes all professional psychological appraisal.

For the psychologist, children in this group are puzzling and need careful watching. In a young baby signs of comprehension which are independent of motor skill must be detected. One baby may show that he perceives an object, a rattle (T:V:1,2) or a pellet (T:V:8) only by bodily agitation or stiffening. Another may fix his gaze on an object or strain in the direction of the object. Attention, sustained interest, and spatial comprehension can be studied in situations where the baby can show anticipation by the same means. Frequently the baby's gaze is unsteady or limited by visual difficulties; E must then make sure that the object to be perceived is in his line of vision. In spite of their general passivity, some of these babies, like Bobby, give reasonably sure evidence of adequate visual perception in noticing, following, and finding objects (T:V:1,2) or in retrieving them (T:V:4). They may see objects nearby, but because of poor head control may be unable to observe those at a distance. They may therefore occasionally appear inattentive and aloof. Beginnings of verbal ability may be indicated by responsive babbling or later by some "words." However, even without vocalizing the child may often show awareness of words by some definite change in expression or attitude. It is easy to underestimate a very young child under these circumstances. It is equally easy to overestimate the child's comprehension of object relationships because his passive responses to an object are usually less differentiated and more ambiguous than would be true if manipulation were possible.

Occasionally a baby as sheltered as these may respond only to a familiar voice and not to a strange one. Another may ignore an otherwise cherished toy because he is awed or uncomfortable in the unaccustomed test situation. In the records under discussion, estimations of intellectual potentiality proved reliable only when all such considerations were taken into account.

Considering the degree of motor handicap involved, it often seems legitimate for a psychologist testing a baby of this age to base an encouraging judgement on reliable success in only a very few test items. Total lack of response to any situation, however, justifies a more sceptical attitude about the baby's ability. Definite prognosis, positive or negative, must be postponed.

For the group as a whole, a few of the more common features at this age are the noted passivity and friendliness in some babies, and heightened irritability and fretfulness in others. Fear of being dropped when carried is described in a fair number of cases. Bodily insecurity can probably be at least partially explained by the lack of bodily experiences. Lack of satisfactory interpersonal physical contacts may also be responsible for the apparent slowness of personality development noticed in a large number of children. Often it is accentuated by the children's deficiency in means of expression. None of these babies talks as yet. Like much younger infants, some can show through crying or smiling only whether they are comfortable or aware of changes around them. Various records note that the baby recognizes foods by sight or notices which person handles him. Several children are reported to respond to words in one way or another or to like certain pieces of music.

Meager as these observations from daily life may seem, in many cases of this group they prove to have more predictive value than performances on standard tests. Children who did not show any signs of such everyday comprehension developed slowly all through the years. Negative responses in standard test situations proved to be less reliable indices.

In the preschool years the demands for psychological evaluation increase. The majority of children in this group are examined at four or five years of age; only a few come for earlier appraisal. Up to this time parents and pediatricians alike are still concerned mostly with physical rather than psychological problems. In many cases the child's mental ability is still not questioned at all. Often any existing doubts are pushed back or dismissed, and delayed psychological development is explained by the child's lack of opportunity. There are fewer parents in this group who are seriously worried about a possible mental defect than in any other group of severely handicapped cerebral palsied children. In some cases the pediatrician seems reassuring because he still tries not to be pessimistic about the intellectual potentialities of the young child. However, as school age approaches, some educational planning becomes desirable, and it seems advisable to base this on a psychologist's advice.

Speech difficulty and limited motor power are foremost in the minds of those parents who still contemplate a normal school situation. Speech problems range from total lack of speech in some to poor articulation in others. Motor difficulties range from total failure to walk or even sit independently to unsteady athetoid gait and shaky manipulations.

As regards behavior, almost all of the most severely handicapped children are described by their families as placid, friendly, or "good as gold"; some seem to be easily disturbed by changes of routine. The most mobile children are said to be responsive, energetic, and "in on everything." Frequently their enterprising spirit compares but feebly with the energy and curiosity of normal children at this age. But their efforts, together with the precarious results, often make them appear surprisingly daring. Serious behavior complaints are relatively rare at the preschool age. Only a very few rather neurotic mothers of less damaged children reject the child's intense and willful manners, apparently mostly because the child's drooling and his chaotic movements seem repulsive to them. With his body mechanism so seriously impaired, there is at this age little danger that any child in this group will become too independent and challenge parental protection and authority.

Means of expression are, in general, very limited. Efforts to use words or gestures are frequently encouraged but hardly ever restrained, as they might be in normal children at this voluble age. The majority of the children discussed here show some comprehension of language. While the parents' comments on the degree of understanding may vary, none doubt that the child can hear. All have some evidence that comprehension of language equals comprehension of visual clues; the child seems to understand and to remember things he hears and sees. He connects people with their names, he knows foods, anticipates events, recognizes favorite radio programs by their theme tunes. All such signs confirm to the parents that the child is participating in daily events and sharing their life. They may often be content with achievements which would do credit only to a much younger child. Signs of communication, often imperceptible to strangers, contribute frequently to the most intimate mother-child relationship which is naturally prolonged through the child's continuing need for complete physical care, as it is in Bobby's case.

The psychological examination during the preschool years shows a number of characteristic features. Most of the children are somewhat slow in adjusting to the test situation. Depending on the degree of physical disability, they may seem lumpy and remote until the position is found from which they can best and most freely operate. At first they often become entranced with the difficult task of just handling the material which is presented and pay no attention to what could be done with it. Their restricted eye movements frequently make them appear oblivious of people around them. Contrary to children described in subsequent chapters, however, they often learn within a few minutes to establish some relationship with E and to deal with objects more appropriately. They pick up clues from demonstrations or follow verbal explanations and directions. However, even those able to produce some speech rarely attempt to talk spontaneously until rather late in the examination. At this age most children of this group appear more egocentric, socially immature, and emotionally dependent on their families than do normal children. After the initial period of aloofness, many of the children are described as responsive. Some at first do not enter the situation actively, but look and smile. Others become overexcited, eager, and persistent, and then become more tense than they usually are. At this stage, as in earlier and later ones, severely handicapped children are as frequently underestimated as they are overestimated. The seriousness of the motor disability can mask efficiency in understanding some of the test materials.

Also, lack of familiarity with a word or an object may simulate lack of reasoning ability. But an examiner may also easily overlook an inaccurate verbal concept or an undifferentiated matching of forms if the motor requirements of the task seem to tax the child unduly. For this reason the proxy method is preferred in those tasks that demand manipulation but essentially test comprehension.

The records indicate that many children of this group show a higher level of performance than might be expected from their immature social attitude. In spite of the more or less serious speech disability, verbal comprehension is adequate or even good in a large number of cases. Also, in spite of the motor difficulties in handling materials, many of these children are able enough in the area of perceptual discrimination. Especially children with pure extrapyramidal involvement show adequate form comprehension in formboards (T:IV:5,6), Montessori cylinders (T:IV:4), blockbuilding (T:I:2), matching and sorting (T:VI), and good reasoning ability in these as well as in all kinds of verbal tasks (identification, T:IV:5,9,10). Patients with a mixed type of palsy may, like the others, be good in tasks that test vocabulary at these younger age levels (T:II:3,6,7), but fail where reasoning and comprehension rather than learned associations are called for. They also have more of the disabilities in form comprehension usually connected with pyramidal injuries (discussed in the chapter on Paul).

Statements about attention spans vary. Some children are described as persistent but easily fatigued, others as having short attention spans. However, it is very difficult to judge persistence of attention accurately in a child of this age. Factors such as interest, physical effort, and motivation interact, and the role of each is not easily determined. Simple, short, and well-defined tasks such as memory for pictures (T:II:8) and Decroly matching game (T:VI:4) are most suitable for the purpose. The majority of children enjoy the often totally unfamiliar activities. Like normal children of their age, they have as yet no ability to judge what they can and cannot do.

The psychological examination tries to reveal the maturity of comprehension underlying the child's activities, regardless of his technical limitations. It also judges his readiness to adapt to new situations as they arise. In this group, appraisal of both reasoning ability and learning ability is basic for the evaluation of a child's developmental level. The psychological examination often has to rely on only a few test items, and it can be dangerous and premature to base a definite, far-reaching prognosis on such meager evidence. But since the psychological study at this age is commonly but one in a series of several to follow in subsequent years, it seems to serve a useful purpose. It helps the adviser to appraise the current situation and aid in planning. To determine whether or not the child is intellectually and emotionally ready for a new learning experience is only one among many other purposes. Many parents, having devoted several years largely to the physical care of the child, are eager to hear suggestions about how to widen the child's range of experience. Many welcome discussions about how to encourage psychological development in a child who appears to make only barely perceptible physical advances. The question of institutionalization or boarding away from home frequently arises at this age in this severely handicapped group. The psychologist helps by discussing the advantages and disadvantages of such a step in the light of the family situation.

Between the ages of six and ten these children present new problems. Some have gained in the ability to walk, though they may still be dependent on help much of the time. The more severely handicapped ones have acquired some means of locomotion. They may use a walker, or may roll or creep on the floor, but they are still essentially helpless. Expressive speech still is a problem to most. A few are able to talk clearly enough, but do it very slowly; many speak not only slowly but with defective enunciation. Aside from their physical situation, these children again present mostly educational problems to their parents. Many families who in earlier days fought, often belligerently, for recognition of the child's intellectual potentialities now feel more or less rewarded by the enthusiastic and optimistic attention the child now receives from home teachers, therapists, or neighbors. The majority of children in this group get some instruction and have learned to read a little. Some of the less handicapped attend special classes with the understanding that their physical limitations, rather than intellectual deficit, make this placement necessary.

In many cases parents and teachers request advice because they want to give the child the best opportunity rather than because they are in doubt about intellectual potentialities. Relations between the child and his family are, in most cases, very close. Still in need of much protection, these children are not apt to rebel at this stage. Many are described by their families as pleasant and content enough in everyday life, but easily overwrought when challenged for an achievement. Often a severely handicapped child seems to become tense; often this is due more to his efforts to live up to his good reputation than to his fear of failure. A less disabled child is apt to be less overtly confident, since he generally has already met frustrating competitive situations.

At this age, as in earlier years, the form of the psychological examination is determined by the degree of physical helplessness and speech difficulty. More methods are now suitable since the children are older. Some who are unable to use their hands can now be examined by verbal methods alone. If their speech is too seriously limited, they can be judged by their actions in test situations. They may express their comprehension through nonverbal activities which they can execute themselves or by proxy. Some of the most severely handicapped children succeed in expressing their ideas in the test situation by eye movements, turns of the head, or by agitation of the whole body. As shown in Bobby's examination, there is a variety of methods which can be successfully adapted to almost any child's situation. Again, as at younger ages, it is preferable to depend on a few well-documented procedures rather than on a series of equivocal results.

The examination is always geared to exploit any possible avenue of communication in order to determine what the child understands of his surroundings, and how and to what degree he interacts with people and objects around him. In spite of motor limitations, these handicapped children have generally established more means of communication than they had before. Many of them expect to be understood by others than their immediate families. They now communicate more freely with E and also show more interest in her reactions to them. At the beginning of the interviews most of the abler children are no longer socially aloof as they were in their younger years; instead they are tense and full of anticipation. Many are agitated and over-responsive; others are apprehensive, observant, and ready to look for clues.

Regardless of speech difficulty, verbal ability is generally high in this group. Good vocabulary is apparent in vocabulary tests (T:XII) which, depending on the case, may be used in various adaptations. Some children can deal satisfactorily with concrete as well as abstract words; others deal significantly better with concrete words. In a small number of children some uncommon classifications or some failure to differentiate verbally animals, tools, etc., seems to attest to a lack of experience. Comprehension of meaningful language and reasoning ability, shown in such tests as similarities (T:IX:2) or similarities and differences (T:IX:3), are usually better in this group than in any of the others discussed. Performances in tasks which depend largely on visual imagery and everyday observations, such as verbal absurdities (T:IX:6) and comprehension (T:X:2,3), are uneven. Apparently they vary with the degree of physical and social experience of each child. Compared with their earlier years, these children now have learned more factual material through schooling, television, and radio. As before one finds that in spite of technical difficulties caused by their severe motor impairment, many children in this group show adequate comprehension in tests involving formboards (T:IV:6–9), recognition of designs (T:VII:2,9), memory for designs (T:VII:1,2,4,5b), or block designs (T:VII:7,8). The correlation noted earlier between pyramidal involvement and difficulties in the area of form comprehension and thought persist at this age level. Children with pure extrapyramidal palsy show no irregularities in form comprehension except those imposed by motor restrictions, while those with mixed types of palsy are apt to function more like other pyramidal (hemiplegic or tetraplegic) groups.

While the distribution of ability in the various areas of functioning remains relatively constant, the social attitude differs significantly from that of earlier years. In spite of their dependence on those close to them, many of these children show an increasing interest in performing for others and have gained more experience in social contacts. Their situation still remains unique. With speech slow and locomotion precarious at best, all their means of interaction are limited and they still must depend largely on the good will of others in listening to them, coming to them, or waiting for them. They lack the social give-and-take of life through which normal children learn their social habits. Even the ablest children of this group seem to be more mature in their knowledge and in their verbal patterns than in social wisdom and sensitivity. Some of them appear somewhat demanding, others overenthusiastic, aggressive, and occasionally slightly inconsiderate.

Thanks to their serious and obvious physical difficulties, children of this group and at this age level meet with indulgence and sympathy from most adults. Often their eagerness and courage seem touching, and their persistence a moral virtue. The harder they try, the more praise and encouragement they are apt to receive from parents, teachers, and relatives. Many of the children are under constant pressure to try for goals which are beyond them. At this stage children are rarely able to judge for themselves how much they can achieve. They accept the assignment to "try their best" perhaps more conscientiously than normal children at their age. They thrive on the approval which they get for their efforts, if not for the actual results.

Often it is an important role of the psychologist to clarify the situation and to help modify some pressures. Many parents, however, are so impressed with the discrepancy between the child's physical and mental powers that they are bound to overemphasize and develop the latter without being aware of the cost to the child in nervous energy. In some rare cases, on the contrary, an alert child is not given enough opportunity to learn and to use his available abilities. The psychological examination may help to better his situation and to relieve his boredom.

From eleven years of age on the problems of children in this group increase. The physical situation has, in most cases, not improved as much as the family may have hoped. With advancing age, some of the physical aspects become more conspicuous and less acceptable. The most severely handicapped children who have to be carried or supported become too heavy for their mothers, who are now often worn out. In the more mobile children, awkward movements and unsteady gait may become grotesque in this preadolescent period, while they may occasionally have given a puppet-like charm to the younger child. Slowness of action and speech may frequently be accepted from a younger child, but becomes difficult in a lively group of growing siblings or efficient adults. Many families are able to suppress growing negative feelings; others admit them. In most cases, loosening of the closest emotional ties between the child and his parents is regarded as a natural development inherent in the age and is frequently welcomed because it is normal. In a smaller number of cases, such loosening has not yet taken place; the ties remain abnormally strong. Families dread thinking of a time when they will no longer be able to give the handicapped child the needed protection. In many cases another psychological appraisal is requested in the early adolescent years to help in making new plans.

These examinations show that many of the children in this group have become increasingly aware of their limitations and of the restrictions of their life situation. Frequently the children complain of being treated "like a baby," whereas the parents comment about moody, demanding, or disgruntled behavior which was not previously apparent. Some children who in earlier years were praised for their neatness and their desire for order have now become embarrassingly critical observers of their mothers' daily doings. Meticulousness pervades many areas of living. Some of the older girls take anxious pride in their painfully neat appearance or in their overpolished social graces. Others, boys and girls alike, use carefully chosen expressions and phrases and self-consciously try to draw attention to their assets rather than to their difficulties. Those who in younger years were ready to try whatever was proposed to them now have learned to judge better what they are capable of doing. In the test situation they may refuse politely a task which would spell failure. Or they may with a half-hearted effort demonstrate to E that it is impossible for them to comply. Often an over-civilized attitude seems to hide much insecurity and discomfort in social situations which appeared pleasant to them before. Some of the children who talk relatively easily try to keep control of E's attention with conversation. Some try to express their high hopes for improvement but do not sound convinced.

The assets of this group are in the verbal field at this age as they were in earlier years. This is true even of those whose speech is laborious. Most children of this group know many words and do best in vocabulary and abstract words (T:XII). Many now read fluently. Their stock of information is often excellent (T:XI:10), and many use this factual material well when it is needed. Their comprehension tends to be better in tests of abstract reasoning, such as similarities (T:IX:2,3) and some comprehension questions (T:X:3), than in tests calling for a quick appraisal of a situation. Their physical condition seems responsible for a deficiency in experiences usually acquired in everyday life that is revealed by practical questions (T:X:2 and IX:14) and tests of orientation (T:IX:7). With reasoning problems (T:IX:2,8,9), which at this age level require more thinking and less practical experience than before, several of the children achieve higher ratings in reasoning than they ever did before. However, communication has become more of a problem than before. Frequently, scanty speech no longer suffices as a means of communication. These children now often seem to keep their thoughts to themselves. Some show relief when their meager expressions are picked up and understood. Reading and listening become for the abler children more satisfactory means of contact than talking. Several in the group like to write long, elaborate letters; a few write poetry with complex and unusual word constructions. Most of the children operate best on the verbal level at this age.

Again it is noted that among children with pure extrapyramidal palsy imperfect performance on form comprehension tests can generally be traced to motor inability rather than to perceptual difficulties. Block designs (T:VII:7,8) and object assembly tests (T:IV:11,12) are easily solved by most of the older children and young adults of this category. However, those with mixed pyramidal and extrapyramidal palsy seem to have more difficulty in form perception. They tend to make reversals in memory for designs (T:VII:1,2,4), block designs, and object assembly tests.

The psychological examination at this age is conducted along the same principles as at younger age levels. The degree of comprehension is evaluated, and the individual's ability for interchange and communication is defined, regardless of the technical difficulties which his physical disability imposes. But after this is done, the psychologist must also try to determine how the individual can use this potential ability within his actual situation. She tries to judge how the child has done this in the past and attempts to foresee his future development under given physical and social circumstances.

Based on such considerations, the best advice is that which combines kindness with realism. Often it is more important to try to ameliorate an immediate situation than to expect far-reaching, radical, new developments from the future. Among the few possible helpful suggestions for alleviating an adolescent's frustration and loneliness is a change of environment. Group life or group activities with equally handicapped individuals seem welcome at this age, although they are only rarely available. Most children no longer want to be soothed by insincere optimism, but want to discuss their situation in realistic terms; many families must now be convinced by outsiders that the child has acquired insight into his own situation. He can, perhaps, be helped to live with it, but cannot and should not be encouraged to entertain false hopes and unrealistic expectations.

Extrapyramidal Lesion, Athetosis Dysarthria, Auditory Defect

Jimmy has a moderately severe athetosis, dysarthria, and auditory difficulty. His main problems are his motor difficulties and his inability to communicate. Though Jimmy has adequate mental potentialities, he is, because of his physical impairment, slow in emotional, intellectual, and social development. He does not fit well into the life pattern of his family; his inadequate adjustment there takes new forms at each stage of his development.

As a baby Jimmy's development is unsatisfactory from all angles; he appears retarded because he is unable to move properly and cannot express himself or understand other people as normal children his age do. His mental awareness is masked by these difficulties. At four years of age he is able to get around, but has unsatisfactory relationships with people. Since he does not communicate and does not understand what others mean, he finds life threatening and fights for his rights. At seven he is learning to get along better. He has found ways to communicate by nonverbal means if need arises. He is gaining more confidence. Thanks to his reasoning ability, he understands his environment better. He still is not able to interpret language adequately and this inability makes him a puzzle to his family. At twelve he has become a lonesome, awkward boy who has learned only the most necessary speech, which is not very intelligible. He still understands very little only. However, through his ability to observe and to reason, he has gained more experience and has become more emotionally stable. His competence and good intentions have become more obvious to more people than before, but in spite of this he is not accepted easily in any group.

Jimmy's complicated situation has not been easy to understand for those around him. Professional advisers have been as puzzled as his family. Varied therapeutic and educational plans have been tried and found wanting. This uncertainty has had its impact on the child and on his family. All through the years psychological appraisal has had to be based on judging both the child's emotional-social development and his comprehension from nonverbal matters only.

Using Jimmy's case as an illustration, this chapter presents a description of the psychological study of a child with moderately severe athetosis, dysarthria, and auditory difficulty. This detailed account of repeated appraisals shows how at each stage Jimmy's behavior and performances in test situations together with descriptions and clues supplied by his family develop into a psychological picture which helps the psychologist to explain some of the problems that arise at each period. The last section shows how, by comparison with other case records, similar situations and trends are found to be common among children with disabilities like Jimmy's and briefly indicates how the psychologist uses findings and interpretations as a basis for guidance.

JIMMY AT FIFTEEN MONTHS

From birth Jimmy's development has been slower than that of his older brother. He has always been a flabby, hypotonic baby. Only two to three months ago he learned to maintain himself in a sitting position, but he is still not steady. He has just started to creep, but does so in a peculiar swimming fashion. Lately he has shown more active interest in objects; until recently he was aware of objects only when they were dangled in front of him; he did not attempt to grasp them or follow them visually. He is a very quiet baby who does not mind being left alone. Only quite recently has he preferred to be where he can see people. There was a time when he babbled more than he does now; he produces only a few sounds. There have been feeding difficulties; he still cannot chew and eats only semiliquid foods. He has likes and dislikes in food. He recognizes carrots on sight and refuses them with his mouth tightly shut.

His family finds him unresponsive and retarded. They are especially worried about his lack of interest in anything which is outside the field of his immediate attention. He still does not respond to his name or to his mother's voice. The question of deafness has been raised, but both parents are inclined to believe instead that the child is physically and mentally deficient.

In the examining room, the baby is placed in the baby tender where he sits reasonably well, though with a tendency to lean forward. His head is slightly turned to one side and droops occasionally. Jimmy is a sober-looking baby with large, serious eyes. He does not smile readily. He pays very little attention to E and responds only briefly to his mother when she leans over to adjust his clothes. He does not notice that his father enters and calls him from one side of the room.

When the first block is presented to him, Jimmy grasps it immediately with the palm of his right hand (T:I:1). He bangs the block on the table and loses it on the tabletop; he tries to grasp it as before, but cannot get hold of it again. E takes the block and presents it to the child, who grasps it as before. She then presents a second block. Jimmy tries to approach it with his left hand, but cannot get hold of it. While he touches it, he drops the block he held in his right hand. Trying to secure it again, he becomes frustrated and starts to fret. E presents an open box and drops one of the blocks into it. Jimmy, quiet again, picks up another block with her help and drops it in the box on his own. While he repeats this with two other blocks, one of them lands on top of the other. He watches this with interest, approaches, and thereby upsets the structure. He picks up a block and tries to pile it on top of another but does not succeed. He loses the block, looks briefly at the floor to see where it went, but immediately returns his attention to the table.

E then introduces the pellet and bottle situation (T:V:8). Jimmy approaches bottle with his right hand, gets hold of it, but then sweeps it off the table. He tries to see where it went by leaning to the side. E places pellet at some distance from the bottle. Jimmy perceives it and tries to approach it, but he sweeps it off the table and turns back to the bottle. E attracts the child's gaze and drops another pellet into the bottle. Then she turns the bottle so that the pellet falls out. Jimmy watches it when it drops on the table. He continues to show interest when the procedure is repeated. In a third trial, he no longer looks at the bottle while it is being turned; instead he fixes his gaze on the tabletop, where the last pellet dropped. Clearly he has learned to expect the new pellet to appear there.

E decides to try him on Gesell's three-figure formboard (a wooden board with three holes cut to fit three forms: circle, square, triangle; T:IV:5). E presents the board with the round block inserted. Jimmy pats the round block with his right hand. E helps him grasp it. He holds on to it briefly, but drops it; it lands near the round hole. E places it in the hole while the child is watching. On repetition, Jimmy gets a more secure grip on the round block; clearly he directs it toward the round hole, where it again falls out of his hand. When the formboard is rotated, Jimmy stares at the square hole, shifts his glance to the round hole, and tries to move the round block toward it. He has recognized where it belongs, though he loses it in mid-air.

Presented with a picture book, he grasps a page immediately, starts turning it, but cannot hold on to it long enough to turn it all the way. He shows no interest in any of the pictures. E substitutes a sturdier picture book, with pictures mounted on cardboards (T:II:1,3). With some help, the child is now able to turn one page and then the next. In this book he sees a large red balloon and fixates on it. Another page is turned for him; he glimpses the picture of a large toy dog and looks at it intently. E asks, "Where is the doggy?" Jimmy does not respond. He gets ready to turn the next page. E stops him, pointing to the picture of a baby. Jimmy looks at it. E: "That is the baby, where is the doggy?" No response. Jimmy's mother speaks up for the first time, explains that he never responds to questions of this kind and surely does not understand language.

E, wondering about Jimmy's hearing, introduces a bell with a handle, approximately four inches high. E rings the bell before Jimmy has seen it. There is no response. When the bell is shown to the child, he tries immediately to grasp it by the handle; he pushes it along the table. E waves and rings the bell, while Jimmy is looking on; then she removes the bell to the floor out of his sight. He turns to where it disappeared, but gives up. E again rings the bell from its hiding place; no response. She brings it up to the tabletop. Jimmy becomes agitated and reaches for the bell. Placed on the floor to sit, he can maintain himself for a brief period, but his position is precarious. He leans forward; he looks ill-at-ease, with legs stiff and wide apart. He seems better off when placed against his mother's legs. Trying to study the child's responses within a wider area, E introduces a ball.

With his head drooping, Jimmy does not see E and does not respond when she calls him. He notices the ball only when it rolls between his legs. He tries to get it, and, without looking up, he feebly pushes it back. When ball is again thrown to him, he notices it only when it comes near. E: "Give it to me"; no response. His mother repeats, "Give it to me" and holds out her hands. He tries to lift the ball up to her.

The session is closed. Jimmy's father approaches from the back with, "Time to go home, Jimmy." He receives no response until he bends down to pick the child up, says, "Say bye-bye to the lady." He explains that Jimmy's reactions to this kind of invitation are irregular. He gets no response to his repeated "Say bye-bye to the lady." Only when Jimmy notices his father's hand waving does he imitate him feebly with his right hand and smile down for the first time from his father's arms.

COMMENT

Analysis of Jimmy's behavior during this short observation period indicates that his situation is a complex one and that several sets of problems are involved.

He has poor motor control; when dealing with objects, he seems to want to do more than he can accomplish (blocks, formboard). Nevertheless, his approach, gestures, and frustrated attempts show comprehension adequate for his age level in many areas (blocks in box, formboard, pellet and bottle). There is a considerable discrepancy between his responses to visual and to auditory clues. In several instances, he showed no interest in the auditory aspects of a situation, but responded immediately when he perceived it visually (bell, father, ball). This behavior suggests the possibility of difficulties in auditory perception. His almost complete lack of sound production, after an early phase of undifferentiated babbling, may also point in this direction, though motor difficulties (dysarthria) may also be a factor. Besides lack of vocalization and comprehension of auditory signs, there is also a general paucity of communication. Since his features remain immobile much of the time and his general motility is impaired, it is not easy for him to express his feelings and desires. He also does not respond easily to the social gestures of others. All this makes him appear immature, unresponsive, and withdrawn.

However, there is evidence that Jimmy's life circumstances have much influence on his behavior and complicate an already difficult situation. Both his motor and probably his auditory difficulties restrict his field of action. With his poor sitting balance, his drooping head, and his unsteady hands, he is unable to investigate and learn to understand his world as normal babies do. He needs a great deal of warmth and encouragement. However, Jimmy's family has probably fostered neither enterprise nor communication. His mother is a rather restrained person. It is not easy for her to give vent to her feelings; she is not a woman who indulges in sentimental and spontaneous gestures or who, from nearly imperceptible signs, guesses a child's feelings and reactions. She used to be gratified that he was a "good" baby and did not need much of her time. She has always been worried about his motor development and has taken conscientious care of his feeding problems, but she still thinks of him as an inscrutable creature with whom social intercourse is impossible.

In the light of these impressions, it is not easy to make suggestions for Jimmy's care. One would like him to have more opportunity and human contact, and as little frustration as possible, to develop the best of his abilities. E hopes that her hypothesis of hearing difficulty may be substantiated through the hearing test. Jimmy's parents may be able to accept such a defect more easily than a diagnosis of general retardation, which they expected. However, good social-personal relations are of primary importance for the training of a hard-of-hearing child, and satisfactory substitutes for these are not easily found. His motor difficulties will continue to be a disadvantage and will make him less attractive to his family; this may complicate his training considerably.

JIMMY AT FOUR YEARS

Jimmy, now age four, is an awkward little boy who as yet does not talk at all. He lumbers hastily, runs into things, and falls. He does not seem to know how to stop. Frequently, he appears eager and determined, and not very friendly. While waiting for E in the playroom, he goes up to another child and grabs a doll she is holding in her hand. He retires to a corner to study it without paying any attention to the upheaval he has created in the room. His mother apologizes, shrugging her shoulders without talking to Jimmy. She seems embarrassed but resigned to this sort of behavior and shows no particular surprise about it.

She reports about life at home. Since her last visit here she has had two other normal children. Jimmy has grown up in the midst of a certain amount of confusion. Time has slipped by, and with all her other duties his mother has not had much time for Jimmy. She has come to realize that the child is competent in many ways. His lack of speech and his general behavior continue to be very disturbing to her. She finds him difficult to handle and impossible to reason with. He gets into trouble around the house and has broken many things. He does not know his motor limitations and seems determined to get into situations which he is unable to handle. On his "good days" Jimmy likes to be helpful around the house. He knows where things are; he knows, for example, what his mother needs in order to bake a cake and eagerly collects it for her. On his "bad days" he may try to bake a cake himself, which usually results in bedlam, spankings, and tears. He can be mean to his siblings; his three-year-old brother is frequently afraid of him. His mother describes life with Jimmy in a half-humorous, detached way; she still talks about him as if he were an unpredictable, strange little being. "If he could only talk so I could get through to him." His lack of speech and his failure to respond to language seem to both parents much more disturbing than his motor difficulties. Ever since two early hearing examinations (at sixteen and twenty-two months) showed inconclusive results, the parents have never been sure whether or not the child hears. (He seems to be aware of the sounds of radio and TV, occasionally hears bells, but still does not respond to language.) The question of a severe mental aberration still lingers in their minds.

The psychological examination is requested at this time in order to throw more light on this difficult situation. Jimmy's parents and their pediatrician hope that it will help explain and remedy Jimmy's behavior difficulties. With school age approaching, some educational plan will soon be necessary. The question of schooling away from home is in his parents' minds. His mother expresses some concern that Jimmy's behavior may have an ill effect on his brothers. She also thinks that he may need specialized care.

Led by his mother, Jimmy enters the examining room. She seats him at the examining table, where he finds:

BLOCKS AND A BOX (T:I:1,3)

Without delay, Jimmy starts to throw the blocks into the box, forces the cover of the box on top. His mother, afraid that he may break the box, tries to help Jimmy and shows him how to be more orderly. Thereupon, Jimmy gets up and walks to the door to return to the playroom. His mother jumps up to prevent this; Jimmy resists. Holding on to the doorknob, he slips to the floor; he protects his buttocks with his other hand and seems prepared for a scene and a maternal spanking.

E, who has stayed in the background until now, suggests that Jimmy be allowed to roam as he pleases. Jimmy, apparently accustomed to unexpected turns of events, wanders into the next room, but returns immediately and finds his mother and E in conversation. Continuing to talk, E casually produces:

Seguin Formboard (T:IV:6)

The child seems to be curious, and approaches. E turns the board upside down. Jimmy does not blink his eyes when the wooden insets drop on the table with some noise. He picks up the star and hastily places it in square hole; he grabs the triangle which he places in the lozenge recess. When E removes it, Jimmy tries to stop her and wants the inset back. She shows him the round form instead and places it in the round recess; then she offers him the oval. Jimmy, somewhat more relaxed, takes time to look around the board and places the oval correctly; also picks up rectangle and does the same. He ignores E, who offers him the next inset, and instead picks up one of his own choice. His grasp is awkward, but he is able to place all insets except the lozenge, which he tries to put angle first into the hexagon hole. He is about to become impatient when E tries to help him by placing this inset in the correct hole. He pushes her hand away, removes the piece, and puts it back. There is no vocal exchange between E and child.

Mare and Foal Picture Board (T:IV:13)

Jimmy seems interested and grasps one lengthy piece (leg) immediately; he is clumsy and holds the piece in his fist. He tries to force it in the wrong lengthy hole; after a while he approaches the correct hole, but has difficulty turning the piece. An oval-shaped piece (grass) is tried in another roughly oval spot (sheep) but is later transferred. His first impulse is to try to match pieces of roughly similar shape. E gives no overt help, but sees to it that pieces remain arranged so that a minimum of sideways turning is required. (Judging by his trials and errors rather than by his motor performance, his comprehension compares with that of normal children at four-year level.)

E points to horse, asks, "What is this?" Points to chicken, inquires again. There is no response. E: "Where is the horse?" No response. E: "Where are the chickens?" Jimmy ignores the questions; he hands the board to E and motions for new material.

DECROLY MATCHING GAME (T:VI:4)

Intending to keep the small cards, E gives Jimmy only the large ones. However, he tries to grab the first card from her hand. His mother pulls at his sleeve and admonishes, "Not so rough, Jimmy!" He shakes her off. E places the card showing the ball; hastily Jimmy takes the cards which are handed to him. He uses the first ones to haphazardly fill all of one large card; he shrugs off E's attempt to show him. He becomes intrigued when E offers train. Jimmy places it correctly and E applauds ostentatiously. Jimmy smiles for the first time; from now on he peruses the field carefully. E removes the wrongly placed cards. Then she offers star and square; Jimmy responds correctly. When she offers flag, Jimmy puts it on umbrella; he then looks sidewise at E. She points toward the correct place; Jimmy accepts the suggestion. From here on he places all correctly except for pear on apple, and ship on triangle. (Performance at approximately four-year level.)

E gets the continued impression that Jimmy is interested simply in the shape of things and not in their meaning. This is difficult to prove with this procedure, but his errors seem at least to point in this direction. The next task should determine Jimmy's ability to match by a different principle.

COLOR-FORM SORTING (T:VI:5)

A set of plastic blocks consisting of disks, triangles, and squares in blue, red, yellow, and green; similar to the Weigl-Goldstein-Scheerer material.

To test his ability to sort colors E chooses this material in preference to the cardboard color matching material (T:VI:2) or to ordinary blocks (T:I:6). The first may lead to frustration because of Jimmy's poor motor coordination. His reluctance to accept help from adults would render any proxy method unsatisfactory. Blocks are being avoided for the moment because Jimmy may not have happy associations with them, owing to the somewhat stormy events at the beginning of the examination.

COLOR MATCHING. Presented with a green, a yellow, and a red disk, he makes no mistake in matching them with another set of green, yellow, and red disks. The same procedure is repeated with triangles and squares. He enjoys the activity and has no doubts about what to do.

FORM MATCHING. Presented with a disk, a triangle, and a square in blue, he matches them with relevant shapes without error (a yellow disk with blue disk, or yellow square with blue square, or yellow triangle with blue triangle, respectively).

COLOR OR FORM MATCHING. Presented with a green disk, a red square, and a blue triangle, he places a blue square with the red square, and a red disk with the green disk; similarly, when presented with a red disk, a green square, and a yellow triangle, he again matches a yellow disk with the red disk, and a green triangle with the yellow triangle.

It is difficult to ascertain whether or not Jimmy actually makes a conscious choice between the possibilities of matching forms or colors. It seems again as if he gravitated toward the choice which seems more natural to him, the choice by form.

PICTURE BOOK (T:II:1–3)

Jimmy turns the pages fast, looking at only one picture on each page. E asks, "Show me the dog"; no response. E: "Where is the chair? the ball?" No response. Jimmy closes the book and wants to get up.

MATCHING OBJECTS AND PICTURES (T:VI:10)

E produces small toy objects from a box; she places a toy dog on the picture of a dog. Jimmy, again interested, stands the dog up and wants to see more of the objects. E offers a toy green chair. The open book shows a yellow chair, among other objects. Jimmy examines the green chair he holds in his hand. E motions to him to put it on the yellow chair picture. He complies and wants the next object. E offers him a red spoon. The page now open shows a metal spoon, among other objects. Jimmy handles his spoon, aligns it to the edge of the page. E points to the pictured spoon; Jimmy tries to cover it with his red one. Meticulously he endeavors to match the shapes of both. E offers a green car. On the open page is a blue car. Jimmy is pleased to get the toy car. He looks at the book; he glances over the picture of the blue car, does not seem to take notice of it. E points to it. Jimmy obediently places his small car on top of the larger picture, picks a red car out of the box and places both side by side, again carefully aligning the two toy cars with each other. E offers round watch. There is a clock on the open page, among other objects. Looking over the page, Jimmy does not register response until E points to clock. Jimmy fits watch on top of clock, which is as round but not as large as watch; not content, he tries instead to place watch on picture of ball which is nearly the same size.

When E offers blue cup, to be placed on page showing green dishes, Jimmy does not seem to know what to do with it. When offered a small pink spoon, to be placed on page showing metal spoon, Jimmy handles the spoon but again does not know what to do with it. When offered a bracelet watch, to be placed on page showing clock, Jimmy gives no response. E points toward clock. Jimmy obeys for a moment, then seems to become uninterested and gets up to examine the objects in the box.

MATCHING OBJECTS (T:VI:9)

The objects to be matched are a green car, a white cup, a red spoon. When presented with the key object, a pink spoon, Jimmy places it with the red spoon without hesitation. When presented with a red car, he places it with the green car. When presented with the pink cup, he hesitates toward the pink spoon, then decides to place it with the white cup. The next objects to be matched are an orange car, a dog, and a round watch. When presented with the key object, a red car, Jimmy correctly places it with the orange car. Also correctly places key object, a cow, with the dog, and third key object, a bracelet watch, with the round watch.

Obviously, Jimmy recognizes all objects presented to him and classifies them properly when dealing with them concretely. However, he does not seem to appreciate the similarity between an object and a picture of a like object, unless the picture is of identical size and shape (red spoon, watch).

It was noted in earlier phases of the examination that Jimmy is more interested in shapes than in content and meaning; he responds to form qualities rather than to functional or conceptual aspects. For Jimmy a picture is not necessarily a symbolic representation, but a form of a certain size, shape, and perhaps color.

During the last part of the interview, Jimmy has lost his fear of being thwarted or interfered with. He no longer grabs things away from E but accepts her cooperation; he seems attracted by the activities. Though well aware that he might become upset again at the slightest provocation, E dares to introduce a new type of task. It will require more give and take between her and the child. The material will probably be less attractive to Jimmy and may prove fragile in the hands of this tempestuous child.

ANIMAL PICTURES (T:II:10)

MATCHING. Jimmy wants to hold on to the cards all by himself. He soon becomes interested in the task and understands immediately. When, as a nonverbal form of demonstration, E uses two fingers to point with each to one of a pair of animals, he imitates this motion. He chooses four of the pictures correctly. His errors are bear for pig and squirrel for cat; in both pairs there is a superficial resemblance because of the similar posture of the animals. (By Revised Stanford-Binet standards, Jimmy passes on three-and-a-half-year level.)

PICTURE VOCABULARY (T:II:7)

Jimmy is to express the meaning of the pictures by gestures. E demonstrates hat and airplane. Jimmy seems amused by her gestures, but does not seem to relate them to the pictures. He wants to get hold of the cards himself and collect them in his fist. He dog-ears the cards; E tries to restrain her apprehension that he may destroy the fragile paper.

To knife (later, car and spoon) there is no response except for Jimmy's consistent attempts to grab pictures. E tries to demonstrate, but both she and the child become increasingly tense. Mother starts squirming. E interrupts task. Jimmy clearly has shown no interest in describing any of the pictures by gestures and has not understood what was wanted of him.

BLOCKS (T:I:1,2,5 AND FIGURE 1)

One set of yellow and one set of green blocks.

Spontaneously Jimmy starts an alternating row of one green, one yellow; after six placements he continues all yellow.

FOUR-BLOCK TOWER. Jimmy takes over, piles three blocks in a wobbly structure; tower falls. He starts over again but his movements are clumsy and the tower falls again. He gives up and makes a horizontal row.

SERIAL PATTERNS. E demonstrates that Jimmy is to place one green, one yellow, etc., by tapping rhythmically. He pays no attention at first, but continues placing blocks haphazardly. Then he becomes aware, understands, and places four blocks correctly.

STRAIGHT BRIDGE. E demonstrates; no response. Jimmy continues to handle blocks as before. E repeats demonstration; no response.

OBLIQUE BRIDGE. E demonstrates. Jimmy tries to straighten

the top block of the model. He does not respond to invitations to copy either of two models. E starts to put blocks back into boxes. Jimmy starts experimenting with remaining blocks. He now tries to place a block on top of two others in an oblique position. Though he cannot place it correctly, his trials indicate that he has become intrigued with the problem of an oblique position versus a straight one. He seems tired; E closes session.

COMMENT

At four years of age, Jimmy is still handicapped by obvious motor difficulties which make him appear clumsy, unsteady, and somewhat heedless. His performances in the test situations show that he has adequate intellectual abilities in many areas. His blockbuilding, in spite of his motor difficulty and lack of immediate cooperation, indicates discrimination and learning ability nearly adequate for his age. His performances on formboards show good form comprehension. In many activities he shows interest and attention spans appropriate for his age. His greatest difficulty is in communication; language is neither used nor understood. His means of expression are most primitive; also, he understands only concrete signs. He has difficulty interpreting expressive gestures, pictures, or any other kinds of symbolic representation. He acts insecure and unhappy. He has very little confidence in people, likes to be independent, and is wary. However, it is obvious that under favorable circumstances he can learn to be more cooperative and amenable.

The interpretation of these characteristics is difficult and complex and can at best lead to varied hypotheses. At this stage, none of them can be reliably tested. Still, they may provide a few clues for future planning for Jimmy.

As before, there is ample reason to believe that Jimmy has difficulty in auditory perception. A serious hearing loss could fully explain his complete lack of language. Even a moderate loss would hinder speech development if the child had not enough satisfaction from sound reception and not enough motivation for communication. Jimmy has not had optimal opportunities. With his family busy and not overly warm and affectionate, he has had to fend for himself from his early days. Competition with his siblings has been on unequal terms. Another puzzling trait contributes toward making Jimmy isolated and lonesome in his world: he has apparently more than ordinary difficulty in recognizing signs and symbols. Whether or not combined with a hearing loss, such a disability would make language development very difficult.

To help in educational planning, another hearing test seems to be in order. Whatever its results, Jimmy must first of all develop a desire and a need for communication and social exchange. A more serene personal attitude and better relationships with those around him are basic needs, though not easily fulfilled. When E meets Jimmy's parents for a long interview following the examination, they are relieved to hear her good opinion of Jimmy's intellectual potentialities. They show interest and some candor in discussing the probability that Jimmy's undesirable behavior may at least be partially due to frustration. They make an attempt to understand the difficulties which this curious and independent child may experience because of his inability to communicate and his motor disability. Because it seems to her unfair to her other children, his mother agrees only hesitatingly to forego punishment for accidents caused by Jimmy's clumsiness.

JIMMY AT SEVEN YEARS

Jimmy, now seven years old, still walks awkwardly with a mildly athetoid gait. He has poor head control; his head is held cocked to one side. Owing to his jerky locomotion and dissociated movements, he still appears heedless often. He gets around with some speed, but does not seem to look where he is going. He still does not talk at all; the few spontaneous sounds he makes do not appear to be words. As yet he does not respond to the spoken word.

His complete lack of speech is the family's greatest puzzle and concern. They find him generally easier to handle and less stormy. He continues to be independent and dislikes pressure. He still gets stubborn when suddenly interfered with. His mother, who communicates with him through simple gestures, finds him now as reliable, if not more so, than her six-year-old. He is somewhat of an outsider in his home. He stays on the fringes when the family gathers with books or songs. However, when alone with his father or mother he seems to enjoy being with them and helping them.

The question of his hearing has never been satisfactorily settled. The confusion about it has continued unabated and has added to the parents' general insecurity and their uncertain feelings about the child.

After his last visit here, a hearing test showed a moderate hearing loss. The child was fitted with a hearing aid, to which he was supposed to be trained in a small nursery group for children with auditory difficulties. His attendance there was irregular and his adjustment unsatisfactory. He seemed inattentive and aloof and would not join in the daily activities. His motor awkwardness was in his way. His mother was pregnant and found it difficult to go with him. Another hearing test by PGSR (psychogalvanic skin resistance) showed near normal hearing. The hearing aid was discarded. A social worker advised that a play group for seriously defective children be tried, since this was nearer home. There again Jimmy was unhappy and stubborn. His mother felt uneasy about the plan, but let him continue for a while until, to her relief, the experiment was interrupted by the family's move to a smaller neighboring town. There the child has had no special education for two years. According to his mother, he has in general become happier and more secure.

In one of her sporadic efforts to give him more individual attention, his mother recently took him on a visit to relatives in the midwest. While there, she impulsively gave in to her family's well-meant pressure and took Jimmy to an otologist. Jimmy was upset by the trip and frightened by the hospital setting; he behaved very badly. His mother was told that he seemed severely retarded besides having a moderate hearing loss. Return to a hearing aid was recommended only if a psychological examination should prove that the child would be able to wear one with profit.

When E goes to meet Jimmy in the waiting room, she takes a ball along. She knows of his inability to understand any explanations and has heard of his recent experience in the doctor's office. Casually throwing the ball in his lap while she greets his family, she establishes a simple and immediate contact between herself and the child. Jimmy gets up to come with her, while his mother suppresses her surprise. Jimmy runs ahead into the wrong room first. In the examining room he starts on his own to explore the contents of a nearby shelf. But he complies when E invites him to sit down; and he turns expectantly to see what E produces from her cupboard.

Seguin Formboard (T:IV:6)

His grasp is clumsy, he works hastily, never looking at E, but completes the board speedily; he has some difficulty in releasing the inset in the recess after holding it between palm and fingers. After looking the board over, he knows where each piece goes and decides on the spot before moving the inset to it. His method of search is a mature one.

FIVE-FIGURE FORMBOARD (T:IV:7)

Jimmy picks up both pieces of the oval, holds them together, and fits them into the proper hole. He picks up the two smaller pieces of the cross, knows how they go, fits them correctly, and looks for the third piece. He places the large piece of the circle correctly, knows that the smaller part will fit in, but tries it the wrong way. E suggests he turn it over; no response. E repeats suggestion. Jimmy continues in his effort. E helps by turning the small piece without placing it. Jimmy takes the suggestion and places the piece correctly. He picks up both pieces of the hexagon, knows their correct spot, but has difficulty positioning them; then he turns the pieces back and forth, persisting in trying the long side of inset against the short side of the hole. E assists in making the necessary flip. Jimmy watches and seems determined to place the second piece himself, but is again unable to flip it over though he seems to try. E helps. Jimmy has difficulty in positioning the two triangles that form the square. He accepts help with one, places the other. When only square and hexagon are removed for repetition, Jimmy has no hesitation or difficulty.

In these nonverbal tasks Jimmy has been able to be active without interpersonal communication. This has helped him to adjust. He still likes and expects to work independently. He accepts help, but never counts on it. He does not respond to the spoken word. His working methods and his errors indicate that his form comprehension is similar to that of children of five to six years of age. His motor disability is obvious, and seems at least partially responsible for his difficulty in turning some of the insets properly. His motions are not flexible enough and do not allow him to experiment freely with the range of spatial relationships inherent in the task. The possibilities of additional disorientation in directions due to possible perceptuo-motor disability must, however, be kept in mind.

PICTURE ARRANGEMENT (T:IX:10)

DOG. E presents cards without demonstration. Jimmy seems pleased and proceeds to use the cards in the order of presentation (tail, C; trunk, B; head, A). He tries to match the black outlines carefully; apparently he does not notice what the cards show. E demonstrates with motions added to words; she outlines the head, body, legs, and tail of the dog. On second presentation, Jimmy imitates immediately.

MOTHER. Jimmy is correct. He is still trying to carefully match the lines, too. He seems interested in making one whole picture.

TRAIN. Jimmy arranges tender in front, engine in back (ONIR). E demonstrates the correct order. Jimmy shakes his head, and rearranges the cards as before, indicating that the engine pushes the tender. Then he rearranges cards as E has done, and gestures that the engine is pulling and that this is not right; so he rearranges them in his original version.

SCALES. Jimmy inspects pictures carefully, indicates the suitcase, then arranges them in the order of presentation (he looks at the scales, A; he walks away, C; he is on the scales, B). He carefully aligns the horizontal lines which indicate the floor in the picture. E tries to explain with words and gestures the actions of the man in the picture. Jimmy looks blank.

FIGHT. Jimmy makes fists, indicating a fight, then pushes the cards together again in the order of presentation (the loser is carried out, Z; he is being knocked out, Y; they start fighting, X). He seems interested only in fitting lines again.

During this test situation, Jimmy has started to communicate with E; reasonably expressive motions make his view known. In this test situation, however, it remains impossible for E to make him understand that the emphasis in Scales is on construction of a story rather than of a picture. (By WISC standards, Jimmy's raw score is equivalent to five years six months to five years ten months level.)

Jimmy would like to see more pictures. E decides, however, to stop here. She has been tempted to exploit Jimmy's present interest in picture materials on the spot and to introduce other picture tests. However, Jimmy appears geared to fitting lines rather than to looking at the content of the pictures. Since verbal explanations have no effect, it seems more prudent to proceed with different material in the hope of breaking up his mental set. This will avoid any danger of contaminating the results of other situations by his tendency to persevere. However, she makes a mental note of some rigidity in Jimmy's functioning.

BLOCK DESIGNS (T:VII:7 AND FIGURE 13)

After the blocks have been shown to Jimmy, E shows Kohs Card A. She demonstrates how to place the blocks. Jimmy is to repeat the same design. He arranges the four blocks in a square, but pays no attention to the colors. E repeats her demonstration by placing three of the blocks. She indicates that Jimmy is to place the fourth one. He does. Then E breaks up the arrangement so that Jimmy can repeat the design on his own. Instead, Jimmy copies her last motions; he picks up several of the blocks at once and drops them back on the table in disarray.

CARD I. Jimmy pays no attention to the checkerboard pattern of the model. He places unselected blocks apparently for the sole purpose of picking them up afterwards in order to again drop them all on the table as before. He seems to consider this activity good fun. E joins in and takes her turn at picking up and dropping some blocks on the table, as he does. She notes that in comparison with earlier years, Jimmy shows more interest in imitation and social exchange. However, he still likes to set the tone and to direct the proceedings. Having asserted himself now, he seems ready for more serious tasks; thus E arranges for him a model of the same design made of blocks. Jimmy is to copy it. He arranges two red blocks side by side, tops them with one blue block. E points toward the model, indicating that he made some mistake. Jimmy responds and tries to rearrange his blocks. Being awkward in handling them, he upsets all of them inadvertently; discouraged and bored, he begins to play with them as before.

CARD II. Instead of using the card, E presents the design as a model made of blocks. Jimmy works at his copy; he ends up with an inverted design: two red sides on top instead of below, two blue/yellow sides below with dividing diagonals parallel instead of meeting in an angle.

Several interesting points emerge from observations of the last two test situations: reversal in copying the last design seems to confirm some disability in spatial orientation which was tentatively noted in his handling of the square and hexagon in the five-figure formboard. Noteworthy also is Jimmy's failure to understand relationships between printed designs and blocks. He does not seem aware that the printed colors of the designs are meant to be replicas of the sides of the blocks and that he is asked to copy the printed color arrangement with the block material at his disposal. Similar difficulty in dealing with representative material might be recognized in the picture arrangement test where he matches lines to lines, and barely understands the main themes (but not individual phases of events). Such disability to interpret properly what he sees is noticeable also when he copies E's manner of disarranging the blocks and fails to understand that the disarranging had meaning only for destroying an existing block pattern.

• The design blocks seem to have left Jimmy disappointed and ill-at-ease. To provide a happy ending with that material, it is used for:

Blockbuilding (T:I:2 and Figure 1)

Oblique bridge. (Copy from model.) Jimmy is correct, but slow because of clumsiness.

Six-cube pyramid. (Reproduction from memory.) Jimmy objects to the removal of the model, indicates emphatically that it must stay. E's efforts to dissuade him fail; she gives in and leaves the model on the table. He copies it covertly.

Six-cube steps. (Copy from model.) Top step is too high. E points to model; no response.

Paper and Pencil (T:III)

Jimmy holds the pencil clumsily and weakly. He starts to make marks on the paper, then produces spontaneously a large J (for Jimmy). Though its two parts are disconnected and cover the entire sheet, it is still clearly recognizable. Jimmy seems pleased and proud of it.

Copying Forms (T:III:5 and Figure 2)

Cross. His cross is clumsily drawn, but recognizable. He tries to improve it by adding to the horizontal bar.

Diagonal cross. Jimmy eyes the card doubtfully, he shakes his head, but responds to E's encouragement. He starts correctly with a stroke in northwest to southeast direction, but is unable to maintain this course. A crossbar is drawn from west to east. The end product resembles his previous straight cross. However, it seems obvious from his behavior that Jimmy intended to make it differently. He is not pleased with the result. He studies the model again, traces it in the air, and tries to correct his production without much success.

British flag. Jimmy clumsily draws a rectangle with a diagonal cross inside. He tries to add a vertical bar to the cross, but his unsteady and shaky stroke spoils his attempt. He gives up, discards the pencil, gets up, and pushes the paper off the table. He seems ready to leave. He returns to the table when he sees E reaching for:

Mare and Foal Picture Board (T:IV:13)

His motor difficulty interferes with the free turning of some of the insets. However, he completes the task without error.

Serial Patterns (T:I:4,5)

E places one green block, one yellow block, one green, one yellow, etc. Jimmy understands immediately and finishes the whole row. When E places two green, one yellow, two green, one yellow, Jimmy begins to repeat the preceding alternating pattern. E points to the model again. He understands and continues to place all blocks correctly from here on, until he has nothing but yellow blocks left. He pushes these aside, obviously sure that he has completed the task requested of him.

Recognition of Forms (T:VII:9 and Figure 15)

FROM MEMORY. He is given five different designs, presented one after the other; he identifies three of the five correctly. His two errors are errors of reversal.

MATCHING DESIGNS. The same five designs are presented to him one by one and left for him to match with the design on the large card. He matches four correctly; one error of reversal.

Picture Vocabulary and Memory for Pictures (T:II:7,8)

E places three pictures side by side. Using the first two pictures she demonstrates how to describe them by gestures; she points to the top of her head for hat and imitates motion for automobile. Jimmy, pointing to the knife, makes the motion of cutting. E repeats all three gestures, pointing each time to the corresponding picture.

THREE PICTURES. (Hat, automobile, knife.) E screens all pictures, removes knife. Jimmy seems amused. When E questions him by gesture as to which one is missing, he immediately makes his cutting motion.

FOUR PICTURES. (Airplane, flag, foot, telephone.) E provides the gestured sign for the first two pictures. Jimmy himself invents the last two. E removes telephone. By gesture, Jimmy correctly indicates which picture is missing.

FIVE PICTURES. (Coat, cane, chair, fork, ball.) Jimmy finds gesture signs for all. E removes coat. Jimmy indicates that fork is missing. The same series of pictures is presented again, and the chair picture is removed. This time Jimmy indicates correctly.

Children who communicate normally would at approximately five years of age know as well as Jimmy does now which picture is missing. However, allowances must be made for him, since he has to find and to remember a sign to establish communication between himself and E. This complicates the task and is a distracting factor.

PICTURE COMPLETION (T:IX:12)

Without waiting for explanations, Jimmy points to the picture of the table and shows that a leg is missing. For coat, he points to the picture of the man's head, as if to indicate that the coat belongs to the man. For cat, he shows correctly that the cat's tail is missing. For bird, he points first to the feet, shakes his head, and indicates correctly the missing wing. When the picture of the coat is presented again, he correctly indicates the missing sleeve. For head, he seems uncertain, indicates hands and also points to part of the face, but his choice is somewhat vague. (By Revised Stanford-Binet standards, he passes on five-year level.)

COMMENT

At seven years of age, Jimmy continues to present several problems which combine to make him a severely handicapped child. His motor difficulty is obvious and disabling, but his complete lack of speech and his inability to understand language are his most serious problems. They make him appear lonesome, willful, and perhaps odd to those who meet him casually. However, his ability to make contacts has improved considerably since he was last seen. He is still on his guard and independent with people. However, he seems more interested in communication than he was before. He has learned to watch gestures, but still does not observe facial expressions. As in earlier examinations, he shows a lack of comprehension in the areas of meaning (picture arrangement, block designs), though he has improved. His comprehension appears at its best in concrete situations (blockbuilding, serial patterns). He continues to do well enough, in general, with forms and shapes (formboards, copying British flag), though he is handicapped by motor difficulty and a tendency toward reversals (copying forms, block designs, recognition of forms). Also, he is occasionally somewhat rigid and cannot shift his mental set easily (picture arrangement, serial patterns). His nonverbal comprehension ranges from slightly below five to a good six-year level. All auditory stimuli are entirely excluded from his field of attention. Again the question of hearing emerges as a crucial one. Jimmy, who is not especially interested in communication and emotional exchange with others, would suffer more seriously from even a moderate hearing loss than a child with a happier disposition and no physical handicap. To develop speech, in spite of considerable difficulty in the differentiation of sounds, would probably require stronger motivation for social contact than Jimmy seems to have at this point. His difficulty in appreciating meanings raises the question of congenital aphasia. In his case it might be added to a hearing loss. It would remain difficult to decide how much of his speech difficulty would be due to the one and how much to the other.

Whatever the diagnostic definition may be, Jimmy must, if possible, be encouraged to find social exchange more and more gratifying and to pay as much attention as possible to auditory stimuli. A good speech therapist would stimulate his speech and make communication worth while for him. This would for the moment be most important for his personality development, even if reading, writing, and arithmetic might have to wait for a time. However, postponing all academic training would present difficulties, too. Considering Jimmy's precarious position in the esteem of his family, it would not be desirable to have his brothers get far ahead of him in school. It would re-enforce the suspicion in his environment that Jimmy is not capable of learning; this in turn would be reflected in the attitudes he encounters.

An ideal specialized educational program for Jimmy would include speech and auditory training together with beginning primary work adapted to his needs. Before learning to read, he would have to get more notions about the meaning of language in general and words in particular. Manual skills, such as writing and drawing, would have to be minimized. His poor motor control would make both difficult and would easily undermine his shaky self-confidence.

However, it is not easy to set up even a moderately ideal program. There is no specialized audiological or aphasia center and no organized school program which he could join. Even if an expertly trained private teacher were available in his home town, his parents could not well afford her for any length of time. Still less could they think of having him away from home at one of the few existing specialized training centers. This is apart from the fact that, from the emotional standpoint, separation from home would appear to be the wrong plan.

A makeshift program seems to be the best choice under the circumstances; the public school will provide a home teacher for Jimmy. She is said to have had some experience with deaf children and seems to know methods for auditory training. Jimmy may do better with this individual program than he would in a group; nevertheless, it means that he will continue to miss proper companionship. He will still be an outsider, and his family finds it hard to accept him on those terms.

JIMMY AT TWELVE YEARS

Jimmy has become a rather gawky, tall boy with an awkward gait. He seems shy and apprehensive when meeting strangers, and ready to avoid contact whenever possible. He wears a hearing aid. He talks, but only sparingly, and is difficult to understand. Though he has learned to lip-read to some extent, he does not easily raise his eyes to those who talk to him.

Since last seen here, Jimmy has continued in a series of educational adventures. He has for the last few years been in a special class where he is said to do reasonably well. At home in the midst of his large family, Jimmy has been able to hold his own as the somewhat remote member of the household. He likes to be in his room in which he jealously guards various collections of stones, woods, and sundry items. He has a cat of his own on which he lavishes more attention than on any member of his family. He often appears moody, but his brothers and his parents know how to avoid his impatient reactions. He may refuse to come to a meal, but later comes to join the family after dinner. His mother does not make an issue of such eccentricities. He spends much time helping an elderly neighbor in his garden; he carries heavy loads and mows the lawn; he likes plants, but is frustrated when, through his clumsiness, he injures delicate parts. He has no friends his age; occasionally he joins in a baseball game in the street; he pitches doggedly with increasing frustration and irritation when things do not go well. Other children have stopped teasing him long since. They know that though he is usually quiet, he can hurt them when he is enraged. His teachers are alternatively impressed and disappointed by him. He reads silently in a second-grade reader; he matches words to pictures and shows other evidence of reading comprehension; however, he does not like to read and does not do so for pleasure. He does not easily join in social activities within the class. He likes to do arithmetic and has recently finished a fourth-grade workbook.

The unevenness of his performances has caused his teacher to wonder whether a special class is the right place for him. Such a question is not a new one in Jimmy's academic career. Shortly after his last visit here five years ago, he started with the home teacher then proposed by the school department. Jimmy made good progress with her; he learned some lip reading and some fundamentals of reading. He started to talk. He was devoted to this teacher for the two years during which she taught him before she left the town. Another home teacher from the school department did not work out. Jimmy did not like her and was sullen and difficult. Since she had no experience with children with hearing difficulties, it was decided that he would be just as well off in a special class where he would have more opportunity for social contacts.

There is some question whether Jimmy should perhaps be entered in a residential school for deaf children since he has made so little progress in speech. Again, as before, the psychological examination is requested as a basis for appraisal and future planning.

Jimmy sullenly follows E; he looks around her room with suspicion. When sitting down, he shrugs his shoulders. E is not certain whether this is an involuntary athetoid movement or a genuine shrug of dislike or dread. Remembering Jimmy's pleasure and skill in puzzles on previous occasions, E produces:

FIVE-FIGURE FORMBOARD (T:IV:7)

Jimmy goes at the task without any hesitation. His grasp is still clumsy, but his arm movements are better coordinated than they were. His motor ability seems improved.

CASUIST FORMBOARD (T:IV:8)

He proceeds without any difficulty. Quickly discovering the size differences, he needs no trials to pick out the right pieces. Jimmy seems edgy and a bit disdainful. He pushes the completed board away as if hoping that when this task is done he may be free to go.

LINCOLN HOLLOW SQUARE FORMBOARD (T:IV:9 AND FIGURE 3)

A board 7½ x 10 x ½ inches, with a 4½ inch square cut out to fit eight combinations of three or four pieces each. There are eleven pieces in all.

He shows a similar attitude in the first four easy combinations of this test. He seems to relax and to become more interested as he meets difficulty. He has to study for a long time how to do the last combination. E helps finally by pushing one of the pieces in its place. Jimmy smiles for the first time with an "aha" reaction and completes the task, but later removes all pieces once more and repeats the task without help.

OBJECT ASSEMBLY (T:IV:10,12)

Three separate figure formboards are presented without indication of what they are to represent.

MANIKIN. (Human figure with trunk, head, two legs, and two arms.) Jimmy puts all pieces together correctly without any hesitation. (Six points.)

PROFILE. (Profile of a woman's head, a large skull with a square cut out to fit two pieces which form the ear, a small piece to fit at the base of the skull; three pieces together form eye, nose, lips, and chin.) Jimmy is slow in manipulating the pieces, especially the small one at the base of the skull. He inverts the position of the ear pieces so that the ear is upside down. (By Wechsler-Bellevue scoring, he earns five points for accuracy and one point time credit.)

HAND. (Mutilated hand from which the fingers and a large section of the palm have been cut away.) Jimmy hesitates a little, then tries to fit the long edge of the thumb piece next to the long side of the hand; later he matches the edge of the index finger with the straight edge where it belongs. He still does not seem to notice that it is meant to be a finger of a hand. He inspects the structure critically, then one by one fits the straight edges of the separate fingers to the edges on the palm. Three of the four fingers are not in their correct places. When he has finished, he looks sullen and seems mystified about what the structure is meant to be. (One point; total score: thirteen points; weighted score: six.)

PICTURE ARRANGEMENT (T:IX:10)

NEST. (A bird flying to its nest, W; a nest with eggs, X; young birds in nest, Y.) This sample series is shown to him first in the order XWY. He apparently studies them carefully, oblivious to E's verbal explanations ("They are in the wrong order; if you put them in the right order, they make a sensible story.") The correct order, WXY, is demonstrated to him. E points to the essential parts of the picture cards. Again he studies the pictures carefully.

HOUSE. (The foundation of a new house, P; a house half-built, A; a finished house being painted, T; presented in order APT.) He places the cards in the correct order. (Two points.)

HOLD-UP. (A masked man holding up another man at gunpoint, A; a policeman arrests him, B; a court session, C; a prisoner in a cell, D; presented in order DABC.) After studying the cards briefly, Jimmy arranges them correctly. (Two points.)

ELEVATOR. (The closed top of an elevator shaft, L; the top partly open with elevator in sight, M; two men appearing in the shaft, N; the two men in full view with the Little King emerging from the elevator, O; presented in order OLMN.) Jimmy recognizes the Little King, smiles, and arranges correctly. (Two points.)

FLIRT. (The Little King riding in a car, J; a woman walking and carrying a bundle on her head [on a card smaller than the others], A; the Little King ordering his chauffeur to stop, N; he leaves his car, E; he walks with the woman and carries her bundle on his head, T.) Jimmy puts J and N together first; he lines up the cards carefully, discards card A, adds E and T, and seems to puzzle out what to do with A; then he fits A neatly in the middle (JNAET). (Three points.)

FISH. (The Little King fishing with an empty bucket next to him, E; he catches a fish, F; he fishes again, the fish he has caught shows in the bucket, G; he catches another fish, H; he shouts in the direction of the water and leaves the dock, I; a diver with a fish in his hand doffs his headgear to the Little King, who walks off, J; presented in order IEJFHG.) Jimmy looks puzzled, does not make sense out of the picture. He starts to assemble those cards which resemble each other (E and G—both show the fish line in the water; F and H—both show a fish wriggling on the line). His final arrangement is EGFHIJ. (One point.)

TAXI. (A man carrying a bust of a woman, S; he hails a taxi, A; he is shown in the taxi from the back holding the bust in his arms, M; he turns around, U; he blushes, E; the bust is seated in the opposite corner of the taxi, L.) Jimmy starts correctly with SA, then obviously finds little sense in the remaining pictures, of which three (MUE) are very similar. Final arrangement is SALEUM. (One point.) (Total Wechsler-Bellevue score: eleven points; weighted score: ten.)

PICTURE COMPLETION (T:IX:12)

E points to the table and shows that the leg is missing. Jimmy understands immediately, and points correctly to all missing parts.

PICTURE COMPLETION (T:IX:12)

Jimmy points correctly to the missing parts in the following pictures: for girl, nose; for man, mustache; for card, diamond; for crab, leg; for pig, tail; for boat, smokestack; for watch, second hand. He makes an error in the third picture: for man whose ear is missing, he points instead to missing body. He also misses on knob for door and shakes his head, indicating that he does not know. For pitcher (water falling out is missing), he shows that the water line in the pitcher should be higher; for mirror (arm missing), he points to something on the chair; for man (tie missing), he points to a small gap in the outline of the sketch; for sun (shadow missing), he points to the roof of the house; for bulb (base thread missing) and girl (eyebrow missing), he shakes his head, unable to find any part missing. (Total Wechsler-Bellevue score: eight points; weighted score: seven.)

Jimmy, though at first apprehensive and reticent, seems to have become interested enough in the test situation. He has accepted E and tackles the tasks presented to him willingly enough. Up to now there has been no social exchange between Jimmy and E except for some actions and gestures in lieu of instructions on E's part, and some indicating signs on Jimmy's part (picture completion). His desire to remain independent is still noticeable. It shows in his general attitude, and particularly in his half-hearted acceptance of help in the hollow square test. His tendency to avoid involvement with people also may show in the picture completion test where he does better in pictures which concern objects rather than humans. Again, in picture arrangement he is more at ease with series which do not contain interaction among people. While he now pays attention to the content of the pictures, he still shows an interest in structural aspects of the pictures. He still lines up the cards side by side; when he has doubts about how to arrange the pictures because he does not understand some of them, he resorts to matching cards which have some resemblance. He puts together both pictures which show the Little King's car (Flirt, J and N) or both pictures which show the line with the bait below water level (Fish, E and H). He also places the smaller-sized card (A) in the center of the series (Flirt) flanked by JN on the left and ET on the right.[1] He always lines up all pictures carefully and does not consider his task complete before he has arranged a neat row. Similar tendencies are seen when he finds the picture of the man incomplete because the outline shows a gap (picture completion), or when he fits the edges of the fingers without noticing that they form a hand (object assembly).

In spite of these peculiarities, his score has not been depressed by his lack of speech or inability to respond to language. His poor motor

[1] Size difference between card A and cards JNET has been omitted in WAIS.

coordination lowered his score in one instance only (object assembly, in profile). There he probably forfeits some time credits owing to his slow motions. While his point scores are irregular, the prorated score based on the three subtests of the Wechsler-Bellevue Scale would give him an average rating on the performance tests.

Since the examination has been going reasonably well up to this point, E now plans to give Jimmy as complete a formal test scale as possible. She will at least do all performance tests of the Wechsler-Bellevue Intelligence Scale, and also perhaps try some of the verbal items of the same scale. Together with samples of his academic achievements, numerical test results will probably be most helpful in planning further management. For administrative reasons, educational authorities usually favor such material when applications to public institutions are made.

Anticipating that Jimmy might enjoy block designs more than paper-and-pencil work or academic tasks, E decides to introduce the harder tasks first, and to keep potentially easier ones in reserve to use when needed as boosters for Jimmy's morale.

Digits Symbols Test (T:III:7)

A printed series of isolated numbers, each one to be associated with a special and different symbol which is to be drawn with pencil in a square above each number; the symbols are demonstrated at the beginning.

Jimmy looks doubtful at first while E demonstrates. Then he starts; he holds the pencil awkwardly, and is slow in applying it to the paper. He looks back to the models each time he places a symbol and makes no errors. However, he is apt to round out angles or to produce crooked lines where straight ones are demanded. He finds it difficult to stay within the square; he tries to erase pencil marks which go beyond the lines. The process is a slow one. He finishes thirteen markings within the time limit of one and one half minutes. (Score: thirteen points; weighted score: three.)

Writing Name (T:III:2c and XI:9)

Again he shows his poor hand control. He writes his first name, James, slowly in a small, cramped style; he uses a somewhat more relaxed, wider stroke with his second name. He adds spontaneously printed letters which read "Class for De—t" with an f between e and t, which he erases and tries again. Apparently he is trying to print "Class for Defectives," which, though surprising, is apparently routine for him.

Memory for Designs (T:VII:1 and Figure 4)

DESIGN FROM FORM M, IX-YEAR LEVEL. Correct except for poor motor control. He tries to improve his design to show that he meant the inverted square to reach the sides of the outer square.

DESIGN FROM FORM M, XII-YEAR LEVEL. As before he draws awkwardly, but his designs are correct. He tries to improve rounded corners. Jimmy seems to enjoy his painstaking efforts; he traces his lines several times. His manners are less rigid now; he has started to loosen up. Occasionally he looks at E to see what she thinks of his productions. She takes advantage of this apparent improvement in relationships; she will try a task which will involve more communication than before.

Repeating Digits (T:VIII:5,6)

DIGITS FORWARD. E, giving three digits forward (five, two, eight) tries to enunciate very clearly; she also points to her lips, inviting him to repeat what she says. He seems to remember speech lessons, looks at her, and tries to repeat the digits she pronounces. His reproductions can be recognized as correct by the sound of the vowels mostly. For five digits forward, E says, "Nine, six, two, five, eight." He reproduces the sequence correctly, as before. For six digits forward, E says, "Five, two, six, three, nine, one." He reproduces "five, two, six, nine, one." To "three, nine, two, seven, one, eight," he responds "three, nine, seven, eight. . . . "

DIGITS BACKWARD. E says "Six, one, nine." Since he does not understand directions, he keeps repeating the series forward. E tries to use her fingers for explanations; he imitates the finger movements only. E interrupts task. (By Wechsler-Bellevue standards, weighted score is five. By Revised Stanford-Binet standards, in Form L he would get credit for five digits forward on the seven-year level; no credit for six digits forward on the ten-year level; and no credit for four digits backward on the nine-year level. In Form M he would get no credit for six digits forward on the ten-year level; and no credit for three digits backward on the seven-year level.)

Reading Numbers (T:XI:8)

Jimmy correctly reads individual numbers between one and twenty.

WRITTEN ARITHMETIC (T:XI:3)

To 4 plus 5, 9 plus 5, Jimmy scrawls the correct answers. To 10 minus 6, 25 minus 8, he is correct. When given 8 times 5, Jimmy continues to subtract, scrawls "3." E points to the multiplication signs. Jimmy corrects it immediately. In 329 times 36, he knows the proper routine and goes about it slowly but successfully.

DISSECTED SENTENCES (T:XI:6)

Disarranged words printed on a card must be read in the order in which they will form a sentence.

Words presented as "a-have-dog-I-fine." Jimmy reads the words slowly in order of presentation but sees nothing wrong about it. E points one by one to the words in their correct order. He reads them obediently with considerable difficulty in enunciation, apparently with no understanding. Words presented as "wool-the-was-coat-of-made." Jimmy starts again to read the words in the order of presentation. E indicates the first two words he should start with. Jimmy looks blank and puzzled.

BLOCK DESIGNS (T:VII:8)

He seems to enjoy the task and goes about it with care. He has some difficulty handling the blocks speedily. He does not always seem to get them oriented as he wishes, but tries until he has the blocks the way he wants them. He has one error of orientation in the last W-B design. Otherwise he completes all designs correctly. Because he is slow, he forfeits time credits on all but the first two designs. Also he fails to get any credit on the sixth design; arranging the blocks into the intricate diagonal pattern and keeping them all together in place is motorwise so difficult for him that he exceeds the time allowance by twenty-five seconds. (By Wechsler-Bellevue standards, he gets fifteen points for accuracy and three points for time credit; total score: eighteen points; weighted score: nine.)

PICTURE DESCRIPTION (T:II:6)

MESSENGER BOY. Jimmy inspects the picture, says "bike broke." When E points again to the whole picture, he apparently believes that she has not understood. He repeats "bike broke." As before in other situations which require motor skill or speech, he has a tendency to spend his effort on technique of delivery and to fail in accurate and full comprehension. (No credit.)

E produces paper and pencil, asks Jimmy to draw a bicycle, and points to the bicycle in the picture to make her request clearer.

Drawing a Bicycle (T:IX:14)

Jimmy starts with one wheel, tries to copy the picture which E removes. He continues to draw; the end product is a rough sketch of a bicycle showing accurately enough the relationship between the parts. There are two wheels with spokes; the chain is attached to pedals and rear wheel. E tests Jimmy's comprehension by asking, helped by gestures, why the chain does not go to the front wheel. Jimmy shakes his head energetically and indicates that the pedals keep the chain and the rear wheel in motion.

Comment

The last test showed his adequate comprehension of some of the causal relationships involved in this task. In the second part of the examination, the Wechsler-Bellevue Performance Scale was completed. Jimmy obtains an over-all weighted score of 34, indicating an I.Q. of approximately 90. This score penalizes him for slow performances in block designs, digit symbols, and object assembly. In these tasks his lack of speed seemed due to his motor disability, rather than to poor comprehension. Therefore, his potential score may be estimated as somewhat higher.

Compared with results of earlier examinations, Jimmy has not only held his own, but has improved slightly. His test performances still show characteristics seen before, though these have, in the course of development, taken varying forms. It has been shown how some difficulties in the area of meaning have persisted. His form comprehension, reasonably good in the test situations of earlier days (except for some difficulties in spatial orientation), seems more irregular now. It still is adequate where pure shapes are concerned (memory for designs, formboards, digit symbols), but it is hampered in the more complex test situations when perception of meaning (object assembly) or spatial orientation (block designs, digit symbols) are involved. He no longer has his earlier difficulties in understanding pictorial situations, but he still is more secure in reasoning which is based on immediate observation rather than assumed relationships. Behavior traits observed earlier take on more mature and better socialized patterns of manifestation. He still is secluded, lonesome, and wary, but he appears shy and anxious rather than resistant and independent.

He has become more experienced in social relationships and adjusts to them better and more quickly than he did before. Nevertheless, in spite of adequate general comprehension and "normal" numerical test results, and regardless of the obvious progress he has made, Jimmy, at age twelve, still cannot function on a normal level. He hardly communicates and cannot understand what is said to him. Even when he hears sounds, he is unable to understand more than their crudest immediate meaning. His scant speech is poorly enunciated because of inadequate hearing as well as dysarthria. Though reasonably observant, he has very little knowledge of anything outside his immediate environment. He has learned very little in school.

Educational planning again is a difficult problem. Jimmy would be at a loss in a normal school group on any age level. But he does not get his best chance in his special class, where his teacher, doubtful that it is the right place for him, is unable to find time to give him necessary individual attention. A program involving a teacher at home would, even if Jimmy liked her, isolate him from outside contacts once again. He seems as ready for a school experience away from home as he ever will be. He would learn to adjust to new patterns of living and, at best, have companionship with other handicapped children. More stress on speech development than he has had would be good for him. Though his hearing difficulty is said not to be extreme, he has not learned to adjust to sounds and the use of a hearing aid as fully as is perhaps possible. This might improve, since auditory training and lip reading are usually practiced through the day in a school for the deaf.

Jimmy's parents are still of limited means and should not have more than the necessary medical expenses. Therefore, it is suggested that application be made directly to one of the best schools for the deaf. The parents and their physician support this plan. After all these years, his mother is ready for a change. She thinks that Jimmy is, too! She is relieved that a specialized and well-structured program can be proposed for Jimmy.

However, these plans fail. Jimmy is rejected at the school for the deaf. According to hearing tests there, his hearing difficulty is again not considered serious enough! He seemed sullen and his movements were awkward; his low academic achievements also were against him. It was feared that in more areas than one he might not keep up with other students near his age.

The result is again disappointment for all and confusion for Jimmy and his family. Even now, as in the many previous years, experts, though well trained and well intentioned, cannot agree on Jimmy's condition or on the best plan for him.

Again, as so many times before, only makeshift arrangements can be made for Jimmy. A state clinic for crippled children will give him speech training. He continues in a special class and is scheduled to join a recreational program for adolescent boys with cerebral palsy.

STAGES OF DEVELOPMENT AND THEIR PROBLEMS

Jimmy's psychological development shows trends that have been found to be in some ways characteristic of those children handicapped by extrapyramidal palsy and auditory loss caused by erythroblastosis and who, in spite of motor disability and difficulty of communication, have more or less adequate intellectual abilities.

At fifteen months Jimmy seems weak and retarded motorwise; he does not respond to auditory stimuli. He appears to be altogether passive and unresponsive, although sensitive and easily disturbed, and to have a restricted field of interest. However, many signs indicate that he is observant and understands visually and socially more than he is physically able to show. The casual observer or busy pediatrician would easily underestimate his mental ability.

His poor development is disturbing to his parents, who are disappointed in him. He is neither cute nor cuddly; his immobile, serious facial expression discourages rather than invites affection. Already, at this age, he does not fulfill the demands of his life situation and seems to stand alone against his world.

At four years of age he has no effective means of communication. He goes after what he wishes without requesting assistance. He handles and understands objects well, but he is primitive and unskilled when it comes to manipulating social situations. He is tense, has sudden emotional outbursts, and appears stubborn. His lack of attention to auditory stimuli simulates refusal and social withdrawal. His parents are much confused about him and about his uneven development. They are sometimes concerned about his behavior primarily, then sometimes more concerned about his lack of speech. His motor disability, though obvious, is for the moment less of a problem to them. With the hearing question as yet not settled, they derive only meager satisfaction from his resourcefulness in nonverbal areas. At an age where other children impress outsiders by verbal skill or social graces, Jimmy is not a child his parents can be proud of. Again he does not fulfill the demands of his life situation and seems to be an outsider who is ill-at-ease.

At seven years of age Jimmy still talks very little but communicates better. He is learning to watch social clues. He understands best gestures which are direct and do not need interpretation. He continues to deal with objects effectively enough. He understands their relationships. His practical intelligence, now increasingly obvious to all, has enhanced his standing. His parents have found better ways to communicate with him than they had before. Since they have become able to make him understand, they have found that he has become easier to live with. Jimmy himself feels more secure now with his family. He is less tense and stubborn, and is somewhat more at ease with people than he was. But he still likes to be independent and resists suggestions, and he gets upset easily. He is desperately eager to show his competence, regardless of his motor difficulty. Now his parents' main concern is the social implications of Jimmy's condition. They worry about what influence he may have on his brothers and what the neighbors may think of him. They are much concerned about his chances of getting an education.

At twelve years of age Jimmy still cannot communicate entirely adequately. His language ability continues to be poor. He can express his ideas with crude means only. He deals competently with objects. He understands form and number relationships better than meanings and symbols. He can function well enough in a simple, well-organized world, and retreats from complex situations. He still acts wary and lonesome, though he has become somewhat friendlier and seems less apprehensive than before. His relationships with people are less explosive. His family has found a reasonably satisfactory *modus vivendi* with him. They find it easier to accept him now as a "character." At his age, the display of specific and unusual personality traits is more respectable than were the antics of an uncooperative child some years earlier. The question of adequate training as a handicapped individual, however, becomes urgent as time goes on. The family relies on society to provide this for him, but naturally resents the fact that valuable time is being lost because of uncertainties and conflicting opinions regarding Jimmy's hearing, abilities, and personality.

Analysis of case records[2] of children with similar disabilities indicates that the course of development and the problems that appear are, with

[2] This discussion is based on the study of case records of 20 children with cerebral palsy due to neonatal erythroblastosis. Of these children, 11 had two psychological ex-

individual variations, common for this group, which because of the varied combinations of symptoms presents the most perplexing diagnostic problems for the psychologist and physician alike.

As babies up to two and one half or three years of age these children are, without exception, judged to be defective by their pediatricians. Only in a very few cases do otherwise wary and sophisticated medical men find it necessary to consult a psychologist for confirmation of their diagnosis. All these babies are late in motor development. They are unable to hold up their heads at the proper time. They cannot follow objects with their eyes as well as they should and have more or less serious difficulty in grasping objects. They have expressionless faces and smile rarely or with delay, often with some grimacing. The few babies who are more mobile have primitive, distorted patterns of locomotion not effective enough to explore objects or space adequately. Nearly all children of this group do not vocalize. Their social responses are considered grossly inadequate. Later developments, however, show that the pessimistic appraisal of intellectual potentialities proved wrong when it was based on these symptoms alone.

The psychologist called to study such children must depend on other, less obvious signs. Many of the usual psychological tests for babies are useless because they require greater motor ability than these children have. With these babies, neither hand, head, nor eye movements are always reliable measures of the child's interest in objects or of his comprehension. But the patient observer can, in some way, notice the baby's alertness or dullness, regardless of the handicap. At twelve to fifteen months, the examiner should watch for signs of persistent interest in one object and for the ability to recognize the same object when it has been moved into a different position (T:V:4,7). Does the baby expect

---

aminations, 5 had three, and 4 had more than three. (Total number of examinations was 55.)

Interval between first and last examinations was more than two years in 2 cases, more than three years in 2 cases, more than five years in 9 cases, more than eight years in 4 cases, more than twelve years in 3 cases.

Mental ability at last examination was above normal in 1 case (5%), normal in 8 cases (40%), borderline in 7 cases (35%), below borderline in 4 cases (20%).

Hearing was severely impaired in 2 cases (10%), moderately impaired in 9 cases (45%), seriously questioned in 6 cases (30%).

Hearing difficulties were discovered or questioned below the age of five in 5 cases (25%), between the ages of five and ten in 7 cases (35%), later than age ten in 4 cases (20%).

Motor impairment was severe in 2 cases (10%), moderately severe in 8 cases (40%), mild in 8 cases (40%).

Eleven children showed no effective language communication by the age of six.

to find it in a certain place after it was removed from sight? Does he anticipate where a ball might roll or a pellet drop? Such observations permit some estimate of the level of the child's comprehension of spatial relationships and of objects. If a child who seems responsive to such visual clues lacks similar attention to auditory stimuli, the observer may already, at this stage, suspect some difficulty in auditory perception. A baby somewhat older may show comprehension of objects or lack of it in other ways; he may or may not actively participate by watching when E picks out certain pegs or inserts for placement in pegboards or formboards (T:IV:1,2,4,5). Often such signs of comprehension are minute, but if watched for carefully, they cannot be mistaken or missed easily.

In a fair number of very young children the psychologist can find adequate comprehension of objects and spatial relations when she uses these or similar methods of observation. The same babies fixate on certain pictures in a picture book (T:II:1,3); they no longer merely scan the pages as they did a few months earlier. They indicate by their persistent gaze toward the next page that they expect to see more pictures once the page is turned. They show that they understand how a book opens and have some interest in its content. This may range from pleasure in a color spot in the younger children to recognition of some definite picture in older ones. Despite this interest in pictures, the same children may not respond to the spoken request to "look" at a picture. This behavior symptom should raise doubts in E about the child's ability for interpersonal communication.

The babies in this group often reveal memory and ability to anticipate in delayed reaction tests (T:V:5). In any situation of this kind, the examiner should also observe whether the child is able to maintain interest in one activity or in one sight for any length of time. The psychologist must try to distinguish between persistent, undistracted, constructive attention and dull perseverance. Exaggerated unilateral attention is often due to special physical conditions; visual and auditory disturbances are common in this group. Difficulties of side gaze, together with poor head control, may restrict the baby's visual field. Inadequate auditory perception may make him oblivious to extraneous clues. (In many cases where lack of social response was noted in the early records, sensory losses were later discovered.)

Appraisal of social comprehension must depend largely on the parents' reports. Their observation of the baby's comprehension of daily events often gives the best clues (T:X:1). These descriptions also help to show the parents' attitude; some tend to exaggerate, some to belittle the child's accomplishments; some try to remain ostentatiously objective. None can for long maintain a casually confident attitude, as they might with a normal child. Most parents are much concerned about the physical situation. Feeding is often difficult, and the general care is frequently exhausting rather than rewarding. With their mothers busy and worried and their own activity sphere seriously restricted, some of the babies of this group often seem overly serious, emotionally restricted, and detached. Many babies, on the other hand, are given an especially large amount of attention because of their infirmity; their families try to work with them and improve them. The children's obvious interest in objects is used to make them strain or reach for things in order to practice motor skills. The approval given for achievements with objects, rather than for social responses, may, in some children, help to re-enforce a natural preference for watching objects instead of people. Better comprehension of object relationships than of social interaction is noted in many children of this group.

The early psychological examination, inconclusive as it may seem, is useful in many cases. It may allay or support the pediatrician's early pessimism. It may help the parents to a more optimistic or a more realistic viewpoint, and therefore help to create a better atmosphere for the child. Advice about how to broaden social experience and interpersonal exchange can, at this stage, benefit further personality development.

Frequently, however, children of this group meet a psychologist for the first time only when they are of *preschool age*. In spite of their numerous, still obvious difficulties, they have often surprised the pediatrician and others around them by their unexpected mental progress.

Inadequate or totally lacking language development is the primary complaint. Often these children are difficult in their behavior at home. Both these factors, together with their motor incoordination, lead to questions about their future education. The psychological examination is meant to help in planning.

In the examining room, all these children, like Jimmy, immediately become interested in performance tasks of the pegboard and formboard variety (T:IV:1–7,10,13). Depending on the degree of their motor impairment, they may be able to manipulate the material themselves, or they may actively participate in the placement of the insets. Regardless of their motor disability, the great majority of children in this group can deal well with form material of this kind. At the proper ages, the same children succeed also in various matching games (T:VI:1,2,4–7). Some do very well in these tests; others show some slight difficulties in fine discrimination. All are more efficient in these tasks than in any other test procedures. In drawing tests, they are less consistent (T:III:1, 4–6). Some of the children's attempts show adequate form comprehension, despite a lack of motor skill. In other drawings, one can detect only the most remote similarity to any required shape. With their difficulties in coordination, severely handicapped children can become absorbed in the act of drawing *per se* and forget to pay attention to what they draw. The same children may again display adequate form comprehension in procedures which simplify or eliminate the motor factor (T:VII:6,9).

In all examinations at this age, considerable discrepancy between the child's levels in performance tasks and verbal tasks is noted. Without exception, responses in verbal matters are the lower. Some children cannot talk at all, some can say only a very few, poorly enunciated, single words which they produce when naming objects or pictures (T:II:1,2,6,7,11). Their comprehension vocabulary usually seems poor in differentiating questions about pictures (T:II:4). All children lack conversational speech, and many of them do not have the ability to express themselves by gestures. Even the ablest children of this group, up to the age of six, are unable to respond to more complex verbal comprehension questions which involve word meanings rather than names alone. They may fail in tests requiring identification by use, groups, etc. (T:II:5,9,11) and in verbal reasoning questions (T:II:6 and IX:1,5). They may be equally unable to convey by gesture any idea of their own. Difficulties in comprehending underlying meanings is also shown by the manner in which these children look at pictures that tell a story (T:II:6 and IX:10,11). They are apt to point successively to one feature after another, but in no way try to interpret events or relationships. Their responses to incomplete pictures (T:IX:12) are uneven; many of the children seem to accept the mutilated picture as it is and fail to compare it with any mental image. A lack of communication and of appreciation of meanings is not the only sign of inadequate social development in these children. In most cases, observers also stress the absence of social contact. In some children, this may show in aloofness or poverty of social responses or imitations. In others, it turns into negativism, resistance, and excessive demand for independence. There may be tantrums and erratic, obstreperous behavior, as in Jimmy. Children brought up in friendlier surroundings than his display noncommittal and often inappropriate smiles.

All children of this group are late in walking. At the time of their examination they all are still more or less unsteady and cannot trust their balance as a normal preschool child does. Many still have visual difficulties which restrict their side gaze. These factors contribute to the common impression of breathless, heedless locomotion. In his haste to reach the desired goal, the child ignores all obstacles, whether they are people or things. Eagerness and tension are striking characteristics of children in this group. Some have been like this for a long time, and since babyhood have been egged on by encouragement and the expectations of those around them. Others, who were quiet and much less enterprising before, develop such rather hectic behavior when independent locomotion, regardless of how shaky it may be, allows them to conquer space which was inaccessible before. This stage of uncertain but determined independence is well known in the normal eighteen-month-old child. His cavalier disregard of obstacles, combined with his tiny physique, usually seems appealing then. The handicapped children in Jimmy's group are older and physically taller when they reach this stage. Therefore they appear more awkward and cause more upsets than the normal toddler. They are apt to create apprehension in their elders. This in turn re-enforces the striving for independence in some children, and creates insecurity in others.

Widely varying attitudes surround the children in this group. Some of the parents worry most about immediate physical safety, but at the same time they also question the child's ability to get along later in life. Their fears cause them to be tense and ambivalent in their feelings and in their management. They may be overprotective in one instance and unyielding in the next. Some discourage the child's bursts of activity and admonish him to be more quiet and restrained. Others promote enterprise at all costs and seem to the observer to take surprising risks without becoming perturbed. Mother and child relationships are, in this group, remarkably undemonstrative in general. The tendency to emotional detachment, already observed in babyhood, seems to persist into the preschool ages. Many children are said to enjoy affection, but are unable to give it. The fondest mothers may describe their children as intelligent and independent, but rarely call them cute, sweet, and companionable.

Frequently, the interpretation of psychological findings at this stage can still be only tentative. The level of comprehension shown in performance tasks is an important clue in the appraisal of mental maturity. Inabilities due to motor handicaps must be distinguished from lack of comprehension. Good ability to deal with simple shapes is an encouraging sign at this stage, but does not necessarily forecast skills in all perceptual areas. Discrepancy between nonverbal and verbal areas (high performances in the first and lower ones in the second) allows exclusion of the diagnosis of mental deficiency. Delay in language development may be due to many causes. There may be severe dysarthria or hearing difficulties which interfere with the learning of speech. There may be a lack of comprehension of symbolic or ideational material, often called aphasia. Various kinds of emotional situations may be responsible for lack of social awareness and disinterest in communication. The psychologist must guard against accepting one or another attractive hypothesis to the exclusion of all others. In many cases there may be a combination of all or several of these factors, each one aggravating the other. One may find that an audiologist reports a child's hearing as "diminished but sufficient for speech development." The same child may have a mild dysarthria and possibly some signs of aphasia. Also there may be some question whether the child gets enough encouragement to attempt social exchange in spite of all his troubles. While each of these symptoms may not by itself seem serious, all of them together can well account for the severity of the delay in language development. One symptom alone may fail to give the whole explanation. This becomes clear, for example, when a child with a definite hearing loss does not seem to profit from training methods usually thought to be effective. Uncertainty frequently surrounds the diagnosis of these children. Even so, their advisers must try to avoid conflicting or unclear counsel which is frustrating to parents and damaging to the child. With so many things "wrong," parents like to be told where to use their efforts to best advantage. Should he be taught as a hard-of-hearing child or as an aphasic child? Should they first of all consider his motor difficulties and have him join a cerebral palsy group? Should they have him with normal children his age or younger, or should they protect him from social competition?

The problems of these children require careful, thoughtful handling. The ideal solution and the best plan may be doomed to failure because the facilities available in most localities are inadequate. From the psychological point of view, the most important goal is to teach the child communication through readily available and suitable means and thus allow the parents and the child to gain confidence. At this age most of these children still do best with individual attention or in small groups. They get easily lost in normal school groups and profit most by one teacher's personal interest. Often this relationship forms the first link with the world outside his immediate family.

In the six- to ten-year age group the psychological examination is frequently requested in order to determine further educational plans. Often parents and pediatricians would like to be reassured once again that the child progresses well enough, within his limitations. Behavior difficulties and parental dissatisfactions seem to be rarer at this age level and less urgent than they were earlier.

In the psychological case records most of the children are described as friendlier and more confident than previously. Still eager to show their independence, they are often also more ready to please; they have learned to wait for social clues and to accept some directions. There is, in general, an improvement in social awareness and communication. Simple gestures are more easily understood and produced. Some have learned how to talk, though poor enunciation is still common. The records note an increase in vocabulary, which is demonstrated predominantly in good performances in tests involving vocabulary, picture description, or pointing to pictures (T:II:6,7,11). Failure to respond well to simple differentiating questions (T:II:4), together with defective enunciation, reopens in many cases the question of hearing difficulty. Expression, as well as comprehension, is still deficient in this group if judged by verbal tasks alone. However, as before, comprehension in nonverbal tasks is normal. All children still show their best skills in formboard tasks (T:IV:6–11) and to a lesser degree in picture puzzles and object assembly tests (T:IV:10–12,14). They also, in the main, do creditably in block designs (T:VII:7,8). There is, however, at this age a tendency toward subtle difficulties in perceptual areas which cannot be fully explained by motor incoordination. Many children who in earlier years seemed to be wizards in form comprehension when dealing with simple formboards and matching games now show minor signs of visuo-motor difficulties in the more complex tasks appropriate for this age level. There are hesitations, trials, and errors in size discrimination or spatial orientation. These may be noticed in Casuist formboard (T:IV:8), Goldstein-Scheerer stick test

(T:VII:6), block designs (T:VII:7,8), recognition of forms (T:VII:9), and some phases of object assembly (T:IV:11,12). Several children display a tendency to write from top to bottom rather than from left to right. More flagrant visuo-motor distortions, as seen in cases like Paul and John (who will be discussed later), are characteristically absent in this group.

Many of the children still do better in the appraisal of shapes, form relations, and numbers than of underlying meaning. While improved in the appreciation and use of direct expressive gestures, they still frequently respond to literal relationships rather than to implied ones. The successful assembling of puzzles, for example, is often accomplished by careful matching of edge to edge rather than through *a priori* comprehension. Sequence of position, rather than content of story, is the clue by which they are apt to determine the sequence of events, as in Sun or Clock in picture arrangements (T:IX:10). Similar tendencies show in other tasks calling for pictorial reasoning (T:IX:11–13).

At this age many children tested for hearing show high frequency losses. In other cases, however, the hearing situation remains chaotic. For some children hearing tests, especially those by PGSR, indicate near normal hearing though teachers, parents, and psychologists feel that the child has an impairment. In others, a hearing difficulty is found which was formerly unnoticed, and parents and teachers remain unconvinced of its seriousness. According to hearing tests, some children have more and some have less impairment than behavior and speech development seem to indicate. In several cases, hearing ability varies from one day to another, or from one situation to another. For some, tension increases the hearing loss, whereas relaxation practically obliterates it.

In many cases, the friction noted earlier between parents and children has decreased. By this time, the families of the abler children have had more opportunity to convince themselves of their intellectual assets. Often they have now won more recognition for their child by outsiders, who are not as apt as before to judge him unfavorably because of poor speech and motor incoordination. The increased confidence of their families has given a number of children increased security and interest in social contacts. Even the least able children in this group have done somewhat better than expected. All seem to profit emotionally from the atmosphere of encouragement and increased loyalty which surrounds them at home and at school. Although tension and tenacity still characterize their activities, these are now frequently directed toward socially approved goals, rather than toward egocentric satisfactions. Many still get praise for their persistence. Though this trait often seems at this age to turn into rigidity and stubbornness, this may be a virtue rather than a liability for a child whose handicap frequently exempts him from demands for quick and fluid shifts.

Those children with borderline difficulties are at this age, as always, the least fortunate ones of the group. Marginal deficiencies in motor power as well as in communication and comprehension can create serious emotional and social strain. A child may be able to run, but not fast enough; he may be able to hear and talk, but not clearly and quickly enough; he may also be able to understand, but not well enough. Parents and teachers vary in the quality and subtlety of the pressure they use. Most borderline children react with growing tension and depression. Many are well aware of their own shortcomings and are critical of themselves. Rebellion against others is relatively rare in this group at this age level.

Once again the psychological appraisal must consider all findings from various angles. The child's level of maturity again seems better expressed by his responses in nonverbal tasks than in verbal ones. The noted discrepancy between levels of comprehension in nonverbal and verbal areas needs special consideration. In each case the reasons for the language retardation must be appraised again from all angles.

At this age a child's motor inability often leads to a new kind of frustration, which the psychologist can try to alleviate. The normal child acquires, through writing, a new medium for expression. For the children of this group writing is usually extremely cumbersome; for them it never becomes a mere tool, but remains a painful physical activity. Already seriously limited in means of expression such as speech and body movement, they become once more much discouraged by trying to express ideas in this difficult way. Frequently, neither parents nor teachers have dared to abandon pressure on writing; but all concerned are often relieved to hear that an electric typewriter might help. More controversial than this advice is the recurring question of a hearing aid. Should it also be tried in cases which the audiologist has considered only mildly impaired? From the psychological point of view it seems essential to give the child the chance to hear as much as possible; this might strengthen his interest in language and acquaint him with the social aspects and functions of language, which he may have ignored because of his limited experience with the spoken word. Increased awareness of the possibilities of communication should in turn enhance his chance for social satisfaction in school and at home.

For this group, problems of social adjustment become most prominent from *the age of ten on*. Many children have now reached a more or less happy equilibrium in their relationships within their families. A number have found satisfaction in educational situations. Some have had understanding classroom teachers, others enthusiastic speech teachers. In most cases, however, competition with normal children remains on unequal terms. The question of how to prepare for a competitive life among contemporaries is urgent. Frequently, it is the reason for a new psychological evaluation.

In the case records discussed, the behavior of this group of children is described as predominantly "friendly," "timid," "self-conscious," "tense," and occasionally in less able children, "simple." Communication can be established more easily than before. With children who have hearing difficulties, E, using simple language and unequivocal directions, often feels more or less assured that instructions and questions have been understood. In the majority of children speech, especially enunciation, continues poor. Again vocabulary is frequently reasonably well developed, but is better in concrete words (T:XII) and common-sense use (T:X:2,3) than in definitions of abstract words. Those to whom the opportunity has been offered have acquired a good stock of information (T:XI:10).

A body of knowledge which has been acquired through reading, arithmetic, and social studies is in these cases a reliable sign that the child has been able to learn and may be counted on to do so in the future. Many of the children, however, have learned very little and do poorly in tasks which depend on acquired information. Often the reason is a lack of adequate educational opportunity resulting from prognostic confusion in the past, contradictory advice, and inconsistent educational efforts. Others have learned very little in spite of fairly adequate training. Performances in appropriate learning situations show varying degrees of learning ability. The majority of children now do better in learning tasks using simple words alone or words and pictures (T:VIII:2,3) than in those depending on awareness for subtle spatial relationships (Rey nonverbal learning test, T:VIII:1). As before, none of the children in this group shows serious distortion in form comprehension (block designs, T:VII:7,8) or memory for designs (T:VII:1,2,4), but a number show reversals and confusion in size discrimination in these tasks and in formboards (T:IV:8) and copying complex figures (T:VII:3,5). Reasoning ability is irregular in this group; it varies with the material and the degree and type of impairment. Children with more or less serious hearing difficulty, even with a hearing aid, may often find it difficult to listen to a lengthy sentence. They easily miss some important points in verbal absurdities (T:IX:6) or comprehension questions (T:X:3), but do better when the same problems are given to them in print. Some, who acquired language and reading late, may do best with picture material (T:IX:10,11,13). As before, most children of this group show their most mature judgement in common-sense matters or in situations which offer visual clues.

Among children of this group there is no reliable evidence of a consistent relationship between global scores on verbal and performance scales (WISC, Wechsler-Bellevue). Neither do the individual scores form a consistent over-all pattern. Performance scores no longer are always higher than verbal scores as they were at earlier ages. Once a child acquires speech, skill in dealing with words can become evident even if the child expresses himself badly. Therefore, his verbal scores may improve. Yet, since the performance tasks appropriate for this age level require more mental imagery and comprehension of meanings than do the truly concrete and practical performance tests suitable for younger children, they are no longer necessarily easier now than some of the verbal tasks.

A child with some aphasic signs may have done well earlier in formboards or puzzles, but may not be able to appreciate underlying relationships in picture arrangements now; another may not have understood earlier how to find similarities, but may now be able to produce them in a concrete, realistic, but "scorable" fashion. Relationships between levels of achievement in various areas are further obscured for the group as a whole by technical difficulties which differ for each child. For one, they may be predominantly in the verbal area (dysarthria, hearing), for another, in the motor or sensory field; or the same child may have a combination of difficulties. In some children, these may increase attention, interest, and tenacity; in others, they may discourage attempts to solve especially difficult problems.

Motor and speech ability may, by this age, have improved enough to cheer those who knew the child earlier and who expected too little from him. However, even minor difficulties of this type become of great social importance when a boy or girl approaches adolescence. At this age contemporaries who are normal but at a stormy age frequently show more intolerance and impatience than they ever did before. General awkwardness combined with indistinct speech may be socially more disastrous among the young than the limping or the irrelevant conversation of the hemiplegic. Children in this group are reported to have even fewer friends during adolescence than they had before. They attend very few social gatherings and events, and spend much time by themselves. The abler ones like to read and are often described as "studious." A few can draw and like to do so. Their artistic productions have a somewhat cool and formalistic quality. They are often painstakingly accurate and true to life, but they seem to lack feeling and expression. In several cases, the choice of subjects continues to reveal the previously observed preference for objects rather than for people.

Many of the children at this age are prepared to continue their education for some time. They welcome rather than resent the prolonged protection from life which this entails. As in earlier years, the most dramatic cases are again those children who prepare themselves to struggle with competition because their impairment is not severe enough to qualify them as disabled.

The psychologist studies, as well as possible, the degree of competence and general comprehension at this stage. As in earlier years, this is predominantly achieved with tasks which circumvent the child's handicap in speech and motor skills. It is now increasingly important to determine to what extent his disability has influenced the child's adjustment and may continue to do so. With the end of the developmental period in sight, it is in most cases necessary to assess the present situation and try to appraise how much progress may reasonably be expected in the various areas. Frequently, the psychological study can help the adviser to decide where training emphasis in the remaining years of the educational period would best be placed. In several cases of the group here discussed, auditory training was stepped up at this period. While it seemed to come late, it proved profitable, in spite of audiological findings that indicated a not very severe hearing loss. In all planning, prevention of psychological strain is an all-important goal for these sensitive children. Many of them are very easily embarrassed and discouraged and know their own limitations all too well; many prefer to avoid socially demanding situations and no longer want to be reminded of their motor and social awkwardness. The psychologist finds that it often helps to relieve tension if families can be persuaded to respect the desire for privacy that is frequently noted amongst these handicapped children instead of trying to arrange for social and occupational life that requires more social poise than they can muster.

JOHN

Hydrocephalus, Spastic Paraplegia

John is a child with a congenital malformation of the brain resulting in hydrocephalus and paraplegia. His main problems are his severe motor disturbance and his mental retardation. His assets are his pleasant, simple personality and his facility in using speech. His physical and psychological handicaps create for him a life situation which, though different from age to age, varies less with development for him than for many normal children.

As a baby he seems responsive and humorous; his ability to imitate wins him affection and approval. His physical helplessness masks his lack of initiative and comprehension. At four years of age he talks fluently and seems bright and alert, thanks to his apparent social awareness. His reasoning difficulties remain largely unnoticed; his passivity and lack of enterprise seem natural in a child who is physically as helpless as John. At seven—with his activities still much restricted by lack of locomotion—he is protected from ordinary educational demands. His ability for social adaptation outweighs his lack of comprehension of new situations. He depends on auditory clues rather than on reasoning. At twelve, social and verbal adaptability are no longer sufficient to gloss over his inherent lack of judgement. It becomes increasingly evident that John's abilities permit but modest academic achievements and would not allow him to become self-sufficient even if he were physically able to be so. With his serious motor limitations, he remains protected from the full impact of his mental retardation. He provides and receives emotional satisfaction.

John's imitative sociability and verbal fluency are evidenced in the various psychological interviews through the years. The shallowness of his comprehension and the inefficiency of his reasoning power become apparent with age. At all stages of his development John has an emotionally satisfying role in his restricted circle. His homely gaiety and calm, together with physical helplessness, do not lose their appeal for those around him.

Using John's case as an illustration, this chapter presents a description of the psychological study of a child with congenital malformation resulting in hydrocephalus, paraplegia, and mental retardation. This detailed account of the approach used at various stages of John's development shows how his general behavior and performances in specific test situations are interpreted by the psychologist and help to create a picture of his psychological situation and role in his environment at each period of his childhood. The last section points out how some of the trends illustrated by John are found to be in many ways characteristic of children with hydrocephalus.

JOHN AT FIFTEEN MONTHS

John is an appealing baby with a large head. He cannot sit independently; lying prone or propped up in sitting position, he has limited head control. He moves very little and seems content lying on his back. The baby is very responsive; he vocalizes a great deal, enjoys company, smiles, and is friendly. He delights his family with a number of tricks and a few definite words. His favorite toy is a cradle gym which he enjoys pushing; he can laugh hilariously at the motion of objects attached to it; his mirth is contagious and prompts the whole family to gather around him. He is described as "quite an actor," who loves to imitate.

The psychological examination, with John on his mother's lap, yields rather uneven results. The baby is well up to his age level in the social areas and performs as described below.

He shows no interest in a picture book other than to pick it up and put it in his mouth (T:II:1). When E pats a picture of a dog to attract his attention to it, John imitates her by slapping his hand down on the book; when E removes the book, he keeps on slapping the table. E tries once more to show him the picture of a car; he repeats the sound "ca-ca," turns to his mother, and continues to vocalize as before. When E again says "Car," he repeats it over and over again, obviously enjoying this vocal give-and-take.

However, he does not understand other kinds of social give-and-take games and cannot learn that an object which he is asked to give to E will be given back to him immediately. Instead, he becomes disturbed even after several experiences; he holds on to the cherished thing and does not relinquish it until he loses interest.

He picks up blocks one by one, does not attempt to pile them or combine them constructively. He quickly stops playing with them of his own volition. He enjoys dropping two in a box with a clang after E initiates this activity. He holds the small pellet over the bottle and has difficulty releasing it (T:V:8). Even after the demonstration, he does not turn the bottle over, but continues poking at the pellet through the glass. Later he sticks his finger in the bottle without making any actual attempt at retrieving the pellet. When a moving object is made to disappear behind a screen while he is watching it (T:V:7), he does not learn to expect it at the other end of the screen, but keeps gazing at the spot where it disappeared from his sight. His field of interest seems to be restricted to his immediate vicinity only. His perceptual awareness and comprehension in adaptive tasks rates at approximately the ten- to twelve-month level only, in contrast to the high level of his social skills.

JOHN AT FOUR YEARS

John is now a big child with a large head which he turns with some difficulty. He still is unable to walk, though he can sit independently. He uses his hands effectively enough and talks fluently.

Except for his inability to walk, his parents are delighted with his progress. Having been warned that the child would develop slowly, they are now triumphant about his responsiveness, his alertness, and his pleasant personality. He has talked early, and because of his precocious statements has been found especially entertaining ever since. He has an excellent memory and is proud of displaying it. He can say his prayers and knows many nursery rhymes. He likes television, especially the commercials, which he can recite. He can amuse himself for a long time with one simple toy (a car) and does not need much change of activity. On the whole he likes people better than things. He likes to look at books when he can sing out loudly about what he sees; he does not enjoy a book without an audience. He is content and easy to handle when not crossed. He eats well and likes most foods. He is happiest when on his regular routine as the center of the family's activities. He gets upset and fatigued at sudden changes in anybody's habits; his only fits of temper occur on such occasions. His mother takes him out in a stroller, but finds it increasingly difficult since he is getting heavy to carry. She does not dare leave him unattended outside. He sees other children only rarely.

When entering the examining room, Johnny, carried by his father, says, "Let us see the nice games and the nice lady." Seated in the examining chair, he accepts E immediately as part of the setting. Actually, he does not establish any personal relationship with her. All through his visit, he remains friendly and even tempered in a noncommittal, detached way. While he does not often turn to either his mother or his father, he acts toward E as one would toward an automaton that dispenses and demonstrates toys or that provides clues to verbal responses.

BLOCKBUILDING (T:I:1,2)

John starts out immediately to pile three or four blocks in a wobbly tower. He uses his right hand, but helps with his left; both hands seem effective enough, though somewhat clumsy. While he builds, he chats, "Build a house, Johnny, see the pretty house." When a block falls and E exclaims, "Hop!" Johnny repeats, "Hop" and causes a second and then a third block to fall, saying delightedly, "Hop." E: "Make another house, Johnny." Johnny repeats, "Make another house, Johnny. See the nice house." He piles three more blocks.

IMITATION OF BRIDGE. Johnny looks at model briefly, but continues to pile blocks while repeating E's invitation, "Let us make a bridge now."

LEARNING STRAIGHT BRIDGE. On request, the child places the bridging third block, but immediately piles a fourth block on top. E leaves model for him to copy, saying, "Let us make another bridge like that now." Johnny chants, "Let us make another bridge like that . . . ," but pays no attention to the proposal.

OBLIQUE BRIDGE. E: "I'll make another kind of bridge now, watch me." The model is left. John ignores it. E: "Let us make another one together."

LEARNING OBLIQUE BRIDGE. John places the two base blocks, then tops them with a third block in straight position as he did before. He pays no attention to the position in which this third block should be.

(All his performances in blockbuilding are below three-year level.)

A second set of colored blocks is presented to him. Johnny starts piling green blocks, interested only in using the new color.

SERIAL PATTERNS (T:I:5)

Johnny enthusiastically accepts the suggestion to line up blocks; he picks them up and lines them up as they come, paying no attention to their color but chanting in repetition of E's directions, "One green, one red, one green, one red." E: "Look, here you've got two green together." Johnny continues working as before, but chants, "Two, three, four, seven, twelve." E hands him the correct color. Johnny, after placing it, follows up with two blocks of the same color. He has obviously not understood what he is supposed to do. (Performance below three-and-a-half-year level.)

SORTING BLOCKS BY COLOR (T:I:6)

There is no adequate response to verbal directions alone. E demonstrates, later corrects his first wrong move. Johnny then places eight blocks correctly and seems to understand but starts to continue haphazardly, carried away simply by the pleasure of putting the blocks away. He no longer pays attention to color.

Analysis of John's behavior up to here suggests many clues to be verified in subsequent phases of the examination. His entrance lines, "Let us see the nice games," as well as his other verbalizations, alert the observer to the child's facility in repeating phrases he has heard. His good auditory memory earns him approval which in turn stimulates new achievements in that direction. His choice of a particular phrase is determined by direct associations with the immediate situation. Blocks suggest to him "Build a house, Johnny," and the word "two" invites "two, three, four." The content of his phrases is at best but partially relevant to what he is doing. His words do not necessarily match his actions. While he is doing things, he likes to vocalize, though he does not mean to communicate or to exchange ideas.

John has immature spatial perceptions (blockbuilding, oblique bridge) and is unable to comprehend the inherent rule of sequence (serial patterns). There is correct differentiation between colors (sorting), but difficulty in persisting in one activity to the end. He is easily distracted and stimulated by motor aspects of the tasks *per se* (lining up, putting away). Some of these traits become more obvious in the next test situation.

Seguin Formboard (T:IV:6)

E hands the round inset to the child, asks, "Where does it go? You show me." Child repeats, "Where does it go? You show me" and tries haphazardly to place the inset. He seems to have no idea where it should go. E points to the correct place and from this point on must continue pointing out each hole, since John makes no effective trial but chants each time he grasps an inset, "Where does it go? You show me."

When the Seguin formboard is repeated with only circle, square, oval, and triangle removed, John places circle correctly, later also square and oval. He tries triangle in correct spot, but does not know how to turn it so it will fit into the hole; he repeats, "Where does it go? You show me." (Performance below three-year level.)

Three-Figure Formboard (T:IV:5)

The three insets (circle, square, triangle) are presented to him with each one facing its proper place. Without hesitating he puts all forms where they should go. The three insets are then presented in a pile. He tries briefly to fit the triangle in the square hole, then puts it aside; places circle and square correctly; finally fits the triangle properly, too. When the board is rotated but the insets left on the table as they were formerly, he tries at first to fit each inset in the hole nearest to it, but gradually fits each one correctly. When the same task is repeated in the same arrangement (rotating the board, but leaving insets in place on table), he again tries each time to fit the insets directly into the nearest hole, but finally finds the correct places for all three insets. (Performance at two- to two-and-a-half-year level.)

Pegboards (T:IV:1,2)

WALLIN A. (Board with round holes.) The box containing all the pegs is presented to him. He picks out several round ones and fits them correctly. Once he gets a square peg into his hand, tries it briefly in one of the round holes, but rejects it; from then on he picks round pegs only.

WALLIN B. (Board with square holes.) He continues to choose round pegs only. E demonstrates that the square pegs fit better. After this John correctly chooses square pegs only.

WALLIN C. (Board with round and square holes.) Three round and three square pegs are given to him. He places them haphazardly; he is left with one square peg for a round hole; he removes one round peg from another round hole and tries to fit the remaining square peg into its hole. E helps. John completes the task.

When the same board is repeated John comes out right and has all square and round pegs placed properly. However, in another repetition, he is again left with an extra square peg for a round hole. Apparently he has not understood the correct relationships of hole and peg, but by accident succeeded in the one repetition. (Performance at two- to two-and-a-half-year level.)

This substantiates the previous impression that John's form comprehension is primitive. His responses to the formboard and the pegboards also indicate a tendency to persevere. He has some difficulty in adapting to the shifting demands of the situation. There follows the study of his skills in the verbal field.

MEMORY FOR PICTURES (T:II:8)

THREE PICTURES. (Horse, hat, ball.) John names hat and ball correctly, but says dog for horse. He does not respond to the suggestion to close his eyes. His mother calls to him to attract his attention while E removes picture of hat and says, "Look, which one did I take away?" John turns and without looking at the table says immediately, "The dog." E shakes her head. John: "The hat." E: "Are you sure?" John, triumphantly: "The ball." He has not understood the game, though he seems to have some idea about guessing games. He remembers the pictures he saw, but does not know how to use them correctly in the context of the game.

THREE PICTURES. (Car, block, knife.) John says fork for knife. E removes car. John again does not understand procedure, performs as he did before, but with less enthusiasm; he seems to become bored. (Performance below three-year level.)

PICTURE VOCABULARY (T:II:7)

E picks up all pictures that were used in the previous situation and shows them again to John. He names ten pictures correctly, including horse. His errors are moon for ball, lamp for telephone, fork for knife, cake for soldier's hat, man for coat, coffee for pitcher, and man for arm. (By Revised Stanford-Binet standards, he passes on three-year level, if one disregards the fact that, contrary to directions, John is shown the pictures for a second time.)

Since John obviously enjoys naming pictures, the animal pictures are introduced next.

ANIMAL PICTURES (T:II:11)

NAMING. John starts correctly with cat, continues to say cat for each of the four succeeding pictures. E: "You know, I think this one is a cow!" From here on, he says to all of the following pictures, "Cow, cow," until he comes to the picture of the dog, which he names correctly.

ANIMAL PICTURES (T:II:10)

MATCHING. John is to match animals. E says, "Find me another one just like this." Johnny does not understand what he is to do. The task is simplified by modified directions, such as, "This is my rabbit, where is yours?" Johnny haphazardly points to any picture, but exclaims with emphasis, "Here is my rabbit," or "Here is my cow." He does not understand the task, but he obviously enjoys the social give-and-take that is involved. (By Revised Stanford-Binet standards, he fails on three-and-a-half-year level.)

PICTURE DESCRIPTION (T:II:6)

GRANDMOTHER'S STORY. John says "Kids," quickly tries to turn to the next page. E: "Tell me more." John: "An old woman, there was an old woman that lived in a shoe, she had so many children she did not know what to do." He turns the page.

BIRTHDAY PARTY. John: "Kids. A house." E points toward the window in the picture. John starts singing, "Happy birthday to you, happy birthday, dear Johnny, happy birthday to you." E: "What do the children want inside?" John: "I do not know." E: "Who is inside?" John: "Their mother." E: "Count the candles." John: "One, two, three, four, seven, twelve." (By Revised Stanford-Binet standards, he fails on three-and-a-half-year level.)

PICTURE BOOK IDENTIFICATION (T:II:5)

E: "Which one can you make houses with?" He points to the blocks, says, "A house." E: "Which one do we eat for breakfast?" John points to cup, spoon, cereal, milk, chair, says, "That we eat for breakfast." E: "Which one do we play with?" John says, "That one we play with and that one and that one," showing duck, trumpet, and car, and missing doll, lamb, and top. E: "Which one can we take to play outside?" He points to saltshaker; his pointing is haphazard and he obviously has failed to understand the question. But he tries to comply.

PICTORIAL IDENTIFICATION (T:II:9)

E: "Which one swims in the water?" John: "The birdie, see the birdie." E: "Which one says meow?" John: "Cat." E: "Which one can fly?" John: "Bird." E: "Which one do we read?" John: "Book." E: "Which one tells us the time?" John: "Apple." E: "Which one do you eat?" John: "Stove . . . apple." E: "Which one swims in the water?" John: "Fish." E: "Which one gives us milk?" John: "The mother." E: "Which one shines in the sky at night?" John: "The cat." (Only three of six Stanford-Binet questions would deserve credit; thus by Revised Stanford-Binet standards, John fails on four-year level.)

OPPOSITE ANALOGIES (T:IX:5)

E: "A brother is a boy, a sister is. . . ." John: "Sister." E: "Daytime is light, night is. . . ." John: "Nighttime." E: "A father is a man, a mother is. . . ." John: "Mother." E: "A brother is a boy, a sister. . . ." John: "Sister." E: "She is a girl—a sister." Then E repeats, "A brother is a boy, a sister is. . . ." John: "Girl." E: "A father is a man, a mother is. . . ." John: "Girl." (By Revised Stanford-Binet standards, he fails on four-year level.)

MEMORY FOR SENTENCES (T:VIII:7)

E: "I like to eat ice cream cones." John repeats correctly, then declares, "I like chocolate." E: "What does it look like?" John: "I do not know." E: "Is it green or red?" John: "Is it green or red." E: "Betty made a pretty dress for her doll out of blue ribbon." John: "Betty made a pity dress. . . ."

The verbal tasks show John's ability to recall and to reproduce verses, phrases, or other auditory series by rote. In his repertoire he also has simple word associations, *e.g.,* "peep peep" goes with bird, "meow" with cat. He fails when more meaningful associative connections are required (opposite analogies, picture description). His name vocabulary is not as good as might be expected from his ability to say most anything. He is not able to designate correctly pictures of objects or animals. His naming of objects reveals many diffuse and poorly structured perceptions. There is also a tendency toward primitive concept formation. He names a chair and a spoon with "things to be eaten for breakfast"; he may do this because he has a global concept of things that "belong" to breakfast, or he may be so flighty in his thinking that he is carried away by another stimulus and forgets what he started out to do.

COMMENT

His performance in all these and previous tasks reveals limited comprehension of complex situations. With his reasoning ability hardly on a three-year level, his form comprehension lower, and his verbal facility his main asset only because of his auditory memory, the child's intellectual development at age four seems to proceed at a borderline rate at best.

Altogether, the examination has given a good picture of John's situation. His verbal responsiveness and social graces still earn him most of his successes. John is still fully satisfactory to his family as well as to himself. He seems secure and serene. Apparently he has not yet had much occasion to regret his inability to get around. In a busy household his lack of imagination and his contentment with the simplest activities are considered virtues rather than liabilities. His perceptual difficulties have not yet caused him any embarrassment, since they are not obvious in any of his occupations. For the moment, John's problems are few; his family hopes most of all that he will eventually walk; otherwise there are no special ambitions or plans.

The psychologist's function for the present is to ward off the early encounter of avoidable frustrations. For the time being, his physical helplessness gives John a natural protection. His mental limitations may remain concealed as long as formal schooling is put off. The longer John can feel appreciated, loved, and admired by his own people, the less he may be thwarted later by his physical and mental difficulties.

JOHN AT SEVEN YEARS

Johnny, now seven, is a stocky boy with a large head and thin legs and arms. He can stand and take a few steps alone, but spends most of his time sitting. He is a friendly, mild child with a high, somewhat insistent voice. His family is still delighted with him, though his mother appears to be somewhat more tense than before. Both parents are eager to report about him. They continue to think he is intelligent, but know at the same time that he is not as mature as other children his age. His sheltered life and lack of experience are, in their minds, responsible for the narrow range of his interests. He still has impressive verbal facility and memory for people and places. He knows the neighbors, their pets and their cars and recently recognized the Fuller Brush man, who had been forgotten by all since his last call the previous year. He has become an ardent television fan, and, while he is not able to tell time, he knows without fail when certain programs are coming on. He still does not have much interest in games or toys. When asked what new toy he would like, he invariably asks for a "little car." He has now accumulated quite a collection of vehicles, and his family's enthusiasm about it has taught him to be proud of it. His five-year-old cousin tries to teach him what she learns in kindergarten. John shows no interest in her paper-and-pencil work, but he learns all her songs and poems quickly and, in general, is ahead of her in vocabulary and the use of precocious phrases.

Up to now there has not been any schooling for Johnny; the psychological examination has been proposed to help in educational planning. The question of a boarding school for crippled children has been brought up. His parents are only mildly in favor of the idea but think that for the child's sake they might have to agree to a separation.

Johnny enters the examining room walking slowly at his mother's hand. He seems keyed-up and slightly overemphatic in his attempts to appear joyous. He sits down without hesitation and waits for E to produce the "games." In spite of his cooperative and friendly attitude, he does not appear curious, but remains somewhat remote and uninvolved.

Seguin Formboard (T:IV:6)

He waits passively while the forms are being piled in front of him. He says politely, "This is a nice game you got there," but remains inactive. When the round inset is handed to him, he takes it slowly, looks around the board, finds the correct hole, and places the inset deliberately with some awkwardness. He waits until the next inset is handed to him, then he places it slowly after looking the board over. He finishes the task, but altogether is slower than normal for his age. There are no errors except for brief trials of lozenge in hexagon, cross in star, triangle in diamond. He corrects them spontaneously.

Five-Figure Formboard (T:IV:7)

He appears to be quite helpless and does not know how to begin. The round piece is handed to him. Without conviction, he places it in the oval hole, removes it, and puts rectangle in square, asking, "Does that fit?" E: "Not very well." Johnny repeats, "Not very well," removes inset and places another rectangle in the same spot, while reciting, "Does it fit—not very well." He shows very little affect about his inability to do the task.

E places part of oval. Johnny completes it correctly, then tries the small oval in the square hole, asking, "Does that fit?" E: "What do you think?" He tries to force another larger piece into the same hole without removing the first, saying, "Does that fit—what do you think?" apparently without expecting any answer. E places one part of each form. After this is done, Johnny completes the board correctly, his only hesitations being with the hexagon and the square.

(In both formboard tasks John's approach and methods show that his form comprehension is well below his chronological age level.)

SERIAL PATTERNS (T:I:5)

Johnny is to make an alternating row of red and green blocks; he understands and places six blocks in correct order, imitating E's verbal directions, "One green, one red, one green, one red." Then E points to the green block which is the first one in the row; she invites Johnny to extend his row from right to left. He has a green block already poised in his hand and has no hesitation in placing it next to the first green block; from here on he continues in correct order (red, green). After all blocks have been placed, E says, "Look at them, they are fine. But is there anything wrong?" Johnny scans the row of blocks and does not see any error in two green blocks being next to each other. With Johnny imitating vocally, E points to each block of the row, repeating emphatically, "Green, red, green, red." E hesitates ostentatiously when she comes to the pair of green blocks, but Johnny continues to chant, "Green, red, green, red." Obviously he does not match the names of the colors with the respective blocks.

COUNTING BLOCKS (T:I:7)

Johnny counts first, says, "Twelve." E asks him to count again "to make sure." On second count he answers, "Eleven." When he recounts, he reverts to twelve. He does not seem surprised about the discrepancy in his results. Each count seems to be an isolated task for him. E: "Look, you had twelve first, then eleven, and then twelve again. Which one is correct?" Johnny smiles; as if challenged in a guessing game, he responds, "Eleven." E: "Are you sure?" John: "Twelve." E: "Sure?" John: "Thirteen, fourteen, fifteen!"

ISOLATING SMALL QUANTITIES FROM LARGER ONES (T:I:8)

E: "Give me three blocks." John is correct. E: "Give me five." John is correct. E: "Give me seven." John counts up to seven, but gives only six blocks. E: "Give me nine." John counts to ten, gives seven blocks. (In the Revised Stanford-Binet Scale "counting 13 pennies" and "number concepts" are placed on the six-year level. By these standards, Johnny fails on this level.)

COMPARING CONCRETE QUANTITIES (T:I:9)

E makes a square of four blocks. John copies it correctly. E: "How many do you have?" John correctly counts, "Four." E: "How many have I got in mine?" John counts again, "Four." E: "Yours and mine look just the same; you have four blocks and I have four blocks; we each took four and arranged them the same way, so we each have four."

E arranges five blocks in X shape. John copies and counts his blocks. E: "How many do I have?" John starts again to count E's blocks which she covers, asking, "Can you know without counting?" John looks blank. E: "How many did you have?" He again counts his own: "Five." E: "And mine?" He insists on counting E's blocks and says triumphantly, "You got five." He has not understood that both configurations must have the same number of blocks and he has not learned it from the first sample.

BLOCKBUILDING (T:I:2)

STRAIGHT BRIDGE. Correct.

OBLIQUE BRIDGE. Correct.

SIX-CUBE PYRAMID. John builds two straight bridges placed near each other.

SIX-CUBE STEPS. He omits middle step. He seems to get bored, asks, "Have you got something else?" E: "Let us just try this one." John imitates six-cube steps correctly, and then reproduces another one correctly.

SORTING BLOCKS BY COLOR (T:I:6)

Following verbal instructions, John puts all blocks away correctly in their boxes. He is slow and systematic; he first neatly arranges the green box, then the red one. At the end, he starts spontaneously to count all twenty-four blocks. He begins by pointing to each one in succession, but as he goes on he skips some. Toward the end he counts "Twenty-one, twenty-two, twenty-eight, twenty-nine, twenty, twenty-one, etc."

The examination up to this point suggests that John's form comprehension has improved in the past three years. However, his performances in formboard tests still indicate a considerable lag in this area. His speed in the Seguin formboard and his approach in the five-figure formboard are inferior to those of most five-year-olds. He reaches only approximately the same level in blockbuilding. Up to this stage of the examination, his verbal facility shows mostly in his ease in counting automatically or in his readiness to repeat phrases and intonations. His comprehension of new situations continues to be slow. Basic concepts which children his age usually have acquired are missing; he does not know, for instance, that identical patterns made of identical elements must contain an identical number of elements. He does not easily profit from new experiences and is slow in learning new patterns of thinking. Another difficulty is his inability to appraise visual situations at a glance. This was first obvious in the formboards, but was even more noticeable when he failed to spot his error in the alternating row of colored blocks. His attention spans are short. He still is carried away by auditory clues. He falls back on them instead of exploring a situation visually. He has become more passive and prefers to wait for help rather than to risk difficulties. He still thrives on playful social situations and takes advantage of them whenever he has an opportunity. The subsequent phases of the examination will consolidate or revise these findings.

The child's pleasure in numbers leads E to introduce other test procedures which use them in different ways.

Repeating Digits (T:VIII:5,6)

DIGITS FORWARD. For three digits, E says: "Three, five, nine." John repeats correctly, imitating E's rhythm and intonation. He repeats four digits (four, two, nine, one) correctly in the same manner as before. He also repeats five digits (three, nine, two, eight, one) correctly. For six digits, E says: "Four, five, nine, two, six, one." John: "Four, five, six, one." E: "Two, three, four, five, six, seven." John: "Two, three, four, five, six, seven." E: "Five, two, seven, nine, three, eight." John: "Five, two, seven, nine, eight."

To confirm the impression that John repeats the sounds of the digits only and pays no attention to them as numbers, E introduces a series which contains nonsense syllables: "Three, nine, ex, por, six." John repeats this series in the same manner as he did the others; he shows no sign of surprise.

DIGITS BACKWARD. E says: "Let us say them backwards now. If I say three, one, five, you say five, one, three. Now I say six, one, eight. You say. . . ." John repeats immediately, "Six, one, eight." He does not understand what he is to do. E: "Let us try it again. You try to say them backwards this time, six, one, eight, backwards." John repeats, "Six, one, eight, backwards." Another similar trial fails. (By Revised Stanford-Binet standards, John passes on seven-year level for five digits forward; he fails on seven-year level for three digits in reverse.)

AUTOMATIC SERIES (T:XI:2)

E: "Let us do them forward again. I say, Four, five, six, seven, eight, nine." He repeats this series correctly. E: "Two, four, six, eight, ten, twelve." John: "Two, four, six, ten, twelve, eight, nine." E: "Nine, eight, seven, six, five, four." John: "Nine, eight, seven, six, four. . . ."

Direct counting is for John a familiar automatic series. Like other children his age counting backward or counting by two's has not yet become automatic for him. Such a series does not sound familiar to him, as it would to older persons. When John repeats a series which is automatic for him, he can repeat six digits instead of five as before. Since sounds are all that count for John, he repeats series with nonsense syllables as easily as digit series. If he has taken in a series by ear, he is unable to break it up consciously in order to manipulate it. That is why he is unable to say series in reverse.

Johnny is apparently becoming somewhat ill at ease, and is ready for a change of activity. He asks, "Have you got any more games?" E: "Let us play a guessing game."

MEMORY FOR PICTURES (T:II:8)

THREE PICTURES. (Car, hat, key.) E removes key. John identifies key correctly.

FOUR PICTURES. (Blocks, horse, knife, coat.) E removes horse. With delight, John repeats, "The key is gone."

FOUR PICTURES REPEATED. Coat is removed. John knows this time that the coat is gone.

FIVE PICTURES. (Cane, airplane, ball, flag, hat.) Flag is removed. John: "It is the coat."

FIVE PICTURES REPEATED. Ball is removed. John: "The airplane." He is unreliable and does not really know how to proceed.

PICTURE VOCABULARY (T:II:7)

During this procedure he names thirteen of the seventeen pictures correctly. His errors are: he calls an alphabet block a "B," an arm a man, a soldier hat a birthday cake, and a telephone a lamp. (By Revised Stanford-Binet standards, he would pass on five-year level, if the task had been presented in standard fashion.)

ANIMAL PICTURES (T:II:10,11)

DISCRIMINATION. He matches correctly seven of the twelve animals. His errors are the following: he matches the squirrel with the cat, the pig with the bear, the giraffe with the camel, and the reindeer with the goat.

NAMING. He names eight of the twelve correctly. His errors are the following: he calls the squirrel a cat, the bear a pig, the camel a giraffe, the reindeer a horse.

All the errors the child makes in naming animals seem to indicate that John has poorly differentiated global percepts. He confuses those animals which are presented in similar positions or sizes, *e.g.,* squirrel-cat, giraffe-camel. (While he passes the discrimination test by Revised Stanford-Binet standards on four-and-a-half-year level, he matches and names animals less well than six-year level.)

IDENTIFICATION. E: "Look at the pictures and tell me which one gives milk?" John: "The milkman." E: "Which one eats nuts?" John: "I do. My father cracks them." He no longer looks at the picture card, but settles down for conversation.

PICTURE DESCRIPTION (T:II:6)

GRANDMOTHER'S STORY. E: "What is happening?" John: "They are on the floor." E: "And?" John: "She is telling them. . . ." E: "What?" John: "To get up from the floor." E: "Why?" John: "They should be walking." E: "Why?" John: "To get big and strong." E points toward stove, asks, "What is that?" John: "Supper cooking." E: "What are they cooking?" John: "Tomato soup." E: "How do you know?" John: "I like it." E: "What else?" John: "Chocolate ice cream." E: "Where do you see it?" John: "In the ice box." E: "Look at the picture

again. What is happening?" John: "She is telling them." E: "What?"
John: "To get up."

BIRTHDAY PARTY. John: "A boy, a girl, they are coming to
see him." E: "Why?" John: "He is sick." E: "Why?" John: "He ate too
much ice cream." E: "How do you know?" Johnny notices the birthday
cake, says, "It was his birthday." E: "How do you know?" John: "I see
his cake." E: "How old is he?" John: "Seven." E: "How do you know?"
John: "I know." To E's query, he answers, "I always know and my cousin
is five." E: "Look at the cake." John: "Candles." E: "How many?"
John: "Four." E: "Count them again." John: "Five." E: "How old is
the child going to be?" John: "Five." E: "How do you know?"
John: "Because my cousin is five. She knows how old she is."

WASHDAY. John: "I like these pictures. The dog is running
away with the clothes." E: "And?" John: "He got them." E: "Where?"
John: "From the mother." E: "How?" John: "She washed them." E:
"And then?" John: "He got them." E: "What is going to happen?"
John: "He is running." E: "And?" John: "She is running." E: "And?"
John: "He is going to tear it." E: "And then?" John: "I do not know."
E: "What does he say?" John: "Bow-wow." E: "What is going to
happen?" John: "They are running."

PICTORIAL IDENTIFICATION (T:II:9)

E: "Which one swims in the water?" John: "Fish." E: "Which one
lives up in the tree?" John: "Bird." E: "What do we cook on?" John:
"In the kitchen." E: "Which one can fly?" John: "Birdie." E: "Which
brings Easter eggs?" John: "Bunny."

IDENTIFICATION IN REVERSE. John repeats "Which one brings
Easter eggs?" E: "Do not tell me. Tell me about them." John: "Tell me
about the fish. Tell me about the eggs. I know a song. 'Birdie, birdie,
up in the tree. . . .' "

PICTURE ABSURDITIES (T:II:11)

MAN IN TREE. John: "He is sawing the tree down." E:
"And?" John: "That is all." E: "Anything funny about it?" John:
"Nothing funny about it."

MAN ON SCALES. John: "He is looking at the clock." E:
"Why?" John: "Because. . . ."

CAT AND MICE. John: "Look at the cute picture—a cat
and a mouse and another mouse and another mouse." E: "What are they

doing?" John: "They are talking to the cat." E: "What else?" John: "Nothing else. Mrs. Smith has a cat. Her name is Punky. She is yellow and black. She comes and jumps in my mother's lap." E: "Do you take it in your lap?" John: "I do not like it to jump. I like to look at it, though." (By Revised Stanford-Binet standards, he fails on seven-year level.)

DIFFERENCES BETWEEN TWO THINGS (T:IX:1)

E: "Johnny, you know birds and you know dogs. Can you tell me in which way a bird and a dog are alike?" John: "I know a dog, his name is Skippy. I do not know a bird." E: "Have you seen one?" John: "I do not know." E: "Have you got birds in your yard?" John: "I do not know, you have to ask my mother."

E: "You know glass and wood. What is different about them?" John: "Glass to drink milk out of; wood I do not know. You burn it in the fireplace." E: "In what way are glass and wood different?" John: "You drink out of glass, wood you burn in the fireplace." (By Revised Stanford-Binet standards, he fails on six-year level.)

MATERIALS (T:X:2)

E: "Johnny, do you know what things are made of? What is a window made of?" John: "My windows in my house are made of glass. It breaks." E: "What is a house made of?" John: "I do not know— blocks." E: "What is a book made of?" John: "Made of paper and pictures and pages you can turn."

John asks, "Have you got another game?" E: "Let us play another game with words; we do it together. I start it and you finish it."

OPPOSITE ANALOGIES (T:IX:5)

E: "A father is a man; a mother is. . . ." John first answers, "A mother," then to E's query, says, "A lady." E: "A brother is a boy; a sister is. . . ." John: "Girl." E: "Daytime is light; night is. . . ." John: "Nighttime." E: "The sun shines during the day; the moon at. . . ." John: "Nighttime." (By Revised Stanford-Binet standards, he passes on four-year level, but fails on six-year level.)

PAPER AND PENCIL (T:III:1 AND XI:8)

John: "I know how to write my name." He prints in large letters with a weak stroke. His letters are out of line and distributed all over the page. His N is reversed. E: "What else can you write?" John: "Nothing else . . . I can make my letters and my numbers." He prints in large letters A to G, reversing D and E, and is baffled by G, says, "I do not know any other." John starts to write numbers up to six. He reverses the 6; it swings to the left instead of to the right. E: "Which one is 5?" He is uncertain, points first to the 3, later correctly to the 5. E: "Which one is G?" John: "I do not know; I can't make a G." E: "Which one is E?" He shows the F first, then the E. E: "Which one is 2?" He points correctly, says, "I know that one; it comes right after 1—1 and 2."

It is not easy for John to isolate and designate numbers and letters out of context. He is uncertain about their individual characters.

COPYING FORMS (T:III:5 AND FIGURE 2)

BALL, CROSS, TRIANGLE, SQUARE. All correct and recognizable, though large and drawn with a weak stroke.

DIAGONAL CROSS. He finds this difficult; he starts from the center; he does not like his first production, starts over again, and produces an acceptable cross.

TILTED SQUARE. He draws this square as he did the simple square, but gives an incline to the last side.

MEMORY FOR FORMS (T:III:6 AND FIGURE 2)

BRITISH FLAG. He produces a rectangle with three lines spreading out of one corner. He does not like his production. He asks to see the card again, and it is shown to him.

COPY OF BRITISH FLAG. He now produces a rectangle with a star in the center but not reaching to the sides. E asks, "What else could you make? Would you like to make a picture?" John: "I do not know a picture." E: "Could you make the picture of a man, the very best man you can do?"

DRAWING A MAN (T:III:3)

He produces a large head with eyes, nose, mouth, arms attached to head, fingers, small legs attached to head, later he adds hair. John spends most time on head and features; the legs are added later. It might well be that this expresses a distorted body image in a child whose legs are useless to him. The large head, too, is interesting in view of the fact that John's own head is large and also is probably frequently commented upon within his hearing. (By Goodenough's developmental standards, his drawing rates at four-and-a-half- to five-year level.)

GOLDSTEIN-SCHEERER STICK TEST (T:VII:6 AND FIGURE 12)

A figure which resembles the letter A is recognized with enthusiasm and produced correctly; he also recognizes E and W, but reproduces them reversed. Other forms are distorted in size or are simplified.

BLOCK DESIGNS (T:VII:7 AND FIGURE 13)

CARD I. Correct sides are up, but the blocks are spread out and not arranged in a square. E: "Can you make them look like the card?" He pushes the blocks together so that they are arranged correctly.

CARD II. He does not use blue/yellow sides to build the yellow triangle in the proper row. Instead, he puts two all-blue sides together at an angle, probably imitating the position of the blue outside triangles. Then he places a yellow block underneath, and further down a red block. The final product is T-shaped. It crudely imitates the color relationships, but not the form relationships of the model card. E demonstrates the correct arrangement; he follows.

When Card II is repeated he uses blue/yellow sides, but instead of lining them up next to each other, he arranges them at an angle as he did with the blue sides previously. He places two red blocks together below. Again the end result is not a square, but a loose arrangement with spaces between.

CARD III. Instead of the blue peak with yellow angles made of blue/yellow blocks, he arranges two blue/yellow blocks next to each other, puts a yellow block on top and a blue block below. The end result is an arrangement in cross-form loosely put together. E demonstrates the correct arrangement.

When Card III is presented again he pushes the blocks around haphazardly, apparently tired and bored, asks, "Where is my mother?" The session is closed.

COMMENT

The second part of the examination confirms that John is still retarded in various respects. His form comprehension is still poor as shown in the way he copies forms by drawing or using stick material and in his productions with the block design material. His verbal facility still is an outstanding factor. It shows up mostly in small talk and in repetition of things heard. Though fluent, his conversation continues to be immature in content. His frame of reference is restricted to his own immediate experiences (differences between two things or materials). He talks about isolated factors, but does not coordinate his observations through thinking about them (picture absurdities). Language remains for him a vehicle for social contact rather than for exchange of ideas. Even when making conversation, he seems somewhat impervious and rigid. He enjoys falling back on previously acquired automatisms. The ones he has at his disposal are simple (counting, phrases) and, in general, do not include verbal patterns which might be based on more complex associations (as shown in his failure in opposite analogies).

At seven John seems somewhat more passive and timid than he was at four. Though his social graces still earn him the satisfaction they did earlier, he now has more opportunity to sense some of his difficulties in comprehension. He is no longer as sure of himself. This adds to his aloof attitude and immature egocentric viewpoint. His severe motor handicap has further stunted any tendency toward curiosity or enterprise that would be natural at his age. However, lack of experience alone cannot account for John's shortcomings. His striking perceptual difficulties and his inability to reason effectively point toward intellectual impairment due to brain injury.

As a person, John still seems to get full emotional satisfaction within his circle. He is content and not yet eager to have wider social experiences than he has in his immediate surroundings. He does not seem ready for more yet and would very likely become confused and upset if he had to be in a less familiar environment. Therefore, placement away from home would seem rather premature. However, John seems ready for some training on a kindergarten level. A home teacher will best be able to adjust her program to his difficulties. His academic successes will probably remain rather meager. Since his family will only gradually become aware of his limitations, it would still seem important for John and them to postpone frustrations and disappointments as long as possible. With his intellectual abilities closer to a five-year level than to that of his chronological age, John still develops at a borderline rate at best. Satisfactions must continue to be brought about mostly by his homey, amiable, sociable personality. It is hoped that his happy disposition may help him to stay contented with his restricted opportunities in life.

JOHN AT TWELVE YEARS

John, now age twelve, is a heavy boy with mild, friendly manners. He walks only on occasion, and then very slowly and deliberately. He talks in a high-pitched, slightly attention-demanding voice which seems somewhat to contrast with his passive attitude.

His parents, still devoted to him, have many questions about his education, his future, and his prospects of fitting into life. John still has not been to school; a home teacher comes twice a week and finds that he is good in reading, but that, after a good start, he makes only slow progress in arithmetic. John likes to read for anybody who cares to listen to him; often he reads to himself, either whispering or in a loud voice. His mother thinks that he likes reading for the sake of words and sounds rather than for content. He is not particular in his choice of literature. He reads *Golden Books,* recipes, or crime news with equal pleasure. He is not interested in games or puzzles. He draws poorly, occasionally colors with much precision. In matters of writing, he likes best of all to copy; he does it slowly and neatly, with large letters. He is interested in the routine of the household, but does not participate much in actual chores. Occasionally his mother invites him to mix a cake; he likes this type of activity, but often forgets some ingredients and gets tired before he is finished. He dresses himself, but needs much time for it; he likes to look neat and enjoys compliments about his appearance, his colorful ties, and his shirts. He has a wheelchair which he still prefers to walking. Though he can operate it himself, he does not change location frequently. He spends much time sitting at the window or in the yard, watching the activities of the neighbors. He talks to them, inquires about their health and their doings, and keeps track of what is going on. His amiable interest appeals to people; he is on "hailing" terms with most everybody on his street. John's outings beyond his immediate neighborhood are limited. There are some rides on Sundays, with an occasional dinner at a Howard Johnson's. Though John likes these excursions and looks forward to them, his family finds him quiet and almost timid in strange places. This seems to them in surprising contrast to his usual easygoing, sociable attitude. His parents have made efforts to attract other children to the house; this succeeds best with some younger girls, who enjoy coming. John talks about his "girl friends" and their activities. Usually he is a commenting spectator rather than a participant. When children leave him abruptly for some livelier entertainment, his mother is secretly annoyed and marvels at John's good disposition.

The psychological examination is meant to check on John's progress and to make some suggestions for the future. John has not been told much about the event. His parents were afraid that he would get unnecessarily excited. They have told him that they were going to see a lady who had known him a long time ago.

John willingly comes with E when she invites him into the examining room. He walks slowly; he tries to be friendly, but is obviously apprehensive. His polite "You have a nice room" does not effectively mask his very evident anxiety.

FIVE-FIGURE FORMBOARD (T:IV:7)

John says, "I do not know that game. I do not have many games—not puzzles like that." E hands him one inset. John: "I do not know where that goes." He accepts help with the first inset, but finds the complement piece on his own and places it. He completes the board without difficulty, except for some wrong moves with the cross and hexagon. (Performance, including trials and errors, is on six- to seven-year level.)

CASUIST FORMBOARD (T:IV:8)

John now becomes more relaxed; he starts immediately and with more gusto. He tries several insets for size in different places. (Inaccurate size discrimination also caused error with the cross in the previous test.) (Performance, including trials and errors, is on eight- to nine-year level.)

Johnny now takes the initiative, asking, "What else have you got besides puzzles? Do you have books? I like to read."

READING (T:XI:7)

John knows the book (a second-grade one) and reads it with pride and self-assurance.

E tries to explain to John the purpose of his visit. She tells him that his family has been so proud of him and wanted to show him off. She (E) is an old friend who has known him a long time. She explains that when he was younger, things did not always come easily to him. She wonders whether he may now still find some things harder than others. She will try to get to know him again as he is now; the best way to get acquainted is to do things together. As he may have already seen, she has easy things and harder things for him to do.

Johnny listens and makes no comment. He seems relieved when E stops talking, and turns to:

DISSECTED SENTENCES (T:XI:6)

(a) He reads off the words "A-have-dog-I-fine" in the order in which they are printed on the card. E: "Could you make a sentence?" John: "I have a fine dog."

(b) He reads with pride: "Wool-the-was-coat-of-made," again in the order of presentation. He seems satisfied. E: "That does not make too much sense, does it?" John laughs again as if it was a good joke, looks at the words, and recites, "The wool was made of coat." E: "Does that sound right?" John laughs again, and corrects it to, "The coat was made of wool."

(c) As before, he reads, "Child-the-playing-garden-in-the-is." This time John reads the words and studies them further until he finds the correct solution, "The child is playing in the garden."

It is probably only through E's suggestions that John has found the correct solutions. (Because of this additional help, by Revised Stanford-Binet standards, he fails on nine-year level.)

(d) John reads the words, "For-the-started-an-we-country-early-at-hour," then says with relief, "We started early for the country at an hour."

(e) He first reads, "To-asked-paper-my-teacher-correct-I-my," then, "I asked my teacher to correct my paper."

(f) First he reads, "A-defends-dog-good-his-bravely-master," then, "A defends dog . . . a good master . . . his bravely defends dog . . ." Johnny knows how to read all the words, but he lacks judgement about content or spelling. Therefore, he fails to construct sentences d and f correctly. (By Revised Stanford-Binet standards, he fails on thirteen-year level.)

RECALL OF FACTS (T:VIII:4)

E: "Here is a story about the school concert. Listen carefully while I read it, because I shall ask you questions about it." She reads:

"The School Concert. On December 20th, the children of the city schools held a concert in the auditorium of the high school. All the children had some part in the program. The program consisted of singing by the school choir, fancy marching, folk dancing, and finally a Christmas play. About 620 parents and friends attended the concert. The sale of tickets brought in nearly four hundred dollars." Johnny, with the printed story in front of him, insists on reading aloud with E instead of listening and following silently. She stops once in her reading to remind him to listen carefully.

E: "What was the name of the story?" John: "I do not know." When questioned again, he says, "It is about school, they had six hundred dollars." E: "Try to listen only. Do not read it with me, so you can listen and remember." She reads the story again. This time John resists the temptation to read aloud and listens.

E: "What is the name of the story?" John answers correctly, "School concert." E: "When was it held?" John: "I do not know." E: "Where was it held?" John: "In school." E: "How many people were there?" John: "Four hundred." E: "How much money did they make?" John: "Six hundred dollars." E: "What was on the program?" John: "Christmas play—folk dancing." E: "When was it held?" John: "I do not know." E: "Could you guess?" John: "In summer?" E: "What was on the program?" John: "Christmas play and folk dancing." E: "When was it held?" John: "I do not know."

He remembers various bits of the story, but does not connect them by reasoning. He remembers that there is a Christmas play, but he has no answer for the timing of the concert. He remembers figures correctly, though he knows them isolated from their context only. (With only four "memories" to his credit, John would, by Revised Stanford-Binet standards, fail on the ten-year level, even if there had not been two readings instead of the one prescribed by the standard directions.)

Learning Fifteen Words (T:VIII:2)

A list of words is read to the child who is asked to repeat in any order all the words he can remember; reading of the list is repeated five times, the child being asked to say all the words he can recall, including those he knew after previous readings; the child's productions are recorded, including all words substituted or said twice within the same repetition.

After the proper explanations, E reads the list of words: drum, curtain, bell, coffee, school, parent, moon, garden, hat, farmer, nose, turkey, color, house, river. John repeats: "Turkey, color, house, river." E reads list for the second time. John repeats the first five words immediately after her and while E continues to read the complete list, John keeps repeating the first five words: "Drum, curtain, bell, coffee, school, drum, curtain, bell, coffee, school." When E has finished the list, he can't wait to recite triumphantly: "Drum, curtain, bell, coffee, school."

E: "Try to listen to all of them so you get them all. They need not be in order." John obviously gets tired of this task, starts looking around the room, but controls himself.

E reads list for third time. John repeats: "Drum, curtain, bell, coffee, school." E: "Do you know any others?" John adds "House, river." E: "Any other?" John: "Table, chair, pencil."

John retains auditory series through rote learning, but he has no effective way of retaining more than his auditory span permits. When pushed, he resorts to enumerating objects in sight (table, chair), hoping that they will be accepted since they show his good will. (According to the norms for this procedure, John's score falls between the tenth and twentieth percentiles for immediate recall after the first reading, but falls at zero percentile for learning after the third reading.)

Since John's mood has become a bit cloudy, E decides to boost his courage with a task which she thinks may be easy for him. She introduces:

REPEATING DIGITS (T:VIII:5,6)

DIGITS FORWARD. John repeats several series of four, five, and six digits correctly. He omits two out of eight digits, but does not notice it.

DIGITS BACKWARD. He is unable to repeat correctly three and four digits in reversed order.

(By Revised Stanford-Binet standards, John passes digits forward on ten-year level, but fails on Superior Adult II level. He fails digits in reverse on seven-year level and nine-year level.)

AUTOMATIC SERIES (T:XI:2)

NUMBERS. John is to give the numbers reversed. E: "One, two, three, four, five." John: "Four, three, two." E: "Two, three, four, five, six." John: "Six, five, four, two, one." E: "Two, four, six, eight." John: "Eight, four, six, two."

DAYS OF THE WEEK. John is to say the days of the week. He rattles them off. E: "Which one comes before Tuesday?" John: "Wednesday." E stresses: "*Before* Tuesday?" John: "Monday." E: "After Wednesday?" John: "Thursday."

DAYS OF THE WEEK IN REVERSE. John says, "Sunday, Saturday,

Friday, Thursday, Tuesday, Wednesday, Thursday." He gets carried away again by the familiar auditory sequence and cannot continue saying in reverse words which he is accustomed to saying forward.

MONTHS OF THE YEAR. John: "January, February, May, August . . . I do not know." E: "Which month do we have now?" John correctly answers, "April." E: "What date is today?" John: "I do not know." E: "What day of the week?" John: "Wednesday; that is when we were to see Doctor X (names E)." E: "What is your address?" John: "22 M———— Street, Newton, Massachusetts." (This is correct.) E: "What is Massachusetts?" John: "It is where we are—in America." E: "What is America?" John laughs: "Just America—you want to hear me say the Pledge of Allegiance?" E: "What is it; what does it mean, 'allegiance'?" John: "I do not know. I know . . . how it goes . . . it has something to do with the flag. They do it at school every morning."

Johnny has become much happier since he has been able to shine with recitations which ordinarily win him praise; he brushes off the last questions which might spoil his success. Up to here, the examination has given the following initial impression. Formboard tests yielded some signs of disability in size discrimination (Casuist formboard). His slow approach to these tests probably indicates that his form perceptions are still less precise than is common in children of his age. His inability to memorize facts (School concert), long series of words, digits, etc., shows how much John still has to depend on his auditory skills. These earn him success wherever pure rote memory is required (days of the week, pledge of allegiance). He continues to have considerable difficulty, however, where manipulation and reorganization are required (learning, digits, or days reversed). In the light of his various disabilities, his fluency in reading appears remarkable. One has the impression that this is being brought about by his skill with words. He is able to establish and retain associations between auditory and visual clues. As he has learned to associate faces with names of people, he has also learned to connect sounds of words with their printed visual image. His skill in reading is technical; he does not have equally good comprehension of what he reads (dissected sentences).

Subsequent phases of the examination must investigate his reasoning ability. With John in confident spirits from his last achievements, a series of new activities may be introduced now which may prove less attractive to him than the preceding tasks. Since he has mentioned school and likes to show what he has learned, E now produces

PENCIL AND PAPER (T:III:1)

John spontaneously prints his name and address. He is slow and meticulous, and is pleased with the product.

WRITING ON DICTATION (T:XI:9)

John is very hesitant at first. Before starting to write "This is the Children's Hospital," he decides whether or not he has previously "had" the initial words. He does not take any chance with an unfamiliar word, is not sure about "children," but agrees to write "hospital" when E promises to dictate the needed letters.

John volunteers: "I can draw a house." He draws a large, rather primitive-looking house without any perspective—one flat surface, two windows with a cross each, a door. He starts to cover the house with small squares representing bricks; though he seems at first set to cover the house in this fashion, he gives up after a while and declares that it is too much.

MEMORY FOR DESIGNS (T:VII:1 AND FIGURE 4)

DESIGNS FROM FORM M, IX-YEAR LEVEL. (a) John simplifies the structure by drawing the two uprights which are unequally high as if they were equal. (b) The inner square does not meet all sides of the outer square.

DESIGN FROM FORM M, XII-YEAR LEVEL. (c) Of the three diamonds, he draws the large one only; he encloses the smaller diamond by two uneven horizontals.

John obviously finds these tasks difficult. Therefore, E rejects her plan to introduce the Ellis visual design test and attempts only:

DESIGNS FROM FORM L, IX-YEAR LEVEL. (d) John murmurs "flags" and draws the squares facing in the wrong direction. (e) John insists that he did not see this design long enough; he only had time to look at the "flags." He sounds irritated and reveals mounting tension. The card is shown him again. He draws two squares not properly connected with corners. He does not seem happy; he acts as if he were imposed upon. Once more E shows him the card; she leaves it in plain view for John to correct his design if he wishes. He erases some, then tries to connect the inner square with the outer one, but the relative positions of the squares are still wrong.

(By Revised Stanford-Binet Form M standards, John earns ½ credit each for a and b, thus passing on nine-year level. He fails to earn credit on twelve-year level for c. For d, he earns ½ credit, but none for e, which would mean failure on nine-year level of Form L.)

John's performances in all memory for design tasks indicate difficulty in accurate perception and reproduction. He gets the general idea, but misses on finer points. The drop in the quality of his performance after frustration becomes significant (in e). It shows how important it is to maintain a happy climate if E is interested in appraising the best possible performance rather than the influence of frustration on performance.

E and John engage in some conversation about school lessons with the home teacher. E tactfully suggests that John probably has not had much opportunity to draw pictures and designs because his teacher does not have enough time to give him such tasks. John responds quickly to this offered alibi and agrees that he never has done anything like "this." Sometimes he colors in a book and gets a kick out of picking "nice" colors. He mirthfully describes how he likes to choose "funny" colors; recently he colored a boy's pants pink and made his jacket green with yellow polka dots. His mother and he thought that this was "very funny" and had a "good laugh" about it. "Imagine, yellow polka dots for a boy and pink pants! But I have a pink shirt; many people wear pink shirts. I like nice clothes; my father says I am a flashy dresser. Do you like my tie?"

E suggests that since John is so good at talking and knows many words, he might like to try how many words he knows of some she might ask him.

ORAL VOCABULARY (T:XII:2)

A list of words is to be defined by the child.

E: "What is a bicycle?" Then she asks for definitions of knife, hat, letter, umbrella, cushion, nail. Without any hesitation, John gives definitions such as "You ride it." "You cut with it."

He is completely sure of himself and gives his answers magnanimously in a slightly high-handed fashion; he cannot conceal his pleasure in the easy task. Gradually he comes to meet more difficult words. But an unfamiliar one does not baffle him; he gets clues from sounds of words, or simply uses a word over again. For example: E: "Sword." John: "You *saw* wood with a *saw*." E: "Nuisance." John: "When your mother says 'What a nuisance!' " E: "What does she mean?" John: "When something is gone, when she can't find her glasses." E: "Chattel." John: "It is almost like chapel—you go to church."

(By WISC standards, John's raw score is twenty-eight, which is equivalent to a mental age of nine years two months.)

SIMILARITIES AND DIFFERENCES (T:IX:3)

The child is asked in what way two objects are alike and in what way they are different.

E: "Honey—glue." John: "Honey is almost like glue. Glue comes in a little bottle and it is sticky, just like honey. It sticks. You eat it on your bread." E: "In what way are they the same? What way are they different?" John: "They are both sticky, but you can't eat glue. You use it to glue a thing that is broken."

E: "Pen—pencil." John: "I know something. They both begin with a 'p.' A pencil is longer." E: "What do you mean, longer?" John: "When a pencil is almost new it is longer than a pen." E: "They are the same because they have a 'p' and they are different because?" John: "Because the pencil is longer—it is a longer word—it has more letters."

E: "Banana—lemon." John: "I do not know how they spell." E: "Do not think about how they spell. Just what they are and look like." John: "They look yellow—but the lemon does not taste good. It is sour. You can't eat it; you can make lemonade and you eat a banana. They are good."

E: "Shoe—glove." John: "They are to wear. You wear the shoe and you wear the glove." E: "What about the shoe?" John: "You shine it. You wear it on your feet." E: "And the glove?" John: "You wear it for boxing. I have seen them; great, big ones." E: "How are they the same?" John: "They are not the same like other gloves." E: "How are they the same as shoes?" John: "They are not the same—but you can wear them all."

John's performance gives a good picture of the quality of his reasoning. John comes to find some barely acceptable solution only when suggestions and directions are repeated. He has no system. He follows every lead which comes his way (longer pencil becomes longer word, the glove is worn not on the hand but for boxing, etc.). There is no logical order in the choice of his criteria; interspersed are many extraneous, loosely connected, personal associations.

SIMILARITIES AMONG THREE THINGS (T:IX:4)

Child is asked in what way three things are alike.

E: "Snake, cow, sparrow." John: "The cow walks, the snake creeps and the sparrow is a bird—it flies." E: "How are they alike?" John: "They all walk, but the sparrow flies."

E: "Rose, potato, tree." John: "They both grow." E: "What does?" John: "The rose and the tree. I do not know about the potato. You eat it."

E: "Knifeblade, penny, piece of wire." John: "You can hurt yourself with the blade when you are not careful." E: "And the penny and the piece of wire?" John: "The penny you can buy something with; and the piece of wire—I do not know—you wire things."

John obviously cannot think of similarity among all three items. He thinks of two or only one item at a time, and forgets the initial instructions. With three items failed and the time running short, this task is abandoned.

PICTURE ARRANGEMENT (T:IX:10)

FIRE. Slow (twenty seconds) but correct. (Four points.)

BURGLAR. Correct in fifteen seconds. (Five points.)

FARMER. He places the cards in the order QRTS. (No credit.) His verbal explanation is: "Here he is putting the seeds in his garden (Q); he puts up a scarecrow (R); he takes it to town (T); here he eats it and thinks it is good (S)."

PICNIC. He places the cards in the order GEFH. (No credit.) He says: "He eats the chicken (G); he follows them (E); here he follows them (F), and then they say 'What happened?' (H)."

SLEEPER. He places cards EPRCY. (No credit.) He explains: "He is asleep (E); then he wakes up (P); he eats his breakfast (R); here he runs to work (C); here he is home again and he is tired again (Y)."

RAIN. John forgets that he has to rearrange the given order, EARSMT. Instead, he explains each picture: "He is all wet and just stands there (E); here he is talking to her in the window (A); and she gives him the umbrella, he walks away (R)." John skips the next two pictures (S, M), points to T and says, "Here it is raining hard and he runs." E points to picture of woman who tries to give the umbrella to the man (M), asks, "How about this?" John: "She is talking to him." (No credit.)

GARDENER. He places cards ERIFSH. (No credit.) His explanation is: "He goes fishing (E); and here he is asleep (R); and here he digs in the garden (I), and his wife tells him to do it."

He skips over the last two cards. (By WISC standards, his raw score is seventeen, which is equivalent to a mental age of seven years ten months.)

John's arrangements are interesting and confirm previously noted characteristics of his reasoning processes. Almost always (except in Rain), he seems to have a more or less acceptable "story." However, neither his manner nor his words nor his arrangements themselves indicate the pictures are organized in one coherent context. Events follow by association rather than by causal relationships. He does not consider details and is not puzzled by factors which contradict each other. He is fully satisfied with a superficial relation among some of them.

BLOCK DESIGNS (T:VII:7 AND FIGURE 13)

CARDS I AND II. Correct.

CARD III. For the yellow triangles in the upper corners, he places two all-yellow blocks at an angle, then puts one blue below; he seems bewildered and cannot think what to do next. E demonstrates. On repetition, he succeeds, but he is obviously not interested.

CARD IV. John says, "I can't do these." He pushes blocks around and has no desire to continue. E: "You do not like these much?" John: "I can't do them. I do not like them."

E says, "Let us do things you can do well."

ARITHMETIC FACTS (T:XI:3)

ADDITION. E: "Five and three." John is pleased, and quickly answers, "Eight." E: "Five and four." Again John responds with ease, "Nine." E: "Six and eight." He hesitates a moment, then answers correctly. Also answers correctly to "fifteen and two."

SUBTRACTION. E: "Ten, take away seven." John is correct. E: "Twelve, take away four." He finds the answer more slowly than before, but gives it correctly. E: "Eighteen, take away five." He is correct.

MULTIPLICATION. E: "Five times eight." John solves this problem by using his fingers, murmuring to himself, "One times eight is eight (he holds on to his thumb), two times eight is sixteen (proceeds to index finger), three times eight," etc. He reaches "five times eight," and has the correct answer, forty. E: "Seven times three." John:

"That is three's—I know them. Seven three's is twenty-one, eight three's is twenty-four, nine three's is twenty-seven . . ."

ARITHMETIC PROBLEMS (T:XI:5)

E asks the child, "At seven cents each, what will three pencils cost?" John: "I do not know how to do this, I only know multiplications." E says, "This is multiplication," and repeats the problem, emphasizing seven and three; John is relieved, repeats "Seven three's . . . seven three's is twenty-one." E: "A man earns thirty-six dollars; he is paid four dollars a day. How many days did he work?" John: "I can't do these. My teacher does not have these."

E: "Let us try this one; you will find it easy. James had eight marbles and he bought six more. How many marbles did he have altogether?" John: "That is eight and six, I know, it is fourteen." E: "A boy had twelve newspapers and he sold five. How many did he have left?" John: "Seventeen." E: "How come?" John: "It is twelve and five; that is seventeen." E: "He sold five." John: "He had five left." E: "First he had twelve." (She produces twelve blocks.) "Here, these are the twelve newspapers; now somebody comes and says, 'I want five of these newspapers.' You take five of those away." John does. E continues, "How many does he have left?" John: "He has all those left." He counts seven. "He has seven left." E: "Suppose he had had only five newspapers, and somebody bought three of them?" John: "He would have two left." E: "Suppose he had twenty-five newspapers, and sold eleven, how many would he have left?" John: "That is hard." E: "Is it addition, subtraction, or multiplication?" John: "I think it is subtraction."

John has learned simple arithmetic facts reasonably well, but he has considerable difficulty when it comes to applying these to actual simple problems. He does not recognize at a glance what kind of operation he should use. He still understands number facts best if they are presented in concrete ways.

The session is closed.

COMMENT

At twelve John is still the friendly, overtly sociable child he was in earlier years. He still is passive and nonaggressive. When he becomes disturbed, he shows it immediately. His irritations seem to be directly related to specific causes and can be quickly relieved. There are no obvious signs of hidden and repressed fears. He does not seem to have the emotional reticence of many preadolescent children. His affects seem flat and his reactions direct and obvious. This impression emerges from his attitude and from the form and content of his responses during this examination.

John continues to rely heavily on his verbal ability. He still uses language for contact more than for information. His ability to use words and to make associations easily has allowed him to extend his skills into the reading field. Reading, like language, remains for him an art, but not a tool. Learning, other than by rote and simple association, is still difficult and cumbersome for him, since he has short attention spans and cannot easily organize facts. His reasoning, though better developed than before, proceeds by small spurts. He still is unable to coordinate many factors or to approach several from one angle alone. His form comprehension has remained poor. Intellectually, he has progressed at his previous borderline rate; at twelve he has the reasoning ability of a seven- to eight-year-old and shows characteristic signs of brain injury.

His physical disability has had a decisive influence on his personality development. His physical dependency has kept him in the closest relationship to his parents; his numerous but superficial contacts with outsiders have not, as yet, made him face conflicting responsibilities or loyalties. Underdeveloped physically, he appears without inner drive to rebel against protection. His parents' love and approval still satisfy his emotional needs. Since there has been very little cause for friction, he has remained secure and cheerful. His family understands his simple reactions and has been able either to prevent or quickly relieve causes of irritation. The alibi of his helplessness and lack of experience has allowed them to minimize many of his immature or peculiar traits and to focus their distress on his physical problems. His reasoning difficulties hardly become an issue at home, since he has no occasion for any but the simplest decisions. There and in the neighborhood his so-called good memory wins him prizes. There is no cause for embarrassment when he is with other children because he never competes with them on equal terms. The only area of real difficulty is academic work. There he senses his limitations and becomes unhappy when pressed. However, both his teacher and his parents have through the years managed to avoid frustration through adjustments in program and praise for his accomplishments.

Up to this age John has been able to fulfill the demands of his life situation in spite of his limited abilities. He has preserved his self-respect and has developed a serene enough personality and a pattern of adjustment which fit his situation.

In planning for the future one must consider whether any radical changes would bring gains. Theoretically, John might profit from contact with other children in a special class or even away from home in an institution. This would probably not help him much academically; he works best with individual attention and a specialized program and would find it hard to learn in a group. Undoubtedly, he would gather new social experiences, though not necessarily happy ones. His peculiar brand of social skills would probably be less successful in a group than they are at home and in the neighborhood. If John should find less sympathetic attitudes in more aggressive surroundings, he would become bewildered, confused, and insecure.

John's mental ability will hardly permit him to take care of himself as a physically handicapped individual. He will be happier and make a better contribution to those who must protect him if he is allowed to preserve his equilibrium and use his social graces as best he can. His family are prepared and willing to arrange their future accordingly.

STAGES OF DEVELOPMENT AND THEIR PROBLEMS

John's personality development through the years follows a pattern that has been found to be characteristic of children with hydrocephalus. The same pattern, with some variations, is characteristic also of children with other cerebral malfunctions such as microcephaly, porencephaly, or some types of scaphocephaly.

John is talkative, sociable, and friendly, but has intellectual difficulties which become more apparent as years go by. The smiling *baby* whose outsized head gave him an unusual appearance for his age, becomes a responsive, humorous *preschool* child whose ready phrases and quick associations make him seem bright to the casual observer. He is easily amused; he depends on memory rather than on reasoning power. He has little comprehension or interest in form materials and enjoys only a very few simple play activities. At *seven* his language is fluent but has very little thought content. He has difficulty in learning in new situations. He is less sure of himself than he was and therefore likes to cling to patterns of activity which he knows well. His perceptuo-motor difficulties have become prominent. He still wins praise for his talkativeness and sociable manners and can still impress outsiders with his glib phrases. While his development seems satisfactory on the surface, his immaturity becomes gradually more apparent to people who know him well. At *twelve* John's intellectual difficulties have become more obvious; he is still fluent in speech, but his reasoning difficulties and his lack of comprehension show up even in his language performances, which no longer appear spectacular even on the surface. Though he is able to read, he understands but little of what he reads. His severe perceptuomotor distortions disturb much of his functioning.

John's severe motor handicap has given him some advantages which many other children suffering from similar malformations of the brain do not enjoy. His physical disability is more sadly in evidence than his mental retardation. His restricted life protects him from demands which he would be unable to cope with. Just as he cannot enter into cooperative play situations in his preschool years, so he is unable to start school at the proper age and is spared the necessity of learning at the age when normal children start their first experiences in the outside world. But, at the same time, he can use his social skills in contacts with grown-ups. For John, as for other severely handicapped children, social assets are more important means of satisfaction than they are for normal children. His physical helplessness also shields him in other ways; having faced John's need for permanent protection for physical reasons, his parents are in no hurry to see him grow up. On the contrary, they more or less dread the time when he may be mentally capable but physically unable to be independent.

Children who, like John, are hydrocephalic and mentally retarded, but who are more mobile than he, have somewhat different problems. These may influence their emotional attitude and personality development. Basically, however, there is much similarity in the psychological make-up of many children with hydrocephalus. The study of their psychological case records shows a pattern of personality development like that described for John.[1]

[1] This discussion is based on the study of case records of 18 children with hydrocephalus. Two of these children do not fit the developmental pattern described here; one had a severe pneumonia in early infancy, and the other's condition was complicated by deafness acquired through meningitis. Of the 18 children, 13 had two psychological examinations, 3 had more than two, and 2 had one only. (Total number of examinations was 41.)

At last examination the ages of these children were under six in 2 cases, six to ten in 11 cases, over ten in 5 cases.

Interval between first and last examinations was two years in 4 cases, more than

As babies up to about two years of age they are frequently described as alert, friendly, responsive, and content. They have the usual social tricks at their disposal at the proper ages and say their first words early. They are mostly even tempered, though some are described as irritable in strange situations. Their parents usually have no special complaints. The pediatricans who notice the abnormal growth of their heads are frequently concerned with the physical danger only and have no doubts that the babies have, up to now, developed normally, if not at a superior rate. Therefore, these children are only rarely referred for psychological examinations at an early age. But even in early infancy one can detect a significant discrepancy between abilities in social and adaptive areas. These babies, when left alone in their own company, entertain themselves rather simply with rhythmic movements of hands, feet, or body; they like to bang objects indiscriminately, as much younger children do. When handling blocks (T:I), pellet and bottle, ring and string, or playing with hidden objects (T:V:4,6–8), the same babies often do very poorly. When they are a bit older, they also fail in three-figure formboards, pegboards, and nested boxes (T:IV:1–3,5). The family may report that the child uses some "words" in specific situations. Since E may use unfamiliar materials in an unfamiliar setting, the child may not produce these words during the observation period. Even at this early age attention difficulties can be noticed when the child's interest in a toy dwindles so quickly that it has to be restimulated repeatedly. Around two years of age situations involving retrieving after delay (T:V:5) may be failed. A lack of comprehension of spatial relationships and failure to observe will be the reason, even though the baby seems greatly amused by these games and enjoys their social character. Most of these babies excel in social tricks (T:XI:1) and love to display them; they seem aware of and responsive to their audiences.

The psychologist must at this stage try to unveil and describe the child's liabilities and assets by studying discrepancies among skills in various areas. The child's ability to reason properly in the future is best predicted from his performances in adaptive tasks which may show how well he can comprehend relationships. His social skill and charm, however, may forecast his tendency to be pleasant, contented, and friendly.

---

three years in 3 cases, more than five years in 5 cases, more than eight years in 4 cases.

Mental ability at last examination was above normal in 0 case, normal in 2 cases (12%), borderline in 11 cases (61%), below borderline in 5 cases (27%).

Four of these children were not walking by the age of six.

The psychological evaluation then helps to give direction to the parents' expectations. It leads them to hope for excellency in personality traits rather than in intellectual achievements. The psychologist must be cautious with predictions, especially with pessimistic ones, at this early age. Often these are not yet in order and only undermine the young parents' enthusiasm, create gloom and defiance, and tend to alienate them from the psychologist, who may be needed for future guidance in other phases of the child's development. Mentioning casually and sympathetically some less favorable symptoms which were observed often leads young parents far enough toward a more realistic attitude. However, guesses concerning the far future rarely serve a useful purpose except in special cases, such as adoptions.

For many children of this group *the preschool years* are the most satisfying and proudest of their careers. At this stage they shine in verbal fluency and social graces. Most of them have an impressive vocabulary of "big" words. They thrive on the approval which usually is given to them lavishly. Some have a tendency to talk like grown-ups; they may prefer the company of adults to that of other children, whose activities are apt to confuse and fatigue them. Most of these children are described as sweet and happy. Some still show signs of irritability in strange situations, and a few are described as resistant to new suggestions.

Psychological examinations are usually requested for social reasons rather than because of doubts about mental functioning. The parents are often anxious to discuss what kind of school group would be best suited for their odd-looking and sometimes odd-mannered child. They may rave about their child's good memory, his interest in songs, commercials, stories, and general conversation. However, frequently they themselves have been wondering about his lack of interest in paper-and-pencil activities or games and puzzles. They may describe rather simple and monotonous favorite play activities.

The psychological examination usually confirms such reports; one finds, in most cases, a superficially sociable child. He is delighted to talk and to be with people but he seems essentially uninterested in a give-and-take conversation. Instead of exchanging information, he exchanges verbal patterns. He does not stay with one topic for any length of time, but goes off on a tangent. Such children usually do well on verbal tests such as picture description (T:II:6) and memory for sentences (T:VIII:7). They also may succeed, through quick verbal associations, in opposite analogies (T:IX:5) or pictorial identification (T:II:9). Their performances in oral vocabulary (T:XII:2) or picture vocabulary (T:II:7) may be just about up to age level. Often it seems surprising that they do not perform better in these tests, since they are so fluent in speech and use elaborate words. Many of these same children fail in verbal tasks which call for reasoning and comprehension; they may be unable to succeed in pictorial identification in reverse (T:II:9), memory for pictures (T:II:8), or comprehension of pictured events (T:II:6). Their lack of perceptual skills is evidenced in nonverbal tasks such as formboards (T:IV:2–6,10), mutilated pictures (T:IX: 12), discrimination of animal pictures (T:II:10), or matching forms (T:VI:4,6). Blockbuilding and drawing are frequently primitive (T:I:2 and III:1–6); a tendency prevails to build for the sake of piling blocks or to draw for the sake of making marks. Like younger children, they are apt to have no plan; they make running comments on what they do and rapidly change designations for their productions. Their short attention spans are seen in these tasks, as in many others.

Despite their apparently carefree and happy attitudes, one senses in many children of this group an undercurrent of anxiety; their voices turn tense and insistent and their manner becomes demanding when they suspect any pressure. In spite of their obvious pleasure in contact with people, they like to have it on their own terms. They use the other person as an animated sounding board for their talk, but establish loose personal ties only. Even older children reserve emotional relationships for their immediate families, but with them, too, they seem somewhat rigid and emotionally flat.

For children of this group, global numerical test results are often especially deceiving, since the most commonly used scales favor verbal facility at the preschool age level. Some children reach scores that are within normal limits. However, qualitative analysis reveals their difficulties in reasoning, attention, and comprehension, and suggests caution. Often it is wise to delay school entrance beyond the age at which the child becomes eligible. Immediate failure in academic situations would confuse him and deflate his self-esteem too suddenly. He is not yet prepared for such setbacks since he has, up to now, only been admired for his "brightness." Poise and pleasant disposition, however, are among his biggest assets and must be preserved as much as possible. He may need them later when he has to face more critical and disparaging attitudes from those who will be puzzled by his ways and looks.

Most parents are apt to accept such a view when it is presented to them sensibly. Many agree that personal happiness is all-important. Mothers are frequently delighted to keep so companionable a child at home for a year longer. Only a few may react differently and be ready to thrust him early into a career of competition.

Between the ages of six and ten children of this group meet varying situations and experience varying degrees of difficulty. Some with relatively mild deformities have a certain amount of social success once they enter school. Often they look slightly older than their classmates and appear to act in a somewhat more mature way. Therefore they frequently gain prestige, at least temporarily. Having been the center of adult attention for some time, some children act bossy and demanding; they may even become the petulant leaders of younger groups. In some school settings they have appeal for a teacher who likes their unretiring, precocious manners and their social poise. Especially in schools which emphasize rote learning, some children get along well owing to their ability to recite poems and prayers, and to spell words and repeat arithmetic facts. Other children are less fortunate; their disabilities are more apparent. Some become awed and confused in school. Some are too immature and mild-mannered, so that they remain friendly outsiders and onlookers only. Children who are able to go to school at all are usually in normal class situations at this age. Some with serious motor impairment are not in school, but may have a home teacher.

To their families, most children of this group appear happy, chatty, and easy to be with. Tension and nervousness may be observed in increasingly frequent instances, especially in connection with outside demands. At home, mothers frequently manage to avoid emotional outbursts since immediate causes of strain are usually obvious. Pressure upsets these children easily, whereas affection and praise restore them quickly. Since they are usually not very enterprising except in words, they are not apt to get themselves into tight spots. Their verbal vivaciousness and their interest in neighborhood events still gain them satisfaction and immediate esteem.

Psychological examinations are often requested during the elementary school years for various reasons. In some cases failure in reading comprehension and arithmetic problems worries teachers and parents, who start to raise the question of special class placement. Other children are losing their popularity because they are too bossy and seem to be "poor sports." Others seem to their parents "too good" and too passive for this world. Still others present no obvious problems, but their families remember previous pessimistic predictions made by pediatricians and neurosurgeons. They now want to show or be told how well things have turned out.

The psychologist most frequently finds these children friendly but slightly tense in the examination. Often they have learned to avoid difficult situations better than they did before. They still manage to direct conversation along lines with which they are familiar. They may appear chatty and communicative; they are apt to ask E personal questions of the kind often asked by younger children, but commonly considered "nosey" in older ones. They still prefer verbal tasks to nonverbal ones. They may volunteer to recite arithmetic facts (T:XI:3), spell words (T:XI:9), and the like, but frequently they do extremely poorly with formboards and on object assembly tests (T:IV:7–12). Usually they have difficulty with block designs (T:VII:7,8) and memory for design tests (T:VII:1,2,4). Verbal tests which demand reasoning are difficult for them too. Those which require the organization of varied facts, such as similarities and differences (T:IX:3) and comprehension (T:X:3), are less easy for them than reiteration of learned items of information (T:XI:10) or activation of verbal associations in opposite analogies (T:IX:5). These same children do well in repeating sentences from memory or in memory for stories (T:VIII:4,7); they often reproduce these almost literally, but are unable to explain or repeat in their own words the content of what they recite. There is frequently a significant discrepancy between ability to repeat digits forward and to say digits in reverse (T:VIII:5,6), the latter being considerably lower.

Often one senses a somewhat moralistic note in these children's manners and responses. They often start their explanations in picture absurdities, verbal absurdities, or picture arrangements (T:IX:6,10,11) with "he should" or "he should not." They are apt to see only this single aspect of a situation and thereby show restricted thinking and a unilateral authoritative moral code. Immature children often cling to these longer than normal, but handicapped children especially seem to find safety and approval in mimicking what they believe to be adult standards.

More or less extreme irregularities of mental functioning add up to borderline ratings in a large majority of hydrocephalic children. In some instances, numerical ratings at elementary school age still reach the lower ranges of normal. Rarely do these numerical ratings do justice to the complex difficulties of these children. Their means of adjustment to life situations become less and less effective as they grow older. As they become less able to live up to earlier expectations, they come to sense the loss of prestige that is setting in. Some children may feebly try to maintain it with tools which were useful in earlier life; they remain talkative and undiscriminating, and therefore often appear tactless and out-of-place whereas they seemed amusing when younger. In spite of their superficially easygoing ways, one may note in some a lack of emotional warmth and contact. Others become more cautious and timid. Losing their carefree, outgoing attitude, they become gradually more dull and more repetitive.

When in the following years the pressure of normal school groups becomes too great, special class placement becomes more appropriate for many children. In their home life, many cling to their families. They feel rejected and ridiculed by their contemporaries. Some develop large appetites for which they gain some reputation. They frequently become obese, heavy, and slow in their movements. To families and outsiders, some children may appear to deteriorate, since they seem less well off than they were in their earlier, "brighter" years. In reality, their endowment has not changed for the worse; it is simply that the skills which were effective then no longer suffice. Disabilities which were present but relatively unobtrusive in early years become a true hindrance later on.

The psychologist and other advisers may foresee such developments and through the years try to prepare the family for them. This is often a difficult task. Here, as with some other types of handicapped children (see Rose and Ann) the level of aspiration must gradually be lowered while the child is still more or less satisfactory to himself and to others and before it becomes too obvious that he cannot live up to his previous prestige. He must keep his chances for limited success wherever it can be found. A comfortable and affectionate surrounding climate must be maintained so that the child can continue to develop into a person who is pleasant to be with. This should be an important and worthwhile goal for many of these children, even if they may always need help for subsistence and decision making.

Part One

CASE PORTRAITS

B—Defects Dating from
Later Injury

Defects Dating from Later Injury

Acquired neurological defects present multiple and serious psychological problems in children, whether or not they are accompanied by permanent, visible, physical damage. Such problems are different in general from those caused by congenital or neonatal defects. Meningitis, encephalitis, thrombosis, brain tumors, or automobile accidents suddenly strike a well child; in the majority of these conditions, the child is dangerously ill for a period of time and then recovers physically more or less rapidly. Immense relief follows the acute period of anxiety. Often attention is focused largely on the residual physical disability, which may still require treatment. Some physicians, impressed by the spectacular recovery, are unaware that psychological and developmental difficulties may result. Others, unwilling to alarm a still shaky family unnecessarily, will be quietly on the lookout for possible difficulties for some months to come and will be ready to act on the first signs.

The role of the psychologist is defined by the doctor's attitude. Some physicians and hospitals make it a practice to consult a psychologist soon after the period of acute illness to determine whether or not the child has sustained permanent psychological damage. In some instances, the psychologist is asked to outline a suitable program for the rehabilitation period and to watch for possible signs of difficulties. In many other cases the psychologist enters the picture only when home or school starts complaining of changes in behavior or learning ability. The psychologist may have only a consulting capacity or may actually join the pediatrician in assuming responsibility for future planning and guidance.

Whether her responsibility is diagnostic, prophylactic, or therapeutic, the psychologist is faced with a set of unusual problems. If she is called in soon after the acute period, she may be somewhat awed by the magnitude and subtlety of her task. It is never easy to examine a child soon after an acute illness. As will be shown later, it is even less easy, except in patients with sensory losses, to detect signs of psychoneurological deviations immediately after the impact of the illness. Tempted to share the attitude of relief and optimism of physicians, ward nurses, and parents, the psychologist is apt to dismiss minor symptoms. Weakness, restlessness, anxiety, irritability, or apathy in a child who has just recovered from serious illness may announce future learning difficulties based on neurological damage. However, they may also be rather obvious effects of serious illness, sudden hospitalization, separation from parents, general fatigue, and treatment procedures.

Psychological appraisal of a child some months after the acute illness presents other problems. It is even then not easy to decide whether, in a particular child, symptoms such as restlessness, irritability, short attention spans, and a tendency to become fatigued are merely aftereffects of disease or whether they are signs of neurological disorder. The psychologist must be cautious in appraising possible sequelae and must avoid being an alarmist and possibly jeopardizing the child's and the family's readjustment to normal daily living.

If the psychologist does not enter the picture until a year or more after illness, the appraisal may often be even more difficult; signs of distorted mental functioning, characteristic of brain injury, may then have become more established and may be more easily discernible, but by that time new emotional situations which need careful analysis and consideration may have crystallized.

Regardless of how long after illness the psychological examination is made, the psychologist tries to get a clear picture of the patient's behavior and status now as it compares with behavior and development previous to the traumatic incident. The climate surrounding the child must be carefully scrutinized. Often in such cases it is peculiarly tense. Parents are brought up sharply against a new reality for which they are totally unprepared. Depending on the severity of the case, the child's position within the family may be profoundly altered by a permanent physical impairment. But emotional reactions of the family may take varied forms even with children whose physical sequelae are transient or altogether negligible; some parents may deny any reminder of difficulty after the period of acute anxiety is over; others may be unable to forget the danger and continue to feel concerned and insecure long after all seems well. Others again may be appalled at the sight of an acquired condition which seems to have "blighted" a formerly perfect and satisfactory child. All such attitudes are important for the child, who is bound to react to them. The more fragile he has become nervously, the more sensitive he may be to pressure, anxiety, or rejection, whether or not these were latent before. With an older child, neighbors, teachers, and playmates enter into the picture. They, too, may develop a new set of attitudes tainted by the awe, curiosity, and glamor that accompany spectacular illness. Each child develops some conception of himself. The child who has been injured may feel that the demands of his environment have changed. But often an older child comes to feel that his own ability to cope with life has been altered. He then may be utterly bewildered and his behavior may become overly aggressive, depressed, slow, meticulous, or anxious.

For all concerned, it helps if the psychologist is able to recognize and to describe, as early as possible, any deviations of functioning which can be traced to the illness and which are reflected in behavior. In subsequent examinations, progress can be appraised. On the basis of psychological findings, ways may be outlined in which to handle new situations and educational problems as they arise. This frequently helps the family, patient, teacher, and pediatrician to meet crises and relieve frustrations through the years.

First, information must be collected about the child as he was in the past. If the right questions are asked, it is usually possible to reconstruct some more or less clear picture of the child as he was before his illness. His emotional, intellectual, and social development through the years can be appraised to some extent. At the same time, an impression can be gained about the climate which surrounded the child from the feelings, thoughts, and expectations of those nearest to him.

The following test sketches illustrate how psychological evaluations may reveal the gradual development of children after an insult to the nervous system. All three children described have only more or less minor physical sequelae; each of them was injured at a different age, and, therefore, at a different stage of development. Thus, each one is faced with different situations and different problems.

ANN

Pneumococcus Meningitis
at Six Months

Ann, the first child of young parents, developed normally up to *six months of age,* when she had a severe pneumococcus meningitis with several right-sided convulsions at the onset. She recovered satisfactorily from the acute illness. On discharge from the hospital, she was alert and smiling and seemed observant. She appeared to be quite tense. Except for a slight tremor in both arms, more noticeable on the right, she seemed to do as well as she had before her illness.

ANN AFTER FOUR MONTHS

The first psychological examination, at *ten and a half months* (four months after discharge), shows a pleasant, active, smiling baby alert to her surroundings. She is interested in everything presented to her; she grasps blocks with either hand, but prefers the left. She hits a block on the table with a block in her hand, she pays attention to the pellet as well as to the bottle (T:V:8), and her comprehension of material seems to be on a ten-month level. Her approaches to small objects such as the pellet are somewhat immature; she pokes at the pellet with index finger outstretched without thumb opposition. She does not spend much time with either material and demands and enjoys a speedy change. She can pull herself up to a standing position and has just started to take a few steps with support. Occasionally she has a very slight tremor of her head. An EEG is reported as normal. Pediatrician and psychologist together can assure the parents that Ann's development is progressing satisfactorily and that she can be considered a normal baby. Ann's parents are delighted with her progress. She is the center of attention in a closely knit family where she is the only child. There is apparently a tendency to keep the baby overstimulated through fussing and loving. This seems to explain Ann's apparent tension and overresponsiveness.

ANN AFTER ONE YEAR

Ann returns at the age of *eighteen months,* one year after the illness. To her parents and her pediatrician she seems to be fully recovered. She has been walking since the age of thirteen months. She still walks somewhat clumsily on a wide base, but gets around speedily. In the examining situation she is lively and interested; she likes to play with everything presented to her and approaches things hastily and over-enthusiastically. She picks up blocks (T:I:1) and bangs them vigorously. She puts them in and out of boxes (T:I:3) without ever putting all of them in or all of them out. She does not attempt any block constructions and pays no attention to E's models (T:I:2). She enjoys the pegboards (T:IV:1) in which she tries to fit the round pegs in their holes. When she cannot find the hole immediately, she lays the peg hastily on the board and reaches for the next peg. She does not learn to discriminate between round and square pegs. She fits three of five nested boxes (T:IV:3) correctly, but turns the largest one upside down over the smaller boxes. She seems satisfied with this arrangement, loses interest, and pays no further attention to E's demonstration. In these adaptive tasks, which also test form discrimination, Ann's performances rate only near the fifteen-month level. Ann obviously likes contact with people; she jabbers continually, though she is unintelligible to all except her immediate family. Activities which have social elements are handled better than any others. When retrieving objects from containers (T:V:8), she gleefully reproduces the object E has made disappear before her eyes. Here as well as in the following of simple commands, she performs at approximately an eighteen-month level. When retrieving objects at a distance (T:V:6), she strains eagerly and directly toward them even if they are clearly out of her reach. She does not see or use intermediaries until she has been shown by E how to do it.

Some of the traits noticed in the first examination now seem slightly intensified. She is still tense and has short attention spans; also, she has some very slight difficulties in form comprehension. These symptoms cause the psychologist to have some doubts regarding Ann's future progress. However, she must agree with the pediatrician that these signs would most likely pass unnoticed in a child of Ann's age who did not have her medical history.

ANN AFTER TWO YEARS

Some apprehension about Ann's development increases in the next year's visit; Ann, now *two years six months,* appears to be in excellent condition physically. She looks vigorous and healthy. Mentally, she seems lively, alert, and constantly on the go. In the psychological examination, she appears unduly tense and excitable. She has a high-pitched voice; she talks a great deal but does not use sentences, enunciates poorly, and stammers some. Her name vocabulary proves to be good when she can be persuaded to sit long enough with a picture book (T:II) or with small toys. In general, she repeats what is said to her. She is interested in all materials presented to her, but does not stay with them long enough to investigate them properly. She places forms correctly once in the three-figure formboard (T:IV:5), but does not adjust to the rotation of the board and becomes impatient. She correctly fits round pegs in Wallin pegboard A, and with interruptions and some difficulty also fits square pegs in Wallin pegboard B (T:IV:1,2). She is unreliable in her discrimination between round and square pegs. It is not easy to decide whether Ann's immature performances with form material are due to her impatience or to a lack of form comprehension. One wonders again when with crayon and paper (T:III:1,4) Ann pays no attention to demonstration but scribbles undiscriminatingly and hastily. Then she gets up, presses the crayon on her father, and tries to have him draw a picture for her. She runs away from him before he has finished. Both parents try to persuade Ann to be "good" and more cooperative. They explain with some embarrassment that they are not surprised about her "bad" behavior here, because she is disobedient and "spoiled." Everybody loves her and showers her with affection; she is a charmer and a whirlwind at home. She gets everybody to do what she wants them to and is stubborn in many ways. Her mother finds toilet training especially difficult. She describes how Ann, on certain days, builds up to a "needed" spanking.

There seems to be a good deal of well-meant pressure and confusion of authority around Ann. These may explain quite well Ann's erratic, though cheerful, behavior and her immature actions. Yet the possibility of some cerebral damage cannot be excluded. While E mentions this to the pediatrician, she sees no point in dwelling on this suspicion in her conversation with the parents. Discussion of management problems and how to solve them seems to be of more immediate value.

ANN AFTER TWO YEARS NINE MONTHS

Nine months later, at the age of *three years three months,* Ann has not changed very much essentially, though she has made some steady progress. She is now very talkative, uses sentences, but still has rather poor enunciation. She continues to be slow in adapting to new tasks; she still has inadequate form comprehension. She is happy and pleasant when allowed to do what she pleases, but is very flighty and resistant to suggestions. Ann has had a convulsion associated with tonsillitis and fever. Her parents have become apprehensive, but try to believe that an isolated convulsion with fever may be of no consequence or foreboding. Psychological symptoms of neurological involvement, however, can no longer be minimized, even if some of Ann's behavior difficulties may well be increased by her family's mounting apprehension.

ANN AFTER MORE THAN THREE YEARS

Seven months later, at age *three years ten months,* Ann has a severe cerebral episode with several long-lasting, generalized convulsions, high fever, and a right hemiplegia involving face, arm, and leg. She has an almost complete aphasia, but is still able to say a very few single words which she pronounces badly. During the following four weeks she improves some, gains back more language, and gradually recovers more use of her arm and leg. She is, however, essentially uninterested in her environment. She picks up objects here and there, carries them around, and loses them. She plays with nothing consistently. She is impulsive and primitive in her social relationships. Eager to be near people, she undiscriminatingly either kisses or bites them. She has severe mood swings; most of the time she is bland, friendly, and somewhat airy, but she has sudden severe temper tantrums, apparently without provocation. She has a tendency to run into things and probably has a restricted field of vision. Compared with her status in her last psychological examination, her condition seems severely deteriorated. At the time of Ann's discharge from the hospital, five weeks after the onset of this illness, her mother had a second baby. But Ann goes home and is taken care of with great patience and affection.

ANN AFTER FOUR YEARS

One year later, at age *four years eleven months,* Ann returns. The psychological study must depend on observation rather than testing because she is still extremely active and stimulus bound; she cannot stay with any activity for any length of time. She derives no satisfaction from any one material or accomplishment, but restlessly roams through the room and the hall. Presented with a Seguin formboard (T:IV:6), she picks up a form, places it haphazardly in the correct hole first, and immediately afterwards puts it in a wrong hole. She talks incessantly, occasionally in relation to an immediate stimulus, more often, however, in repetitive phrases carried over from another situation. Though her vocabulary has obviously increased in the past year, she is unreliable in the proper use of names (T:II:7,11). She is apt to call a horse a dog, but immediately afterwards, in a new connection, may name it correctly.

The child's attitude and behavior indicate permanent damage to her learning ability. She has, however, a friendly, happy, and rather charming sociable manner. She must feel secure and happy with those around her. Though she probably is very trying at home, she is apparently still being handled with affection and skill. With another normal child in the picture, Ann's mother can be more relaxed with her, and no longer has to focus all her eagerness on Ann. Ann's hemiplegia is still present, though improving; her intermittent convulsions give her a respectable alibi of illness. Her mother is able to cope more calmly with this distressing situation than she did in earlier years when Ann's rather minor behavior difficulties disturbed her far more.

ANN AFTER SIX YEARS

Ann returns two years later for reevaluation, at age *six years ten months.* She still has a mild hemiplegia and uses her left hand predominantly. She has had some convulsions at monthly intervals earlier in the intermittent period, but these are now well controlled by medication. Her parents find her much improved and are much encouraged. She is in the first grade, with an experienced and understanding teacher, who has known both parents from childhood on. Ann loves school and is apparently protected and made much of by the other children. She still spends much time with her grandparents, whose continued devotion has been a great help all around. Ann's mother is busy with a third baby, but does find that with her sisters around, Ann is better off than she was before. She adores her sisters and likes to be the "big girl."

Ann, looking pretty and angelic, is immediately friendly with E. She sits down without hesitation.

Seguin Formboard (T:IV:6)

She immediately knows what to do, places two forms correctly, then tries another one in a wrong place, but leaves it there without adjusting it, picks up another inset, and places it correctly. She hardly seems to notice when a form does not fit where she has left it. She is hasty and absent-minded, and deals with all the insets in the same way, regardless of their degree of difficulty. Ann keeps on chatting; she is filled with news about her sisters; all of it is reported in a sketchy, disconnected, and repetitive fashion, as, "Susan is a bad dirl . . . she has to stay home . . . she is still a little dirl . . . I am a big dirl," etc. When E tries to interrupt the flow of conversation and to invite her to pay more attention to the formboard, Ann obeys pleasantly and continues with two correct placements. However, this does not last long enough. E now picks up one form after another for her, and asks with each, "Where do you think *this* goes?" Ann repeats the question each time and proceeds to find the correct spot. The same pattern persists through the further stages of the examination.

Mare and Foal Picture Board (T:IV:13)

While some of her trials are nonsensical, in others she brings a piece immediately to the correct hole, but before placing it forgets what she wanted to do. Her performances in these and other formboard tests range from a three- to five-year level. The level of her performances depends on the degree of attention she can muster and on the amount of support she receives to maintain it. She does best with constant re-stimulation.

Blockbuilding (T:I:2,4 and Figure 1)

Green and yellow blocks.

OBLIQUE AND STRAIGHT BRIDGES. She copies the two bridges immediately and correctly.

SIX-CUBE PYRAMID. (In two colors.) She arranges blocks

without spaces in between, later corrects it. She uses two colors, but not in correct arrangement.

SERIAL PATTERNS (T:I:5)

Pattern alternating two green, one yellow, two green blocks.

She comprehends the construction of the pattern and goes on correctly until she runs out of green blocks. She does not become perturbed by this, but continues to add all remaining yellow blocks. E: "Is it all right? Is it all the way the two green and one yellow?" Ann glances at the row and tentatively answers, "Yes . . . no." E: "What could we do to have it only two green and one yellow all the way?" Ann does not think of removing the superfluous yellow blocks, but cheerfully declares, "We will do it all over again." She scatters the blocks and lines them up without any order. She seems pleased to show her good will, but has forgotten the directions. E gets the impression that Ann is familiar with experiences of this kind; she seems accustomed to being asked to improve on some task, yet she has no effective way of correcting errors and cannot learn easily from experience. She offers to repeat "all over" as the only means of mending errors.

Ann's flightiness precludes consistent success in learning tasks such as:

MEMORY FOR PICTURES (T:II:8)

She understands the principle of the procedure. In the first series (consisting of three pictures of which one is removed while she is not looking), she responds correctly. When at a later stage of the examination the procedure is twice repeated with five pictures, she succeeds once, responding for this short moment on a level equal to that of five-year-olds. In between, however, Ann becomes distracted by the pictures. Seeing the picture of the flag, she gets up, stands straight, and explains, "We have one in school . . . boys and girls pledge allegiance to it." Then she flits to the window and starts to look around, saying, "Who lives in that house over there?" Ann is fluent in phrases and acquired verbal patterns. She sounds polite and socially attractive when she makes remarks such as, "You have very nice games," or, "What a lovely view you have from your window."

Her good vocabulary can be seen in other tasks, such as:

ANIMAL PICTURES (T:II:11)

NAMING. She names all of the twelve pictured animals correctly and without any hesitation.

Her difficulties in reasoning are obvious in several instances. Especially illustrative is one of her responses in:

PICTURE ABSURDITIES (T:IX:11)

CAT AND MICE. Ann: "It is a cat and her kittens." E: "What about them?" Ann: "They are playing." E: "Are they tiny kittens?" Ann: "No, they are mice, three little mice." E: "How many are there?" Ann starts counting correctly to five by putting her finger on each mouse. However, she continues to make the round to eleven. E: "Which is the biggest mouse?" Ann points to the cat. E: "Which is the smallest one?" Ann points correctly to the smallest mouse. E: "Which is the biggest mouse?" Ann again shows the cat. E: "You know, you said before that this is the cat; the others are mice. Which is the biggest of them?" Ann points correctly. E: "Which mouse has the longest tail?" Ann points to the cat's tail. When asked for the the biggest mouse, or the longest tail of a mouse, Ann follows her immediate impulse and responds either to "tail" or to "biggest" without paying attention to any of the restricting qualifications. She has obvious difficulty in thinking of several things at once.

MAN IN TREE. Ann: "He should not climb, he may break his arm." (By Revised Stanford-Binet standards, Ann fails on seven-year level.)

Simple, egocentric projection, in general typical for younger age levels, can be seen in Ann's performances toward the end of the examination, when the newness and the attractions of the situation start to wear off.

PICTURE COMPLETION (T:IX:12)

E shows picture of coat with sleeve missing, asking, "What is missing?" Ann: "A button . . . a buttonhole." To picture of cat with tail missing, Ann responds, "Somebody to play with." To bird with wing missing, she says, "He wants to see his Mommy." To face of man with mouth missing, she says, "He wants to go home."

Interpreting these responses as a wish to get away and look for her mother, E invites Ann to bring her mother to show her what she has been doing. Ann responds with enthusiasm and proudly shows her mother into the room. She now gladly consents to:

DRAWING A LADY (T:III:3)

Much scribbling and erasing ensues. The final product has a head, eyes, nose, arms, hands with five fingers each, legs, feet, and some scribbles later interpreted as buttons. It resembles in many ways drawings of human figures commonly produced by children at about five years of age. It shows unusual features, however; it is scribbled in a hectic, disorganized fashion; also, the number of fingers on each hand is correct, while other important features are completely omitted. This indicates irregularities of functioning.

The examination has shown the child's assets and liabilities. Though sociable, sweet, cooperative, and pleasant, Ann is flighty and unable to stay at one task. She is constantly distracted by new ideas or outside stimuli. While she follows these divergent clues, she is at the same time often rigidly persevering when started on a line of thought and is unable to get away from it. In thinking as well as in perception, she has difficulty in combining multiple facts into a coherent whole. Her form comprehension and her ability to evaluate spatial relationships are much impaired. The combination of her good auditory memory and her ability in social imitations provides her with verbal expressions which help her to appear at ease and well-poised to the casual, uncritical observer. However, her development is progressing only at a borderline rate, with her best abilities at present approximately on a five-year level.

COMMENT

Ann's development from her early illness on has been one of gradually accelerating deviation from normal; her second bout of illness at age three intensified difficulties which seemed latent before. Traces of many of her present psychological symptoms were manifested earlier.

Hyperactive, tense, and impulsive behavior was noted a long time ago. As a year-old baby, Ann liked a quick change of activities; she did not like to stay with one thing for any length of time and was easily attracted to new materials. At eighteen months, she impulsively went for objects clearly out of her reach and did not bother to get them through intermediaries. She had little or no satisfaction in completing a task, either at eighteen months or at three years of age. Difficulties in fine coordination first appeared when, at nearly eleven months, the baby approached the pellet with index finger only and when, at eighteen months, she did not easily fit pegs into holes in a pegboard. Motor and attention difficulties combined also in her inadequate performances at two-and-a-half years, when, instead of drawing horizontal and vertical strokes, she scribbled in all directions. In the same task she also probably showed some lack of comprehension of spatial orientation when she failed to adjust to the rotation of the formboard. Her failure to discriminate between round and square pegs at eighteen months foreshadowed future difficulties in form discrimination; these difficulties became more apparent in her inferior and irregular performances with formboards later on.

Ann's attractive, easygoing, and sociable disposition was noted through all examinations. There were times when it was slightly endangered, and it could have easily changed when her parents started to become baffled by her poor behavior and began to discipline her. However, they soon understood that they had more success with Ann if they treated her with more leniency, less confusion, and less high standards. In spite of her limitations, which became more apparent with age, the child could continue to function happily. Slow but definite intensification of latent psychological inabilities are not uncommon symptoms in acquired brain injuries, especially in children who, injured early in life, have otherwise only minimal or nonexistent physical difficulties.

Measles Encephalitis
at Five Years

Rose, second child of young and intelligent parents, had, at the age of *five years three months,* an encephalomyelitis with prolonged coma and subsequent inability to walk; the latter lasted four months after the onset of illness. The process of recovery was slow in every respect.

Before her illness, Rose had developed normally. She was cheerful, lively, and rather a tomboy. She was responsive, warm, chatty, and gay. She was easygoing and friendly with people, and hardly ever required a reprimand at home. She was scheduled to enter kindergarten the following fall. Just lately she had become interested in making letters. Her parents did not expect her to have as scholarly tendencies as their older son had; Rose seemed to them more practical, active, and down to earth than he had been at her age.

ROSE IMMEDIATELY AFTER ILLNESS

Rose is seen by the psychologist three months after onset of illness, at *five years six months,* when she is still in the hospital ward. She sits in a wheelchair with a vague smile, looking pretty but blank. She seems to watch the ward activities foggily, but shows no affect or facial mobility. Nurses report that occasionally Rose cries quietly when surrounded by the least bit of confusion. With her bland facial expression, Rose usually does not give them any warning. When E approaches her, she responds slowly and automatically to simple questions on her name and address.

She cannot, on request, name the members of her family or her pets. However, when names are mentioned to her, she acknowledges happily those which are correct and shakes her head to those which are not.

Asked to count (T:XI:2), she smiles blankly and does not seem to understand what is wanted of her. When E starts to count, "one, two, three," she very slowly but without hesitation continues up to fifteen. Asked to count the (four) buttons on her dress (T:I:7) with E pointing to them, she starts out several times, touches some twice, and gets confused. Her hand movements are still weak and she has a slight tremor which interferes with her attempts at blockbuilding (T:I:2). She handles the blocks idly, trying to pile two on top of each other. She tries to copy the six-cube pyramid, seems to know how to do it, but gives up when her wobbly structure starts to topple. She sorts blocks of three colors by proxy (T:VI:1,2), but obviously becomes very tired. The session is interrupted by E.

The examination shows that the child reacts to some simple stimuli appropriately. She can, through immediate association, activate some previously learned verbal patterns (personal information, counting); she does not produce speech spontaneously. She perceives block structures and colors adequately for her age.

Within a few months, the child has improved considerably. She delights nurses, doctors and (after discharge) her parents with her rapid gains in speech and more appropriate responses to situations which arise. However, she still has little spontaneous conversation and is content with the simplest or no play activities.

ROSE TWO MONTHS AFTER DISCHARGE

Another psychological examination, at *five years eight months,* brings forth more clearly a psychological situation vaguely outlined in the first observation. Rose now can activate more previously acquired patterns if she receives the appropriate clue. She seems to react to more and more such diversified stimuli.

She can name animals (T:II:11) adequately for her age, though occasionally she hesitates in finding the correct word. She identifies pictures of animals and other objects (T:II:5,9,11) accurately by their various attributes. She knows which parts are missing in mutilated or incomplete pictures (T:IX:12), but in several instances she points to them and cannot name them. However, she can mobilize the proper verbal automatism and succeeds on a six-year level in opposite analogies (T:IX:5).

When asked to draw a lady walking in the rain (T:III:2), she enumerates various parts, as "eyes, arms, umbrella," each time jotting some mark on the paper. None but the umbrella is recognizable; none is set in relation to any other. With her motor coordination still poor and her stroke weak, she is absorbed in the task of applying pencil to paper and forgets what she is drawing. When she copies forms (T:III:5) and later when she works with formboards (T:IV:6,7,13), it is difficult to distinguish lack of attention from lack of appreciation of forms.

Inability to adapt to unfamiliar thought processes is marked in memory for pictures (T:II:8), which she fails even with three pictures. She does not understand how to "guess," but is attracted by one of the pictures left in front of her and names it instead. Visual stimuli interfere in similar ways with reasoning in pictorial identification in reverse (T:II:9). Like a very young child, she keeps pointing or naming the very thing she wants E to guess, *e.g.,* "Where is the fish?"

Measured in terms of numerical test results, Rose's mental age is between five years six months and six years seven months, which corresponds to an I.Q. of approximately 100. This, however, in no way describes her lack of effective mental power five months after onset of illness.

ROSE AFTER ONE YEAR

Seven months later, or one year after onset of illness, Rose, now *six years three months,* returns for a follow-up examination. Her parents have been delighted with her progress; she now moves around freely. She talks as well as before her illness, and more than she did then. To her parents she seems her old, cheerful self again, essentially unchanged, but livelier and more easily excitable. Her mother finds her occasionally stubborn and restless, but thinks that this may be due to lack of organized activity. It is difficult to keep Rose interested in any one thing for long. The child finds many things to do, but never seems to finish what she has started. Her mother describes some "silly," impulsive, thoughtless actions (emptying a cup of milk on the floor, or wetting in a closet). She "pesters" her older brother, who adores her "in spite of it," and, like her father, "lets her get away with murder." Both parents think Rose might well enter kindergarten the coming fall.

Rose looks chubby and healthy. She talks hastily and somewhat breathlessly. In spite of her vivaciousness, her facial expression remains immobile, with a bland, friendly, but somewhat frozen smile.

Seguin Formboard (T:IV:6)

She starts out to put the forms back where they belong, and asks, "May I take this home?" She hardly waits for the negative reply which she seems to have expected. She continues, "My father is going to get me one like this." She quickly completes the board without difficulty, and gets up from her chair.

Mare and Foal Picture Board (T:IV:13)

Rose hastily places two pieces correctly; she picks up a third one, brings it to the right spot, but does not take time to fit it properly; then she goes on to the next piece, but leaves it on top of the board next to the correct hole. E suggests that she put them in "nicely." She complies, but her thoughts are already elsewhere: "Did my mother speak to you?"

Five-Figure Formboard (T:IV:7)

She has no difficulty with the cross. She tries to fit triangles into the hexagon. E helps by removing one. Rose places another identical one in the same spot and leaves it there. She places the oval and circle without difficulty. Then she tries to fit part of the hexagon in the square, gives up, saying, "Can I go to school?" E: "Let us finish this first. We'll talk later." Rose has no objection, goes on and completes board with E placing half of square and hexagon. (Performance below five-year level.)

Conventional Manikin (T:IV:10)

Rose reverses arms as well as legs. Neither one of them fits properly in its place. Rose: "It's a people." (Performance at four-year level.)

Counting (T:I:7)

E: "Count his buttons." Rose: "Ten." (Correct.) E: "How many would he have if he lost one?" Rose: "Eleven."

Opposite Analogies (T:IX:5)

E: "A father is a man, a mother is a. . . ." Rose: "A mother." E: "A brother is a boy, a sister is a. . . ." Rose: "A sister." E: "In daytime it is light, at night it is. . . ." Rose: "Dark." E: "The sun shines during the day, the moon at. . . ." Rose: "Night." E: "The snail is slow, the rabbit is. . . ." Rose: "A rabbit." E: "A dog has hair, the bird has. . . ." Rose: "Feathers." E: "Rabbits' ears are long, rats' ears are. . . ." Rose: "Little." E: "Snow is white, coal is. . . ." Rose: "Cold." E: "Wolves are wild, dogs are. . . ." Rose: "Good." (By Revised Stanford-Binet standards, Rose fails on six- and eight-year levels, though the response "feathers" is correct and of good quality.)

QUESTIONS ABOUT MATERIALS (T:X:2)

E: "What is a house made of?" Rose: "Wood." E: "What is a book made of?" Rose: "Paper." E: "What is a window made of?" Rose: "Glass . . . Guess what! Jim broke a glass from a picture!"

DIFFERENCES BETWEEN TWO THINGS (T:IX:1)

E asks in what way two things are different. E: "Wood—glass." Rose: "The house . . . my doll house needs painting." E: "Bird—dog." Rose: "Dog is made of . . . birds have feathers, dog has shaggy hair." E: "Slippers—boots." Rose: "Boots are made of rubber." E: "And slippers?" Rose: "I do not know what rubbers are made of." (By Revised Stanford-Binet standards, Rose fails on six-year level, but she obviously has some good ideas and tries to find answers.)

Rose looks around and out of the window and sees smoke coming from a nearby building; she asks, "What does the smoke come from, a train?" then adds, "My mother and I came to Boston by train."

MEMORY FOR PICTURES (T:II:8)

THREE PICTURES. (Hat, horse, car; car is removed.) Rose states correctly that "the car is gone."

FOUR PICTURES. (Knife, boat, flag, key; boat is removed.) E: "Which one did I take away this time?" Rose: "The horse." She seems to find the game amusing, but though she has seen the new pictures and repeated their names, she is still thinking of the previous series. E shows her the picture of the boat in her hand.

SAME FOUR PICTURES REPEATED. (Knife is removed.) Rose, taking her clue from the previous setting, quickly and with assurance exclaims, "The boat." She has not noticed that the picture of the boat has this time remained on the table.

FIVE PICTURES. (Airplane, cowboy hat, block, coat, ball.)

While she is looking at the pictures, Rose asks, "What can we do now?" E: "Let us finish this game; I am going to take one away again, and you guess which one I took." E removes block, asks, "Can you find out which one I took?" Rose does not seem to study the remaining pictures, but she looks briefly and immediately says, "The block." It is difficult to say whether she just guessed correctly, or whether this time she recognized the situation at a glance.

SAME FIVE PICTURES REPEATED. (Ball is removed.) Haphazardly, no longer interested in the matter, Rose says, "Airplane"; she gets up, goes to the window, says, "Do you see airplanes from here? My Jimmy went up in an airplane."

This procedure leaves E uncertain about the reliability of Rose's performance. If Rose could not understand at all, why did she seem to do all right immediately in the first series? Did she misunderstand, or did she forget in between? Was she not interested, or was the large number of pictures too confusing for her? All that is clear after this procedure is that Rose is distractible, inattentive, and irregular, but she names all pictures correctly. She would have passed the picture vocabulary item from the Revised Stanford-Binet (T:XII:1 and II:7) on the five-year level.

Following up on appraising her vocabulary, E presents:

ANIMAL PICTURES (T:II:11)

NAMING. Rose willingly comes back to the table. She names all animals, but picks them out at random and names some twice. She names a squirrel correctly once, later calls it a cat. Reindeer is once a dog, later a deer.

Here Rose knows as well as most six-year-olds how to differentiate animals by name, but she is unreliable and irregular and intersperses names which seem based on primitive perceptions.

PICTORIAL IDENTIFICATION (T:II:9)

To E's questions, "Which one swims in the water? Which one tells us time? Which one gives us milk? and Which one do we read?" Rose responds correctly.

IDENTIFICATION IN REVERSE. E: "Now you ask me, make me guess." Rose: "Which one is in the sky?" E: "You mean the moon?" Rose nods, but does not seem convinced; she keeps looking at the bird, which obviously she meant. E: "Ask me another." Rose now points to the clock, asks, "What is that?" E: "Do not show me; that makes it too easy. Ask me about it the way I did." Rose: "Which one swims in the water?"

She has obviously not fully understood what she should do. She is unable to reflect on what she did just before when she responded correctly to the questions. When E explains again, she takes the request to do "the way I did" literally, and repeats E's first question.

All through the latter part of the examination Rose has been cheerful and seems to enjoy herself. She is not at all self-conscious, but rather self-assured. She appears accustomed to being appreciated and smiled at. She remains charming and somewhat airy. The extreme irregularity of her performances is obvious. She is at the mercy of immediate associations which constantly interfere with glimpses of comprehension that are adequate enough for her age. Her immediate perceptions become entangled in bits of information or memories, or remain fleeting impressions and steppingstones for her fluent conversation. They do not become properly integrated or assimilated in broader contexts. Rose's inability to structure perceptions into newly organized patterns is evident also in the following test procedures.

COPYING BEAD CHAIN (T:I:5)

With the child looking on, beads are strung in a pattern of two round, one cylindrical, two round, one cylindrical, etc.; the child is asked to make an identical chain.

Rose is delighted with the beads. She starts immediately to string them on the string offered to her. E repeats suggestion that she "make it just like this one." She chooses beads as they come to her fingers, not bothering to follow the pattern. She stops with six beads on her string. She compares it for length with the model, but makes no comment on the fact that her chain is the shorter one. "Just like this one" may at some moment have meant to her "the same length," but, her bead string done, she pays no further attention to what she is measuring and seems satisfied.

GOLDSTEIN-SCHEERER STICK TEST (T:VII:6 AND FIGURE 12)

IMITATING SQUARE. She tries to copy it correctly. When one of the sticks she has first chosen proves to be too short, she corrects the error spontaneously.

IMITATING TRIANGLE. She picks three sticks, two of them shorter than those of the model. She arranges them in an irregular triangular shape with gaps between them.

REPRODUCING FROM MEMORY. She is shown various designs, including shapes of W and double-pointed arrows. For each form she uses the correct number of sticks, generally of proper size. However, she arranges them in shapes which show gross distortions.

BLOCK DESIGNS (T:VII:7 AND FIGURE 13)

CARD I. She places three red blocks angle to angle in one diagonal line, then adds a blue block at the side of the red one. E demonstrates. On repetition, Rose has learned to arrange the blocks in a square, but she pays no attention to color. E demonstrates again and leaves her model on the table to be copied. Rose copies correctly.

CARD II. Rose places three blocks (a red one, a yellow/blue one, and a blue one) all in one horizontal row and tops it with one yellow/blue. E demonstrates. When invited to repeat, she has lost interest and places some blocks at random. E demonstrates again and leaves her model on the table to be copied. Rose no longer shows any interest; she is ready to quit. She does not respond to E's suggestion that she do this "just once more."

In both situations, Goldstein-Scheerer sticks and block designs, her reproductions represent some diffuse perceptions characteristic of the design which she is to copy. The arrow becomes a rod with four appendages, the W a collection of sticks arranged in an angular shape. The red blocks touching at an angle in the red/blue checkerboard design stress the diagonal direction which stands out most of all for her.

Similar primitive perceptual configurations are represented in the following procedures.

COPYING FORMS (T:III:5 AND FIGURE 2)

CROSS, SQUARE, TRIANGLE. These are copied correctly, as were similar simple forms when copied with stick material.

TILTED SQUARE. Copied as a diffuse form with four large angular protrusions, probably representing the corners.

BRITISH FLAG. Copied as a square with two vertical and two horizontal lines inside crossing each other. The same design subsequently copied from memory is a roughly drawn square; inside are two lines and a half-round mark. Asked what the latter represents, Rose says airily, "The holes in between."

In paper-and-pencil work, Rose's stroke has much improved in strength since she was seen last. She handles the pencil without difficulty now. The fact that she is able to draw a triangle and a square, but not a tilted square and a British flag, would rate her on a five-year level. However, her difficulties cannot be expressed by success or failure alone; the specific distortions of her last two designs point toward the same gross distortion in form perception which was noted above.

LADY WALKING IN THE RAIN (T:III:2)

She draws a crude figure with arms, legs, eyes, etc. Arms are attached to the body in the mid-line; separate round lines near the neck indicate the shoulders. An umbrella is indicated above the head of the figure. (Performance at approximately five-year level.)

PRINTING NAME (T:III:2c AND XI:9)

She prints her full name (Rosemarie) without a mistake.

Rose has become tired; she starts to dart out of the door to "tell my mother something," but is easily persuaded to climb on E's lap to look at some pictures with her.

PICTURE DESCRIPTION (T:II:6)

GRANDMOTHER'S STORY. Rose: "She is telling them a story— three little bears went walking one day. . . ." E: "Who is telling the story?" Rose: "The old woman . . . she lived in a shoe . . . she had so many children she did not know what to do . . . come on (pulling at the page), turn over."

BIRTHDAY PARTY. Rose: "School days, happy golden school days." She looks at the picture again. "Happy birthday." She starts singing: "Happy birthday to you, happy birthday to you, happy birthday, dear Jimmy."

WASHDAY. Rose: "Hey, you dog, stop doing that to my washing."

PICTURE COMPLETION (T:IX:12)

Her responses to pictures of table, coat, and cat are all correct. But to picture of man's head with mouth missing, she says, "He needs another sleeve," and to bird with wing missing, "He needs feathers."

PICTURE ABSURDITIES (T:IX:11)

MAN IN TREE. Rose: "He is going to fall off; he is sawing it where he is sitting; he is going to break his neck; there is a stone down there; he will hurt himself."

MAN ON SCALES. "He is so fat, he can't even step on the scales."

CAT AND MICE. "The mice are eating up the cat." E: "Are they?" Rose: "The cat is eating up the mice."

Session is interrupted.

Rose's volatile chattiness is again demonstrated in these last situations. The pictures cause her to reproduce immediate associations which have emotional appeal for her, *e.g.,* reference to falling "on a stone," or being fat (at home Rose is being gently teased for her chubbiness), or cats and mice do not get along. She has only these patterns to fall back on; she brings them out haphazardly without bothering to see how appropriate they may be to the specific occasion. Such familiar associations, however, go a considerable distance in helping her to solve some of the tasks presented to her. For example, she senses immediately the danger of staying on a limb which is being sawed off and understands the main theme of other pictures. However, she does not notice that the cat and mice are unduly friendly with each other. Yet her responses add up to some creditable performances. (By Revised Stanford-Binet standards, Rose passes on six-year level in picture description. She fails on seven-year level in picture absurdities, since she has to her credit only one point instead of the two required for passing.)

Attitudes which she displays in the test situation also direct her daily activities and emotional reactions at home. Her parents confirm this by their descriptions. Rose is, in many ways, back to what she used to be before her illness at age five. She knows approximately the same facts, produces the same automatisms, and uses the same interpersonal techniques which worked well for her then. She has, as yet, not enlarged her stock of experiences or developed new behavior patterns, and this is her most important problem. She is unable to modify her old patterns or to form new ones. Her "stubbornness" is a lack of plasticity which prevents her from assimilating new facts, adjusting easily to new circumstances, and controlling her immediate emotions. Because her perceptions remain isolated and are not properly embedded in the contingent field of factors, the feelings they arouse have a sharper and more immediate impact on her actions. Her sudden "silly" reactions (turning over a cup of milk) are caused by this immediacy of response to impulses at the expense of well-established social habits and tabus which had long been useful to her.

Considering all her difficulties, it would seem that early school entrance would present some hazards. However, her parents would like to try it, and the prospective teacher knows the situation. The family has handled Rose in her prolonged convalescence skillfully and kindly; their advisers seem well justified in trusting their judgement and supporting their plan. Absence from home for part of the day may lessen opportunities for friction which might arise as time goes on. In a new environment and on a new stage, Rose may be able slowly to learn to make new adjustments. For the time being, Rose can bring to this school adventure her personal charm and some automatized skills which may help her along in the elementary grades for some time to come.

ROSE AFTER TWO YEARS

One year later, at age *seven years three months,* Rose returns for evaluation. She has spent a year in kindergarten. She is obedient and easy to handle now at home, as well as in school, as long as life goes on routinely without sudden, confusing events. She has become rather quiet; she plays with other children, but frequently is taken advantage of because she is docile and does not know how to defend herself. At the beginning of the psychological examination, she seems the same friendly, easygoing child she was before. She accepts with enthusiasm any task proposed to her. Her interest and efforts fade as quickly as they did in earlier examinations. But the child has learned to control herself better. Instead of openly "wandering out of the field," she continues what she was doing; she goes automatically through the motions without putting herself into the task. Often she seems to have forgotten how she started. She still follows new and loosely connected lines of thought. They are of less egocentric character than before, but frequently lead to repetition of learned patterns which seem to have but little meaning to her. Drawings are better organized and show a firmer stroke and better structure. But they are meager and show poor form comprehension and signs of rigidity. The few printed words which she has learned show reversals in several instances. She is still best at solving problems which can be dealt with in one quick, intuitive glance. She becomes hopelessly confused when she has to do more consistent planning. She seems more upset and aware of failure than she was when seen before. In terms of numerical test results, Rose now has a mental age of five years eleven months, with an I.Q. of 85. Her I.Q. has dropped, but Rose has improved in working habits, efficiency, and behavior. Her former buoyancy has started to give way to timidity and uncertainty.

ROSE AFTER THREE YEARS

At her next visit, at age *eight years three months,* three years after the onset of the illness, Rose has developed into a husky, chubby little girl. She still has the same pretty, doll-like face; she has become slower and more deliberate in her movements.

At the start of the examination, Rose again is entirely willing to do whatever is requested, but her enthusiasm seems somewhat artificial. She is hesitant to start and seems to wait for specific directions. For a while, she talks in a whisper. She no longer talks spontaneously as much as she did. Questions pertaining to the examination are answered directly, without the added fringe conversation of earlier times. Still, Rose seems to enjoy being given the opportunity to talk about personal experiences, such as a recent trip to New York and the adventures of her cat. Her manner of speech now is somewhat long-winded and slightly monotonous, with much emphasis and detail devoted to simple humorous situations. She obviously enjoys contact and company, but there is a rigid and puppet-like quality about her. Her performances in the test situations show that certain traits which were previously noticeable have developed further. In earlier years, Rose seemed to be at the mercy of isolated stimuli which she responded to regardless of coherence. While this trend has now largely disappeared in her actions and in her conversations, it still interferes in subtler form and on a more mature level with her efficiency in learning.

REY NONVERBAL LEARNING TEST (T:VIII:1 AND FIGURE 16)

In this procedure Rose shows extreme irregularities; she learns the positions of the first two boards rather quickly in five runs. After this, she has great difficulty in remembering the positions of the proper peg on the third and fourth boards; when she has almost learned the third board, she remains uncertain about the sequence of the boards. She loses track and can't keep straight which board she is working on. When the procedure is interrupted, Rose's performances, measured quantitatively, show that she has not learned the arrangement of the key positions better at the end of seventeen runs than she had after five runs. For Rose it is almost impossible to see all boards as a unit; she deals with each one separately and is unable to coordinate these various separate experiences.

Coding (T:III:7)

A printed form has five rows of figures—circle, star, square, cross, triangle. A model on top of the paper shows the same figures, each enclosing a special mark; five sample figures serve to introduce the procedure. The child is asked to mark these figures on the form in the same way, placing a vertical line inside the star, a horizontal line inside the triangle, etc.

Rose marks the first three samples with E's help. When she makes a mistake, E describes the task again. Rose finishes the sample correctly, continues with first two figures, a star and a circle, which also correspond to the first two figures of the model. Engrossed in copying from the model, she does not notice that the sequence of the figures on her row no longer corresponds to that on the model row. Though the third figure on her row is a square and the third figure of the model a triangle, she acts as if they were alike, and copies the horizontal line (of the triangle) inside the square. From here on she keeps copying the subsequent marks of the model figures inside the figures of her row, regardless of the fact that the model shows a cross and a square as fourth and fifth figures, and her row has a triangle and a cross. Coming to the end of her row and with no model figure left to copy, she turns to her second row. She looks at her last mark (two vertical bars), then marks the next two figures (a square and a cross) each with an 8, the next figure (a star) with a 0, the next (a triangle) with a 1. When she starts to make a 2 inside the cross, E repeats the directions. Rose now fills the next two figures with the correct mark, then again makes new mistakes. (Scaled WISC score: two)

Rose seems to be carried away by every lead; at first she keeps on copying the model row, later the vertical double bars remind her apparently of the number 11, so she proceeds to mark numbers, etc. She keeps forgetting what she is to do.

Rose, always at ease with language, now has an answer for all verbal questions presented to her within the WISC. They are most frequently associations or automatized responses. These help her along in vocabulary (T:XII:2) (scaled score: six) and opposite analogies belonging to similarities (T:IX:2,5) (scaled score: seven). In factual information (T: XI:10), however, her impulsive answers are not precise enough to earn adequate credit (scaled score: five). In comprehension (T:X:3), she can only find answers to questions pertaining to personal experiences (scaled score: six). With her good auditory memory, she is able to repeat six digits forward, but she is unable to do any of the digit series in reverse (T:VIII:5,6) (scaled score: six). Inability to adjust to sudden shifts in a situation shows in picture arrangements (T:IX:10 and IV:14). She does not know how to change from the puzzle type (A,B,C,D) to the story type (1 to 7) series (scaled score: six) just as she is unable to shift from opposite analogies to similarities.

Rose's mental functioning, as shown in her test performances, is determined by many complex factors. However, the test scores hardly do justice to these. According to her score Rose has "borderline intelligence" (I.Q. 75). The unsophisticated examiner, reading the scores alone, would be apt to say that she shows only marginal evidence of brain injury. The scaled scores of the performance scale show severe irregularities, ranging from 2 in coding to 11 in picture completion. But with object assembly highest and block designs only one point lower than picture arrangement, the distribution does not form the classical pattern of brain injury. Verbal scores taken as a whole are not appreciably different from performance scores as a whole. Contrary to what might be expected, the performance score is slightly higher than the verbal score. It is evident that the complexities of Rose's problems three years after illness cannot be described by or derived from numerical scores.

COMMENT

Rose's development through the years following her illness shows clearly the interaction of constitutional factors and environmental influences and experiences. Rose seems to have been a well-adjusted, healthy little girl before her illness. Her parents were happy, warm, and stable, and were ready to enjoy the development of this second child without tension or overambition. From earliest days, Rose was loved for her personal charm and warmth rather than for her accomplishments. For some time after her illness, Rose's inability to establish new and more mature forms of adjustment remained almost unnoticed in daily life. At her age, just between preschool and school level, her flighty gaiety and chattiness did not shock anyone. For those around her, they were rather promising signs of returning health. For all of the first year after her illness, she met few new demands and did not run into many situations which she could not cope with. By the time she entered kindergarten and started to play again with other children, she had become ready to try some new experiences. Accustomed to protection and friendly support at home, she expected and received the same treatment from her teacher. She was able to get along reasonably well with the old stock of emotional and intellectual patterns, and added new ones at her much reduced rate. These new ways, however, were effective enough to maintain her in her relationships with her environment, even though they seem meager and unsatisfactory when measured against earlier potentialities. One is inclined to speculate that without her illness Rose would have become more enterprising and better organized in intellectual matters, less passive and subdued, and, perhaps, less anxious to be sweet and agreeable to grown-ups. Though the illness may have changed the course and speed of her development in all areas, Rose seems again reasonably well integrated and controlled. The favorable environmental conditions, including family setting and Rose's age at the time of illness, allowed gradual rearrangements of plans and feelings for all concerned. They prevented a sharp break which, under other circumstances, might have been caused by acquired disease and its psychological sequelae.

Head Injury at Seven Years

Jack, the only child of a middle-aged couple, was hurt in an accident at age *seven years nine months,* when his bicycle collided with a trolley car. He was treated for a skull fracture with concussion and stayed in a hospital for two weeks. He returned to school and entered the third grade with his class a few months after the accident. After discharge from the hospital, he complained for some time of double vision and weakness in his left eye. Double vision subsided, but the eye kept bothering him. He had frequent headaches, complained of dizziness, and often vomited when he returned home from school. His teacher found him inattentive and doing poorly, though he had been a "straight A" pupil before his accident.

His pediatrician refers the child for psychological examination six months after the accident. He would like help in deciding whether Jack has actually sustained damage to his learning ability, or whether his symptoms are emotional sequelae which are intensified by the fussing of an oversolicitous mother. The medical findings are not remarkable; there is some slowing and minimal slurring of speech, ptosis of the left eye most marked after fatigue, and an EEG reported as "slow but within normal limits."

Jack had a normal, if not superior, rate of development as a young child. He walked and talked early; he knew letters at four years of age and could read some before entering school. He was the pride of his parents; his mother hoped he would be a doctor; she herself had had a better education than her husband. She had been a medical secretary, while he had gone to work early as a simple laborer and now had his own small business.

The mother had spent much time with the child. He had never been gregarious; before he entered school, he had not often played with other children. Then he had acquired a few good friends with whom he had enjoyed playing. Since his accident, however, he prefers to stay by himself, but does not seem to find much to do except watch television, which his mother fears may increase his headaches. She does not encourage him much to go out to play, since he might get too tired or hurt again. She feels that she has to keep watching his health, his food intake, and his bedtime, and hopes that this will improve his nervousness. She knows that Jack resents her close supervision; he complains that she treats him "like a baby." He is more irritable and disgruntled than he was before. He also seems worried and depressed about his poor schoolwork and the prestige he is fast losing with his classmates. He spends much effort on his homework. Though his mother has never reprimanded him for his poor marks, he has lately taken to concealing his papers from her. She is worried about the situation, but has not told this to Jack. With regard to today's visit to the psychologist, she has not mentioned to him any school difficulties, but has explained that they need a consultation because of his headaches and dizziness. Jack dislikes coming because he doesn't want to miss school and is tired of seeing doctors.

After this information has been received, a plan for Jack's examination emerges. E must first study the child as he appears now. His mental level, his attitude, his working habits, and the quality of his functioning must be investigated. In addition, the examination should reveal independent information about the rate and level of Jack's development previous to his accident. Comparison of quality of learning and reasoning then and now may be significant and, through further analysis, lead to better understanding of the child and his problems. Such a psychological study will also serve as a baseline for evaluation of progress.

JACK AFTER SIX MONTHS

Jack, aged *eight years three months,* enters E's room; he is an attractive child with pleasant manners. He seems somewhat anxious and harassed, but sits down expectantly without any comment. When asked what he knows about the purpose of his visit, he talks about his headaches, but declares politely that they are getting better; he really is all right now, and school is giving him no trouble. He has almost caught up with his class and likes it fine. The teacher has been very nice to him and has helped him with arithmetic after hours. Jack's speech is slow and somewhat hesitant; frequently he has to grope for the correct word.

E explains that Dr. P, his pediatrician, suggested that she might like to help Jack. People, grown-ups or children, often tire easily and more frequently after an accident than before it. Sometimes they find the work hard and get headaches and become worried. Dr. P thought Jack might like to talk about this sort of thing. First they would get acquainted by doing things together.

Jack becomes somewhat more relaxed, and with a warmer expression on his face he admits that he, too, finds some work very hard and that he gets headaches in school when the children are too noisy.

FIVE-FIGURE FORMBOARD (T:IV:7)

Jack seems to like this. He goes about it efficiently, picking up the two triangles and holding them together in midair to form the square. He looks around, but does not see the square hole immediately. Coming upon the oval hole, he lays the triangle aside, picks up one-half of the oval, looks for its companion piece, and fits both together into the proper hole. Then he finds the square hole, wants to place the two triangles, but can only find one for awhile. He seems to know which pieces go together and where. But his gaze often slides over the correct inset or proper place too hastily and he does not recognize it quickly enough. He completes the board satisfactorily, but has taken more time than usual for a child of his age.

CASUIST FORMBOARD (T:IV:8)

He proceeds much as before, trying a segment of the larger circle in the small circle, then finding where it belongs and placing it correctly. After this he discriminates correctly between the sizes of three other segments. However, twice in succession he first grasps one of the wrong size; then he fumbles with the oval, accepts E's help with half of it, and completes it correctly with the proper symmetrical arrangement.

In both these test procedures, Jack is quick and eager to start; he seems confident of his success. When he has to stop and correct errors, he hesitates and seems puzzled and annoyed about it, and shrugs his shoulders tensely.

REY NONVERBAL LEARNING TEST (T:VIII:1 AND FIGURE 16)

Impulsively Jack tries to touch the pegs before E has finished giving directions. When she stops him with a gesture, he makes an effort to

listen attentively, but several times again he shows an impulse to start
prematurely. After the "go-ahead" sign is given, he begins systematically
and carefully. For the first and second boards, he tries the same initial
approach; for the third board, he takes his clue from his previous experience and tries the position which was key position on the second
board. He touches the same peg twice while dealing with the fourth
board. He apparently knows the key positions on boards 1, 2, and 4 on
the second run. There are still trial and error moves with board 3 until
the fourth run when he has learned which is the correct peg. By that time
errors appear again on board 2 and continue on this board until the
fifth run. Apparently unnerved by these errors, he now forgets also
the position of board 4 and needs fourteen moves to find the proper
peg again. Now he no longer appears systematic; he keeps touching
the same pegs tensely and fumbles without thinking. Whenever he finally
reaches the right peg, he barely acknowledges that he has finally found
the one he has been looking for. He uses trials and errors again in the
next (sixth) run, and again needs seventeen moves until he finds the
correct peg. He has, however, retained positions 1, 2, and 3. He succeeds
on all four boards once on the seventh run; then continues to make mistakes on boards 1 and 3 for the next five runs. Finally, he reaches
the goal of three successive runs without errors. (He scores in twenty-fifth
percentile.)

When the boards are reversed he seems uncertain; he acts as if the
whole series and not just two boards had been reversed, and begins by
trying the position of the fourth board instead of that of the second. He
seems unable to visualize the new order of succession, and cannot tell
apart those two boards which were reversed and those which were not.

Analysis of this test situation is interesting and revealing; the
numerical test results are less enlightening than the procedure which
led to them. At first, Jack understood and learned systematically. However, he could not maintain his gains; he was thrown off by his first failure. He lost insight, became confused, and then only very slowly
recuperated his gains with much effort. Later on, again, he could not
maintain them because he did not know how to adjust to the reversed
boards.

Similar fluctuations between quick comprehension and inefficient
performance were noticed in the formboard tasks, where Jack showed
knowledge and facility with form relations, but had difficulty perceiving
some shapes and sizes at a glance.

Jack's attitude in this short segment of the examination seems also of significance. Each one of the three tasks was approached without hesitation. There was no sign of cockiness, or "devil-may-care" heedlessness; he seemed to have confidence in his own competence which appeared justified by his efficient initial approach and partial success. In each of these tasks, this period of confidence seemed to be followed by surprise and puzzlement about difficulties which arose. He seemed annoyed, without blaming the material or E. He acted as if he could not understand why it should happen.

To E, this attitude seems to be of great importance. Jack appears to be a boy with essentially good comprehension, who cannot sustain his effort in a prolonged task and seems slightly slow in perceptual awareness. These difficulties seem to be a new experience for him and have obviously not been a part of his life for any length of time. Such an initial impression must be checked carefully in the next phases of the examination. The next test situation must help to investigate what stock of information and what kind of reasoning patterns Jack has at his disposal. There must also be further study of his learning ability and a more detailed test of perceptuo-motor functions which so far have only been tapped in the formboard tasks.

Opposite Analogies (T:IX:5)

Jack appears to have an adequate stock of normal routine verbal automatisms. (By Revised Stanford-Binet standards, he passes on eight-year level.)

Counting (T:XI:2)

In counting by one's to twenty and by ten's to one hundred, Jack has complete success; no hesitations. In counting backwards, twenty to one, he says, "twenty, nineteen, eighty, ninety," then corrects himself, hesitates, and succeeds.

Arithmetic Facts (T:XI:3)

ADDITION WITHIN TEN. (Such as six plus three.) He finds all problems easy and somewhat below his dignity.

ADDITION OF LARGER NUMBERS. Fifteen plus two is again simple for him, but fifteen plus seven requires more thought; he first answers "Twenty-three," then says, "Oh, no, that is fifteen plus eight, fifteen plus seven is twenty-two."

SUBTRACTION WITHIN TEN. He goes at them with assurance,

but gets somewhat tense; he gives a wrong answer, but corrects it spontaneously, ápologizing, "We have not had those for a long time."

MULTIPLICATION. With three's (five times three, eight times three, etc.) he is immediately correct, says, "We have just had them." With four's (six times four), says, "We are just learning these. I have to start one times four is four, two times four is . . . eight, three times four is ten. . . ." When E questions this last answer, he says, "No, two times four is eight, three times four is . . . twelve," etc.

SERIAL USE OF ARITHMETIC FACTS (T:XI:4)

ADDING THREE NUMBERS. Jack starts correctly with "One plus three equals four, plus three equals seven, plus three equals ten," but when he comes to "ten plus three" he hesitates and becomes confused, says "Twelve, no, fifteen plus three equals sixteen"—gives up in exasperation, saying, "I can't do it, I used to do things like that."

REPEATING DIGITS (T:VIII:5,6)

DIGITS FORWARD. Jack repeats five digits forward correctly.

DIGITS BACKWARD. He fails three series of three digits backward, but succeeds on the fourth trial. (By Revised Stanford-Binet standards, he fails on seven-year level.)

SIMILARITIES AND DIFFERENCES BETWEEN TWO THINGS (T:IX:3)

He understands immediately, finds correct answers for all. At no time does E have to repeat directions. (By Revised Stanford-Binet standards, he passes on nine-year level.)

ORAL VOCABULARY: ABSTRACT WORDS (T:XII:2)

He has some difficulty expressing his ideas, but seems to be familiar with words such as pity, curiosity, surprise, and knows what they mean. (By Revised Stanford-Binet standards, he passes on ten-year level.)

FACTUAL INFORMATION (T:XI:10)

Eleven of his answers are correct and of good quality, *e.g.,* "Columbus— I know—he sailed around the world; he thought it was flat; they only knew later that it was like a big ball." He answers only those questions of which he is sure.

All these performances show a high level of general knowledge. However, Jack has some tendency to become confused when he has to reorganize material. This can be seen in digits reversed, in counting backwards, and in some arithmetic items. It also becomes apparent in the following procedure:

MEMORY FOR PICTURES (T:II:8)

He succeeds immediately when presented with either three or four pictures from which he must identify the missing one. However, he cannot remember all the pictures belonging to a series of five when presented together. He obviously knows that there was a fifth picture which he cannot remember. Unlike some younger children who fail this test, he remains fully aware of the proper technique. It does not occur to him to mention either a picture used in the previous series or else one of the pictures still on view on the table. (Still, in terms of achievement, he fails in this procedure, which is usually within the limits of most five-year-olds.)

LEARNING FIFTEEN WORDS (T:VIII:2)

A series of fifteen words is read and repeated to the child; he is to recite all those which he can remember each time.

There is a quick rise in his learning curve. As in Rey's nonverbal learning test, he learns quickly at first, but again is unable to maintain his first good effort. He cannot easily add to the material which he has acquired in one quick sweep. He repeats eight words after first reading (hundredth percentile), gains only three more after second reading, and again repeats only the same number after third reading (fiftieth percentile); he gains another word after next repetition, but loses it again in last one (twenty-fifth percentile). The number of words said twice increases from one word after the first reading to seven after the second, diminishes after the next two repetitions, but increases to six after the last run. From the third time on, he also consistently substitutes the word "yard" for "garden." These repeated words and synonyms starting in the course of the learning process indicate his difficulty over a prolonged period in maintaining good working control in one and the same task.

Information about perceptuo-motor functioning is obtained from:

Block Designs (T:VII:7 and Figure 13)

Cards i and ii. He reproduces both designs correctly.

Card iii. He fails because he reverses positions of the yellow and blue triangles.

Card vi. He works hard and correctly builds the two red triangles, but is unable to put them together in one structure. He gets fussed at E's suggestion and gives up.

(By Kohs standards, his mental level in this procedure is approximately seven years six months.)

Memory for Designs (T:VII:1 and Figure 4)

Designs from form m, ix-year level. He seems to find the task easy. For b he draws an outer square carefully, encloses in it a well-drawn diamond, but does not have it meet the outer square properly. He is aware of this mistake and tries to correct it by connecting the diamond with the outer square by straight lines. He explains that these are only to indicate that both figures belong closer together. The second design a is poorer and shows only two small squares loosely connected. Jack is obviously dissatisfied and explains that there should be two small squares, but that he cannot remember how they hang together. (By Revised Stanford-Binet standards, he fails on nine-year level.)

Drawing a Man (T:III:3)

He produces a conventional man with jacket and pants, arms and legs in double lines. There is only one minor transparency. He also draws a house. (By Goodenough standards, his mental age is seven years nine months.)

Writing (T:XI:9)

He writes his name in fluent cursive writing without hesitation. On request, he starts to write the word house, but writes it "h-o-s"; he becomes hesitant, starts to erase the whole thing, writes it again with the same error. He becomes puzzled and accepts E's suggestion to write it with a "u." Asked for other words, he volunteers car. When this is written, E suggests dog; he starts to write "g-o-d-y," later reads it back as dog; E suggests to start it new with a "d." Jack immediately complies. Puzzled and somewhat annoyed, he wants to erase "g-o-d-y" but agrees to complete the new version beneath. He declares that he does not know any other words, though he used to.

WRITING ALPHABET AND NUMBERS (T:IX:2,8)

He says and writes alphabet without hesitation, but does some letters in print and some in script. His "s" is illegible and somewhat resembles an "x." Asked to write numbers, he writes 1 to 20 correctly, except for reversal of 9 in 19 which he writes as 91. He does not become aware of this mistake even when E asks whether "everything is all right."

The last group of test situations shows again the contradictory trends noticed in the formboard tasks. There is reasonably good knowledge of shapes and form relationships. He understands how to copy block designs from printed models, and knows that the positions of the blocks must be arranged in relation to each other. In memory for designs, he recognizes immediately the different shapes of the diamond and square and orients both correctly with proper angles but wrong size. His drawings of a man and a house are adequate for a child of his age. He also knows the shapes and combinations of numbers and letters. His mistakes are reversals or a faulty combination of form elements.

Summarizing the impressions gained in the examination, there is consistently good evidence that the child has developed normal patterns of mental activity for his age. However, he has acute difficulties in functioning. He is unable to use his acquired patterns effectively enough wherever reorganization of facts or prolonged process demand an effort which he is unable to maintain. These difficulties of functioning must be of recent origin. Had they been of older standing, they would have seriously interfered with the integration and acquisition of material which Jack still so easily activates now. Also, his performances in perceptuo-motor tasks show only subtle deviations, mainly in spatial relationship. Otherwise they, too, show evidence that development of form perception has proceeded intact and has been essentially normal up to this time.

This last point poses important diagnostic problems. The uncritical observer may dismiss the possibility of "organic" damage too lightly, since the gross form distortions characteristic of brain damage are absent in this case. The consistent tendency to reversals may be interpreted by these examiners as a more or less benign sign of immaturity, or perhaps even as a symptom of regression on an emotional basis. This would also help to explain the consistent learning difficulties.

Such an interpretation, however, appears somewhat dangerous and probably not warranted by the facts; reversals in Jack's case are unlikely to be signs of developmental immaturity. There has been corroborated evidence that Jack learned to read early and was an "A pupil" up to the time of his accident. Children who tend to reversals or mirror writing beyond the normal age seldom acquire skills in writing and reading early in life. Mother and teacher later confirm that the tendency to reversal is new for Jacky, and has been noted with surprise just since his return to school. The question of regression is too complex to be discussed here; somehow Jack's earnest concern and interest in learning, his desire to minimize difficulties, and his generally mature attitude, suggest that his anxieties take other forms than dropping to a lower level in this one particular area.

In view of the history of head injury and the slight physical symptoms still present, it seems most likely that learning difficulty and tendency to reversals stem from a recent insult to the nervous system. In Jack's case, their form is somewhat more subtle than in some other cases of injury. Before his accident, Jack had been an intelligent child and had already reached a certain level of maturity with intact functioning. From the standpoint of personality, he is a well-integrated and controlled person. His reactions to failure and learning difficulties are self-criticism and moodiness rather than the aggressive outbursts seen in more temperamental and less controlled children. E's diagnosis of "organic" involvement needs more proof either through time or events or, if possible, through more investigation. For the moment there is no real possibility for further psychological examination for practical, as well as for secondary psychological, reasons. Jack has become tired; his mother is apprehensive that more visits here may upset him and set him back. The trip to Boston is long and expensive for them. The most pressing problem is how to relieve the general tension and how to spare Jack humiliating situations. Pediatrician and psychologist agree to remove him from school for the rest of the year and to give him time for more convalescence. Sometime later in the year he may have a home teacher who can help him fill the gaps in his school learning at his own new, slow speed.

JACK AFTER NINE MONTHS

On a return visit three months later, Jack, now *eight years six months,* looks happier and more relaxed. His speech is still slow. He seems to enjoy the quiet life at home, but has lately started talking about wanting to go back to school. His mother thinks that the time for a home teacher has come.

In a short review examination, Jack's situation shows no spectacular improvement as yet.

Learning Fifteen Pictures (T:VIII:3)

After the first presentation, he retains seven (seventy-fifth percentile); after the third presentation of the pictures, he knows eleven (fiftieth percentile); after the fifth he reproduces twelve (twenty-fifth percentile). There are still many repetitions and one words substitution (fork for knife).

Benton Visual Retention Test (T:VII:4 and Figure 8)

DESIGNS 1, 2, 3. Correct.

DESIGNS 4, 5. Correct for order and gross form, but reversals in direction.

DESIGN 7. Correct, as above, but the triangle is equilateral instead of right-angled.

When he tries to memorize designs 2 and 3, he names the figures "zero-zero and a little square," or "square-zero and a triangle." (His score is three, which equals low average.)

Ellis Visual Designs Test (T:VII:2 and Figure 5)

He has much difficulty with the irregular figures. (Score: three points, well below twenty-fifth percentile.)

Block Designs (T:VII:7)

He fails on Card III and on the following designs, as before. (By Kohs standards, his mental age is seven years six months.)

Verbal Absurdities (T:IX:6)

When trying to find what is wrong with the statements, Jack reasons on the basis of over-all impressions.

To statement about a young man with a cane and his hands in his pockets, Jack says, "It was not true that he had a cane, he could not hold on to one."

To statement about a father's letter enclosing money, recipient to send a telegram if letter not received, Jack says, "He did not receive the letter, he could not know."

To a marching soldier complaining that everybody is out of step except himself, Jack says, "Everybody out of step, that means him too."

To a kindhearted man with heavy bag sitting on horse and carrying a bag on his own shoulder to make it easier on horse, Jack answers, "He made the horse carry everything, him and the bag."

A man digging a hole does not know what to do with dirt; a neighbor suggests he dig another hole to put it in. Jack: "That would be too big a hole."

He does not find the stories either foolish or amusing, but wrong and untrue. He corrects the statements with a slightly moralistic tone which accuses or defends the characters in the stories rather than the stories themselves. (By Revised Stanford-Binet standards, Jack gets credit for responses to first, second, and fourth sentences, so that he passes on nine-year level.)

The reappraisal of Jack's psychological functioning clarifies at this date some points which had come up in the previous diagnostic study. Jack's visuo-motor retention is becoming very irregular. He still can do well enough with material which has some meaning for him. He still can memorize positions and size relationships of shapes which are simple and familiar to him. This can be seen in the Benton Test where reversals continue to be his only source of error. The more complex and irregular Ellis figures, which require new learning and new perceptual organizations, are considerably more difficult for him. In block designs his performances have not yet improved with age, so that with his mental age staying what it was before, it becomes more apparent that Jack is not making progress. In reasoning problems, such as verbal absurdities, Jack still can get along through immediate intuitive appraisal based on past experiences, but he fails where systematic judgement and new constructions and adjustments are required.

JACK AFTER TWO YEARS

Two years after the accident the picture has changed somewhat again. Jack, now *nine years nine months old,* has had a home teacher for a year and has entered school again. On recommendation of his home teacher, he was promoted to the fourth grade, apparently mostly for social reasons. Though his school performances are still meager, his teachers have been sympathetic and have tried to save his self-respect. Jack notices that special considerations are given to him and resents this bitterly. He has become more moody and depressed and insists that there is nothing the matter with him. His mother is very concerned about him. He still has occasional headaches, but her main complaints are his lack of friends, his desire to stay by himself, and his irritability against her. She feels that Jack is unhappy and that she does not know how to reach him.

The psychological examination shows improvement in some areas and more marked problems in others. Jack has improved considerably in his performances in learning tests. Learning fifteen words (T:VIII:2) no longer shows the discrepancy between immediate repetition and gradual learning of new material which was first seen in earlier examinations. On each of the first, the third, and the fifth repetitions, he scores in fiftieth percentile. In these situations there is a general improvement in attitude and control. Only a very few words are repeated twice and there are no substitutions. In the Rey nonverbal learning test, presented with a modified arrangement of the respective positions of the pegs to make the task a new one for him (T:VIII:1), he remembers the proper positions in three trials. He goes at the task carefully; each time he finds a correct peg, he stops to recapitulate this position and those previously found. He uses his index finger to point the positions out to himself. His tempo is slow, but there are only a few errors. (He scores in seventy-fifth percentile.)

Jack's working habits have changed. He is no longer sure of himself; he is apt to approach each problem slowly and with caution; he seems to expect difficulties and tries to guard against them. His performances in the block designs have improved, but his method is cumbersome and slow. He tries each block separately, compares its position with the model, and adds one block to the next in a piecemeal fashion. In the Rey-Osterrieth complex figure test (T:VII:5 and Figure 10), he is most meticulous and slow; he copies each unit with great care, adding line to line. Using his pencil to point out to himself where he is, he counts the bars and dots and compares each unit repeatedly with the model. He ends up with most units represented on the paper. However, he has made several errors in the relationships of the units to each other; some overlap, some are too far apart. Since he has turned his sheet and also the model several times to get better access to the spot where he was working, he has some items reversed because he forgot to turn back either his paper or the model. When at the end he looks at his design, he does not seem to notice the discrepancy in spatial orientation. He seems exhausted. Therefore the procedure is not repeated as a memory test, though this omission probably deprives E of some interesting results. (Score: twenty-two points, well below twenty-fifth percentile.)

After a short interruption, other test items are presented. Jack does better in some of the performance items of the WISC than he does in verbal ones. Thanks to his quick, over-all grasp, he has a score of twenty-four points in picture arrangement (scaled score: nine), and eleven points in picture completion (scaled score: eleven). Since in object assembly he recognizes the familiar shapes of the figures but is slow in bringing the pieces together, he earns a score of twenty points (scaled score: ten). However, in factual information he has only nine fully adequate responses (scaled score: seven); whereas in vocabulary he almost exclusively gives definitions of one-point quality only. They earn him a credit of twenty-two points (scaled score: seven).

Formerly, these two last areas were his strongest field. Since they depend on new learning more than others, the drop in Jack's achievements in these tasks is of great significance. Before his accident, Jack had accumulated a good stock of information through his quick immediate grasp. He could get along on the strength of it for some time. However, with his diminished learning ability after the trauma, he has learned less and has acquired new material less rapidly than before. Even though his learning ability seems to be gradually improving, in this crucial developmental period the lost time cannot be made up. Jack will continue to need concessions because of the sudden break in the rate of his intellectual development.

COMMENT

Jack's personality development during the past few years adds an important factor to the picture. Jack was bright and inquisitive in his early life. He received much praise and emotional reward for skill in reading and for interests which at that time set him somewhat apart from other children of his age. From the early history, one gets the impression of a proud, somewhat lonesome little boy who liked to keep himself assured of his ability to shine. The accident and stay in the hospital were frightening; then later his confusion and sudden learning difficulties came to shake his self-confidence. In the following period, he tried to avoid humiliation by staying away whenever possible from new experiences which demanded new, difficult adjustments. His early air of curiosity and initiative changed into slightly surly passivity and remoteness. His difficulty in expressing himself at times added to making him shy of contacts and exchanges of ideas. He started to feel less comfortable with people than ever before. His family's attitude was obviously another deciding factor. In his early years, the child fulfilled desires and ambitions of his parents, especially his mother. She adjusted to his disability as to an event beyond her power and tried to be "sensible" about it. At the time, her willingness to keep Jack out of school seemed rather admirable to her advisers. However, her apparent acceptance of his shortcomings gradually seriously irritated Jack. Possibly it caused him to relinquish further ambition and drive. A court decision, awarding damages for permanent injury to Jack, added another emotional complication to all concerned. Three years after the accident psychotherapy was attempted in a psychiatric clinic nearby. Jack's emotional problems were obvious; he was given opportunity to air his resentment and feelings of failure. Therapy did not prove a great success, due to difficulties commonly encountered with children with organic involvements. Jack showed little insight into his own problems and had difficulty relating to his therapist. A complete Wechsler-Bellevue Intelligence Test, done there at the same time, showed an I.Q. of 95 (performance score: 99; verbal score: 94). A psychologist described him as "low average, with no organic involvement." This psychologist was unfamiliar with the fact that the intricate interactions of multiple factors involved in as complicated a case as this are not adequately represented by numerical test results. The single fact that total performance scores are higher than total verbal scores does not necessarily exclude psychological damage of organic origin.

Stages of Development
and Their Problems

The case portraits of Ann, Rose, and Jack illustrate how acquired insults to the nervous system are apt to influence decisively the course of a child's development. The psychologist tries to understand the child's psychological picture by studying objective clinical findings against the background of the child's personal history. If she knows that the patient has had an injury at some time during childhood, she may understand certain findings without too much difficulty. Often, however, the psychologist does not know whether the child has ever been injured or had an illness that might affect the nervous system. There may be no telltale physical symptoms. The child may have been referred for psychological study because he seems unable to learn or shows behavior problems, or both. Frequently, it is the psychologist's task not only to discover, describe, and interpret interrelationships of psychological symptoms, but also to determine as well as she can the non-psychological causes of certain difficulties. Nowadays medical colleagues very commonly expect the psychologist to find out whether or not the child has "organic" damage which can be demonstrated through psychological findings.[1] In some cases this may be relatively easy; in others, however, it can be very difficult and sometimes impossible. This uncertainty disturbs younger, inexperienced psychologists more than older ones. They may think that they must have a definite answer and may feel pressed to make a decision even if they are uncertain. Upon meeting such a diagnostic impasse—well-known in medical practice—some may find that

[1] However illogical, the term "organic," meaning "neurological," has come to be accepted. It is often used in instances where as strong a word as "brain-injured" is being avoided, although the difficulty is of neurological rather than emotional origin.

270

they wish that the last generation of clinicians had been less successful in winning a place in the medical diagnosis for those psychological factors of organic origin which are so clearly evident in many cases.

Valuable experience in recognizing relevant psychological symptoms can be gained through the systematic study of children with known injuries to the nervous system. Persons injured during childhood, rather than at birth or immediately afterwards, show a great variety of psychological situations that are of particular interest to the psychological diagnostician. Many different constellations of symptoms result from injuries or illnesses that seem similar in origin. Knowledge about the type of infection and site of cortical injury is often less a determining factor for psychological symptoms than is the severity and timing of the event, the temperament and emotional habits of the child, and the attitudes of people around him.[2]

Even though the most commonly recognized organic signs are often absent or minimal in these children, the sensitive examiner can discover significant psychological developments that clearly point to organic disturbances. The case portraits of Ann, Rose, and Jack illustrate the methods by which such diagnosis is accomplished. This chapter discusses the developmental trends and problems found to be characteristic for children who have suffered during infancy or childhood traumata involving the nervous system.

During the *first two years* of life a baby reacts more violently to infections and accidents, and is more apt to suffer damage to the nervous system, than he would if the accident happened in later years. The degree of this damage may vary from very severe to hardly perceptible. In the most serious cases, the child afterwards remains permanently unresponsive or he is extremely slow in making new gains. It will be obvious to all that this child is severely and irreparably damaged. The psychologist, if called at all, can only confirm the sad truth.

However, thanks to improved medical procedures (earlier recognition of danger, antibiotic drug treatment), such cases have become rarer in recent years. Many babies recover promptly and completely from infections such as meningitis. After an amazingly short time, they seem as chipper as before. The examining psychologist—like everybody else—will find them fully competent in performances of the standard infant

[2] Edith Meyer and Randolph K. Byers, "Measles Encephalitis; A Follow-up Study of Sixteen Patients," *American Journal of Diseases of Children* 84:543–579, November 1952. Also for general discussion of the effects of localization and differences between early and late brain injury, see Donald O. Hebb, *The Organization of Behavior* (New York: John Wiley, 1949), Chapters I and II. Also David Wechsler, *The Measurement and Appraisal of Adult Intelligence* (Baltimore: Williams and Wilkins, 1958), Chapter 13.

scales. Yet some warning symptoms may be worthy of note. These babies may show signs of irritability immediately after the illness or within three months afterward; they may be startled by noises and movements more than usual and overreact to these. Occasionally a child may still seem somewhat tremulous when handling play materials; he may become impatient and annoyed, cry easily, or give up what he has been doing. Another baby may be unduly lethargic if left to his own devices, though he may be more responsive if frequently encouraged and restimulated. An "older" baby in his second year may attack test materials in a rather immature way at first; he may bang, suck, poke, or throw things. Later in the examination he may show sporadically the more mature approach that is appropriate for his age. Such intermittent regression may be observed with blocks (T:I), pellet and bottle (T:V:8), pegboards (T:IV:1,2), and also with techniques requiring the finding of objects (T:V) and reactions to picture books (T:II:1–5).

The psychologist should find out from the family whether irritability, impatience, or lethargy was part of the child's behavior pattern previous to illness. The answer may be that the behavior is entirely new, or that it was present previously but not to the extent it is now. Or one may hear that the baby is just as he always was. Experience shows that all these answers need further clarification; none can be taken at its face value. The emotional tension accompanying the child's illness may alter the judgement of his family. Possibly the symptoms they describe have only temporary significance. They may be only transitory difficulties caused by the fact that the child was ill or hospitalized, was separated from home, frightened, upset, or weak. They may soon disappear through indulgent, intelligent, and relaxed handling on the part of the family. However, the psychologist should not dismiss the symptoms too lightly; while avoiding alarm, she should make a mental note for future reference. Subsequent examinations may show total improvement in all respects; often, however, one later finds that these slight indications of nervous imbalance were the first signs of attention difficulties and perceptual confusion that become more prominent as the child grows older.

Children who, like Rose, had illnesses or accidents *in their preschool years rather than in infancy* have had a chance to develop normally during the very important formative years. They have been able to establish a system of normal reaction patterns. They have made adequate sensory-motor and emotional adjustments, and have learned to reason and use language. The latter, especially, stands them in good stead when they are being examined shortly after the acute stage of the trauma. Even though they are often fatigued, weak, and tense, when clinically fully recovered they respond normally to everyday questions. They may count, recite, and answer without difficulty questions that demand quick responses based on previously acquired associations (T:XI). Some (after a head injury, an acute encephalitis, a thrombosis) occasionally have difficulty finding the correct word when naming simple objects or pictures (T:II, XII); this disability may pass unnoticed in casual conversation. Many do well on the simple formboards appropriate for this age level (T:IV:5,6,13), but they may flounder on those that demand some mental construction rather than immediate perception of well-known shapes. They find it easy to copy or reproduce some well-known geometric forms, but may find the unfamiliar ones much more difficult (T:III:5,6 and VII:6). Frequently, some difficulty in adjusting actively to totally new tasks appears in tests of reasoning ability such as identification in reverse (T:II:9), questions (T:II:6), or memory for pictures (T:II:8). In many tasks they start out with energy and aplomb, but soon lose interest. Their inability to pay attention for any length of time, their haste, tension, and restlessness may render the whole examination somewhat painful and may even induce the examiner to shorten the session. This inability to pay attention may have important clinical significance even if it can be shown that, when he is attentive, the child understands probably as well as he might have without his illness.

As in younger children, the few symptoms that are noted may be mostly transitory; fatigue and tension may keep a child from functioning at his best, may make his movements and pencil stroke weak, and cause his energy to flag. The clinician should remember that good numerical test results and potentially good abilities shown now do not exclude the possibility that permanent irregularities will be more prominent later and may be foreshadowed already by the tense and restless behavior. Again, such symptoms should never be passed over lightly. They indicate that for the time being at least the child still has to be granted concessions and treated with consideration because he is not yet fully recovered, even if he appears to be normal from the strictly medical point of view. If to his family he seems demanding and stubborn, easily upset and overwrought, it is not usually because he has been "spoiled" by the attention he has been given through the period of illness, but because he still is nervous and vulnerable. Observations have shown time and again that undue pressure after trauma may easily result in permanent behavior problems. Often, however, the worst manifestations of the so-called postencephalitic behavior can be avoided through close guidance and emotional protection at this crucial time.[3] A calm and serene environment is necessary to overcome transitory periods of fatigue; it is even more important in cases where (as with Rose) family and child have to adjust to disabling irregularities of functioning which may ultimately turn out to be permanent. After the initial psychological examination, it becomes natural for the psychologist to be the one who gives advice. Follow-up examinations for future guidance and evaluation of progress may be proposed.

It seems that the older a child is at the time of injury or accident, the more complex his symptoms may become—even though the chances of full recovery seem best in older children. *Older children,* when first examined after an injury or illness, frequently show tension, flightiness, and confusion as the most characteristic symptoms. Depending on personality, maturity, and own insight, children seem to have different ways of coping with their restlessness and inability to pay attention.

In the first examination, most of these children, except those who have always had some problems, seem content with tasks that are familiar to them. As in the younger groups, most find it simple enough to respond to certain everyday questions (T:X), automatic series (T:XI:1,2), well-learned associations like opposite analogies, differences, etc. (T:IX:1,2,5). They become less secure when the same task includes more difficult items that demand on-the-spot reasoning and judging. Older children familiar with writing, printing, reading, or arithmetic facts, may still rattle off multiplications and write and read fluently. They may stumble over arithmetic problems or serial use of facts (T:XI:3–5), dissected sentences (T:XI:6), memory for stories (T:VIII:4), content of reading (T:XI:7). School beginners who before illness were still in the process of learning how to make or recognize letters may become confused about the spatial orientation of letters such as "b" or "d," "w" or "m" (T:XI:8) or they may misjudge quantities

[3] See Meyer and Byers, *op. cit.*

(T:I:8,9). Their tendency to spatial confusion may also be apparent in performances with form material, as it was in the preschool groups. In the older children such disability in learning new perceptual entities may frequently be evident in memory-for-design tasks more than in direct copying (T:VII:1–6). The most conspicuous difficulties are again seen in all tasks that require new learning. Aside from the memory-for-pictures test (T:II:8), which is most useful for younger children, learning tests such as the Rey nonverbal learning test (T:VIII:1), learning pictures (T:VIII:3), and learning words (T:VIII:2), have yielded especially significant results. They allow the psychologist to judge quality and level of present learning ability and provide a basis for comparison between past and present performance.

A child who learns and reasons poorly now, but seems to know and have previously understood a lot, must have been more effective earlier in life than he is now. If he had been as distractible and slow then as he is now, he could hardly have assimilated as much information and developed such good judgement about as many things. One may find that in reasoning problems a child does not attend properly to what he is asked. He may respond to only part of the question in similarities and differences (T:IX:3), verbal absurdities (T:IX:6), comprehension (T:X:3), or overlook some of the relevant details in picture arrangements (T:IX:10). He may judge properly enough those factors which he has retained. He may show vestiges of knowledge or orderly approach that do not now lead him the right way, although they attest to well-established work habits that seem to antedate the present ones.

Often this discrepancy between present and previous achievements becomes evident not only to the examiner, but also to the child himself. An older child particularly reacts to awareness of his own failure in specific ways. He may (like Jack) show amazement and discouragement; he may verbalize or show by actions that he finds things much more difficult than he expected. Often this genuine bewilderment can be an added diagnostic sign. The examiner can usually distinguish it easily enough from the disenchantment or the boasting of an overoptimistic child who seems perpetually to deny his own limitations. The child to whom difficulties are a new experience is apt to get annoyed at himself or to find fault with the material or the task. He may tensely and stubbornly try to find solutions, but soon become overwrought and upset, start again, change his approach, and not easily give up. Most pathetic in this way are those children who have aphasic symptoms as sequelae to injury and infection. These symptoms vary in degree of severity from an almost total loss of speech to much milder signs. Except in the very rare cases of purely "motor" aphasia, loss of speech is accompanied by other disturbances of functioning similar to those that are well known in adult patients.[4] Frequently, the child is able to make some casual automatic responses such as, "Thank you," "Please," "I like that." He may respond accurately to requests such as, "Close your eyes," or "Show your tongue," so that his difficulty passes unnoticed in a routine medical examination. The psychologist, however, may find that the child is unable to carry on a free conversation, that he understands some questions and not others. Often he may have more fragments of speech left, but gropes unsuccessfully for certain words. Instead, he may say words he did not want to say. If he continues to try and does not give up in embarrassment, he may produce a distorted or incomplete version of a word or he may seem to stammer. If an older child is asked to write down what he wants to say rather than trying to say it, he may find to his surprise that he is unable to write what he wants, that he makes the wrong letters, does not know how to continue. He may be greatly relieved when he finds that he is still able to write such familiar letter and word sequences as his name and address. He may be able to write the regular number series, the alphabet, etc., but unable to write on dictation isolated numbers, number combinations, or single letters. Yet he may be able to write familiar dates such as "1958" without hesitation. Difficulty in naming pictures, objects, animals (T:II:2,7,10) may be one of the first clues in milder cases. Also difficulty in finding the correct word in tasks such as differences, similarities (T:IX:1–5) often provides clues. Some children may be able to express by gesture what a picture represents or what an object is used for, if they cannot find the proper word for it; it may be significant that they can do this only when the picture or object is in front of them. Such a child seems unable to evoke by gesture the idea of a thing that is not there. He may be unable to match an object and a printed word (T:VI:11); he may be able to copy words he sees but not to produce them spontaneously from memory (T:XI:9). He may copy a design line by line but be unable to produce it from memory (T:VII:1–6). He may sort objects one by one

---

[4] Kurt Goldstein, *Language and Language Disturbances* (New York: Grune and Stratton, 1948). Also Theodore Weisenburg and Katharine E. McBride, *Aphasia: A Clinical and Psychological Study* (New York: The Commonwealth Fund, 1935), out of print.

or in concrete arrangements only, and not comprehend more abstract categories at an age when such sorting normally becomes possible (T:VI:5,12). He may be able to reproduce serial patterns of blocks (T:I:5) if they are started for him, but be unable either to reverse the pattern, to reproduce it in different colors, or to do it on verbal request.

Frequently, the clinician must content herself with identifying and describing some of the many difficulties that might occur. This is not always easy, since aphasia cases with their varied combinations of startling symptoms can be a great challenge to scientific curiosity and theoretical speculations. It is tempting to probe further and to discover the pattern of interrelated factors that cause distortions of language and thought. At the present state of incomplete factual knowledge in this area, most clinicians are forced to restrain themselves and to heed practical considerations. Experience shows that in the majority of children who have some aphasia after injury or infections, the inability to speak is the first to recede spontaneously. Usually rest, relaxation, and lack of emotional strain are more beneficial than speech training. All these children do best if their elders make light of their language disorders and also of all other difficulties that may occur. This protection must begin in the examining situation. Until then, many of these children may remain almost unaware that they cannot express themselves as they did. The less they notice this and other disabilities, the happier they can remain. Therefore, the clinician must see to it that the child does not discover too much, and must reassure him that he will get better soon.

A wait-and-see policy with plenty of patience and concessions is recommended for all children who recover from serious illnesses, but especially from illnesses that involve the nervous system. Most children seem to profit from a prolonged period of convalescence in their familiar surroundings. Whether much impaired or little, they must for some time live quietly and be protected from the strains of normal daily wear and tear. With few exceptions, it seems best to have school children stay out of class for a considerable period of time, and only at a much later date start on a very gradual program. They need much repetition of what was learned previously. Even if they seem about as well as before, they may for some time be unable to progress at their previous rate. Neither may they be able to catch up with what they lost. The fact that recovery means different things in an adult than it does in a child has been stressed repeatedly.[5] The adult has to get back to where he was; the child has not only to get back there, but ahead to where he would have been if development had not been interrupted through trauma.

Many of these children may be greatly improved a few months after illness. To their parents they may seem fully recovered, less fidgety, and more composed than they were shortly after illness. Their previous tendency to quick fatigue may have disappeared or be on the wane. In some cases a home teacher may have entered the picture after the child has had a period of total rest. She too may have noted the progress and feel that the child is ready to go back to school.

In the second psychological examination (*three to six months after illness*) this improvement may show in better attention spans, better learning ability and memory functioning. The child may handle reasoning problems better. Any mild difficulties in finding proper words and names may have disappeared. In drawing and paper-and-pencil work the stroke may be stronger now than it was; all the child's movements and his posture may seem more decisive now.

Amongst those who have not yet fully recovered at the time of the second psychological examination there are of course numerous variations. The children's attitudes, efficiency, moods, may show many individual differences, as do the opinions, feelings and judgements of those who live with them. Often the parents' chief complaint may still be restlessness, mood swings, impulsive actions, exaggerated reactions to frustration, and/or general fatigue. Some parents complain that the child has become difficult to reason with, that he is oversensitive to criticism, noises, etc. Outside he may get into fights with other children, or he may be out of sorts and have his feelings hurt too frequently. Often some of this behavior is blamed on the fact that the child has too much leisure, license, and boredom. Even parents who have been models of patience may become restive and wish that life were back to normal, since there does not seem to be anything physically wrong with the child.

In the psychological examination at this time, these same children

[5] Bronson Crothers and Elizabeth Lord, "The Appraisal of Intellectual and Physical Factors after Cerebral Damage in Children," *American Journal of Psychology* 94:1077–1088, 1938. Also Edith Meyer and Marianne Simmel, "The Psychological Appraisal of Children with Neurological Defects," *Journal of Abnormal and Social Psychology* 42:193–205, 1947.

usually still show considerable disturbance in functioning. Those who had difficulty in speech may be fluent once again, except perhaps for an occasional inability to find the right word. They may seem less vague and restless, and more ready to settle down. They may stay with the same task longer than they did when seen the first time. They may not get up and change the subject as frequently as they did, but they may in the course of the same task still become blank and unproductive. They still have considerable difficulty in learning tasks (T:VIII) and continue poor in reasoning problems (T:IX); they may still see only one aspect of a problem at a time and become confused by more complex tasks. Some may be able to write and draw better than they did, and have more patience for accurate detail. Their stock of information may still be respectable enough and therefore out of line with their present learning disability; but the discrepancy may gradually be less marked. They may get as many items correct as they did before in information tests (T:XI:10) and vocabulary lists (T:XII), but they may not get more now, which causes their Wechsler scores to drop slightly. Similar lack of gain, and therefore drop of score, can usually be noted in block designs (T:VII:7,8) and memory for designs (T:VII:1,2,4,5) though at this point these scores are often not as strikingly inadequate as they are in cases of organic injury of long standing.

Changes in the children's own attitudes are again important items in diagnosis: about this time, and from here on, it is evident that their own shortcomings are no longer a surprise to them. They are aware of the fact that they cannot do well; the older ones know and say that they no longer are as effective as they were. They face each new task with more apprehension than they showed at an earlier time after their illness. There may be varying reactions to failure: some children may be negativistic and resistant, others depressed but resigned to having difficulty, others persist in trying stubbornly and insistently. It is usually not yet too difficult for the psychologist to decide whether a child's difficulties are of relatively recent origin or were present long before the trauma occurred. His own reactions to his situation often give some clues. A child who did not do very well before often seems less acutely disturbed than one who was accustomed to success.

The psychologist's opinion continues to be a deciding factor in the management of the child. Immediately following the illness, she could help to plan for the near future only. Now, at the time of reexamination (three to six months later), a longer span of time must be envisioned and a plan outlined. As conditions diversify, time passes, and children differ, this may become more and more difficult. Many things have to be considered.

The period of more or less rapid improvement may be over; yet the next two or three years—if well managed—may bring less spectacular, slower gains in mental and emotional adjustment. Some children learn gradually to live with their reduced capacity and acquire some insight. Others continue to run into a succession of impulsive, unrelated actions, and keep on getting overwrought and exhausted. Some older ones may find out for themselves that they cannot stand pressure and speed. They learn to be cautious in their approach and come to see that although they cannot understand all at once, they can understand bit by bit. If they are unable to develop new patterns of adjustment, they may easily become overwhelmed by their own confusion and become unstable and unreliable people.

Success in readjustment seems to depend as much on the personality of the individual as on the attitudes of the people around him: a rather formidable emotional and social readjustment becomes necessary for all, owing to the changes in the child's mental power and nervous stability.

The child's concept of himself comes to change gradually. He may develop sensitivities in new areas; he may be easily hurt by things which did not hurt him before. Some incidents may assume outsized proportions because he cannot see them in relation to their background.

Most of the children who still show disturbances in functioning must have concessions of one kind or another. Parents and teachers must understand that the child still needs protection from stress. While this must be an important and stringent rule, it can happen that it is followed too emphatically: some child may find the new attitudes and changed emotional environment very unsettling. He may sense a loss of confidence if nothing is expected of him any longer, and none of the former standards any longer apply.

He may need help in order to see himself in a somewhat different light. However, his personality change is never a sudden break that creates overnight a totally new person with new emotional and intellectual habits. Except in some rare cases of total deterioration, the post-traumatic personality changes that admittedly occur are at first hardly perceptible: they are gradual modifications of reaction patterns that result from the new circumstances of the patient. In practice one may hardly ever expect a total change in a child after illness or accident. Usually, traits already present are intensified: a potentially quiet and passive child may become more retiring and unable to make decisions, while an active, lively child may become more tense, overexcited, and hyperresponsive.[6] To make a new adjustment is difficult enough for the stable, well-organized child, but often impossible for the less fortunate labile one.

The few facts just briefly described imply that the psychologist who tries to appraise a child several years after an accident or illness must first of all try to develop historical sense. She must grope her way back to psychological factors that might have been influential in the past, before and after illness. Only by doing this can she judge changes that have occurred, whether in the child himself or in those around him. This may also allow her to appreciate how parents and teachers have coped with these changes in the past and how well they may do in the future. Compared with this kind of insight test results obtained *two to three years after the incident* itself seem bland and uninformative. They may become more meaningful when seen against the wider background.

Practice shows that after a considerable lapse of time psychological evaluation may yield the most varying results; traces of organic difficulties may be very noticeable in some children, but hardly perceptible in others. The examiner may not find it difficult to detect damage when a seven-year-old like Rose does poorly in form comprehension, is flighty and disorganized in train of thought, but chatters with poise and a good vocabulary. The psychologist may be sure of her ground when in older children total performance scores on the WISC or Wechsler-Bellevue Scale are lower than verbal scores or when block designs (T:VII:8), object assembly (T:IV:11,12), and coding (T:III:7) are below other achievements. However, there are many cases where evaluation is not as simple. Often verbal test results lose more as time goes on, since the ability to learn new things is necessary for regular gains in information (T:XI:11), vocabulary (T:XII:2), and comprehension (T:X:3). Also, organized reasoning ability is needed for the more advanced comprehension and similarities questions (T:IX:2). Block designs (as was seen before) can occasionally be solved well though slowly through patient piecing together of detail to detail. Similarly, coding

[6] Meyer and Byers, *op. cit.*

can be done by painstaking comparison of model and copy, which may result in a slow but accurate performance. Some children who are accustomed to draw may copy complicated forms by methodical adding of line to line or dot to dot cautiously and slowly. Memorizing designs (T:VII:1,2,4,5) for reproduction is probably one of the most difficult tests for all the injured children. Therefore, in the Rey-Osterrieth complex figure test (T:VII:5) a marked discrepancy between a child's direct copy and his copy from memory may indicate organic difficulty. Most learning tasks (T:VIII) also may show difficulties, with older children especially in the learning of pictures and learning of words. Occasionally only, one finds a child who in these tasks depends almost entirely on his auditory memory and thereby succeeds. Attention difficulties are prominent in many of these children. Frequently, one may find them outbalanced by the individual's tenacious desire to stick it out and to try even if he gets more and more rattled and confused. Reasoning problems (T:IX), generally difficult for this group, give uneven results; they are hard if they demand spatial organization (T:IX:7,9), but less so if common sense and everyday knowledge help toward success (T:IX:8,10). Some children reach solutions through a quick, intuitive guess, others through patient piecing together of bits of thinking. True constructive and creative thinking are uniformly difficult for most.

With many children who still show in the examination a higher level of aspiration than they can possibly achieve, the psychologist may feel the constant urge to make as little as possible of any difficulties because she senses the child's uncertainty and despair about himself. The need to spare such a patient's self-respect can hardly be overestimated: at this point—some years after the illness—most children would like to forget what happened to them, even though they may too often be reminded that something went wrong. The situation of these children whose injury occurred when they were older is utterly different from that of children whose injury dates from birth or before. Children in the former group usually have no, or minimal, physical sequelae to serve them as an alibi; the fact that their difficulty is "mental" only often leads to misconceptions that can be painful to all concerned. These children may still try desperately to regain their old roles and social position. Often they must be allowed to find out for themselves what they can and cannot do. Some children by this time know that they must abandon academic ambitions, and for them the adviser can help plan a more practical career that will provide social, emotional, and possibly remunerative satisfactions. Other children, however, want to see for themselves whether they are able, as they had expected, to carry a high school program without undue strain and fatigue.

There is never a ready-made solution for the difficulties that arise for children with handicaps, whether they were injured earlier or later in life. As with all children with problems, the setting is different for each one and advice must be adjusted accordingly. But the leading thought in all planning and guidance must be the assurance and continued protection of emotional well-being. All these children must gain early as much emotional equilibrium as they possibly can get to weather approaching adolescence. Their turmoils, their depressions and rebellions then may be similar to those of normal children, but their sensitivity and vulnerability may make their need for understanding and personal recognition more acute then as well as later.

Part Two

TECHNIQUES

Techniques

In the following chapters are described in some detail those techniques used in the case studies in the preceding chapters. In many instances, these descriptions include reference to original test procedures from which the particular techniques have been derived. Variations and alternatives are suggested. Certain interesting and relevant techniques are included here, even though they are not represented in the case studies.

Test materials, test procedures, and methods to evaluate results are discussed. Where test manuals are commercially available, the reader is referred to these for detailed directions, scoring methods, and scoring rationale. Directions and scoring methods are given in more detail for material that has appeared in periodicals or in foreign-language publications only and therefore may not be easily available to the average reader. For procedures originally part of comprehensive books, some references have been made to the standards published there; the reader is referred to these books for the original and complete texts.

The approximate age ranges for which the individual procedures are most suitable are briefly indicated at the end of each chapter.

I

Blocks

1—FREE PLAY

Use a set of twelve to sixteen one-inch blocks painted a bright color.

1A—SPONTANEOUS PLAY. When a preschool child is being examined, blocks may be used to advantage as an introductory task. The blocks may be spread on the table in front of the child's chair. He may find them there when he first enters the room. Often they may check any apprehension of the child or parents better than words. The child is apt to move toward them spontaneously and to start playing. E can invite the parents to be seated at some distance, while she herself settles down next to the child or opposite him. If all adults seat themselves quickly, the child may feel that everybody has come to stay a while. The situation may be allowed to speak for itself; E does not need to say much or be otherwise conspicuous until the child has become used to her presence.

Note: Does the child approach the material immediately on his own or is he hesitant? Does he expect or invite social interaction? Is his mother satisfied to keep in the background or does she try to set him at ease by talking to him and showing him what to do? Does she realize or does she have to be told that it would be preferable to let him get adjusted on his own terms? Does the child explore the material, or does he know what to do right away? Do the results of his activity produce new plans? Is he orderly or careless, compulsive or hectic? Is he sociable or noncommittal? Relaxed or apprehensive?

1B—SUGGESTED PLAY. If the child does not touch the blocks at all, avoid prolonging this period by starting to hand blocks to him one by one. Frequently, he will accept them and be drawn out of his passive, expectant attitude. With some extremely shy or negativistic children, try only to manipulate the blocks and to push them nearer to the child without handing them to him. It may help occasionally to drop a block near him. This may give him an opportunity to change position by looking at the dropped block or by picking it up and putting it back on the table. E may need tact, ingenuity, and emotional equilibrium to get the child going and to help him establish some relationship to the room, to the material, and to herself. She must remain unruffled and confident that the ice will be broken sooner or later; and whenever this happens she must refrain from seeming surprised, overjoyed, or otherwise overbearing.

At the beginning a young child may turn to play with the blocks, ignoring E by handing one or another block to his mother. E may reach out and ask, "Will you give it to me?" and then invite the child with, "Let us play with these." The use of "we" instead of "you" will emphasize the fact that E intends to be with the child rather than only to watch him.

For the same reason direct note-taking must be avoided, if not altogether, at least in the introductory phases. A grownup who intermittently turns to paper and pencil while "playing" with the child is an unreal, disturbing, and preoccupied companion, and not the casual, warm, and interested person an examiner of young children must be.

2—BLOCKBUILDING

For children from eighteen months to six years old, the following eight models (see Figure 1) may be used in various ways: tower (Gesell[1]); train (Gesell); straight bridge (Gesell and Revised Stanford-Binet Scale, Forms L and M, III-year level[2]); oblique bridge; six-cube pyramid (Minnesota Preschool Scale[3]); six-cube steps; ten-cube steps (Gesell); and gate (Gesell).

2A—IMITATION. Construct the model and say, "See what I am doing." Leave the model in front of the child, push more blocks toward him, and invite him to "do one like that."

2B—FROM MEMORY. Construct the model as above, and say,

---

[1] Arnold Gesell, *The First Five Years of Life* (New York: Harper, 1940), p. 109.
[2] Lewis M. Terman and Maud A. Merrill, *Measuring Intelligence* (Boston: Houghton Mifflin, 1937), pp. 81, 140.
[3] Florence Goodenough *et al.*, *The Minnesota Preschool Scale* (Minneapolis: Educational Test Bureau, 1932).

FIGURE 1.   Blockbuilding models

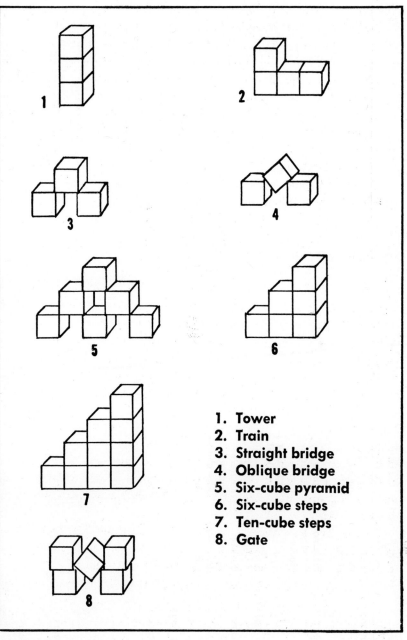

1. Tower
2. Train
3. Straight bridge
4. Oblique bridge
5. Six-cube pyramid
6. Six-cube steps
7. Ten-cube steps
8. Gate

Models 1, 2, 3, 7, and 8 from Arnold Gesell, *The First Five Years of Life* (New York: Harper, 1940), pp. 113, 115, 117–119.

T:I:2. Age norms for blockbuilding

Age	Tower (Gesell, Revised Stanford-Binet)	Train (Gesell)	Straight bridge (Gesell, Revised Stanford-Binet)	Oblique bridge (Informal)*	Six-cube pyramid (Minnesota)	Six-cube steps (Informal)	Ten-cube steps (Gesell)	Gate (Gesell)
18 months	Imitates with two blocks	Imitates pushing						
2 years	Piles more than four blocks	Builds in one direction— vertical or horizontal						
2½ years								
3 years	Piles up without demonstration	Imitates complete with chimney	Imitates	Appreciates difference from straight bridge				
3½ years				Imitates				
4 years			Copies model		Imitates	Imitates vertical and horizontal. Has two instead of three levels		Imitates
5 years						Copies model slowly		
6 years							Tries three tiers but does not succeed	Copies model

* "Informal" standards are those derived from E's experience

"You look at it now. I am going to take it away, and then you make it."

2c—BY COPYING. Use a cardboard screen and construct the model behind the screen. Say, "I am going to build something for you. You look at it when it is all done and then you make one like it." Leave the model in front of the child.

2d—BY GRADUAL LEARNING. Say, "Let us try to do it together." Example (a bridge): say, "I'll take this one and this one and put them like this, and you take two and do the same." Wait for the child to place the blocks; then say, "I'll take another one and put it right here on top. You do the same." When the building is completed, ask the child to do it over again "all by himself." The model may be left in front of the child or be taken away.

One may repeat the learning situation with the same model or with other models. Study the child's ability to remember what was done and to apply it to other similar but varied buildings.

E may vary procedures as the situation requires. She may first gauge the child's level by having him imitate one of the simpler models (bridge). She may try some other models (six-cube pyramid) and ask the child to copy from model (2c). If the child succeeds, she will continue with the same method and more difficult models. If he fails, she may return to having him imitate (2a) or learn (2d).

Blockbuilding as a clinical tool has been popular with many psychologists who deal with children. It permits many observations on general behavior, motor ability, comprehension of material and spatial relations, and ability or desire to imitate and experiment.

In piling blocks, for instance, the youngest children (*fifteen to eighteen months*) do not know without experimentation how far two blocks must overlap to prevent toppling. When building a bridge-like construction, children *between two and three years old* find out by trial and error how far two blocks can be separated and yet support a third one. Difficulties in such constructions may be due partly to neuromuscular immaturity and partly to intellectual immaturity and lack of comprehension of spatial relationships. One child may seem unable to copy a building modelled for him, though he builds it on his own in spontaneous play. Another may, during the observation period, arrive at a certain construction but be unable to repeat it later; his blocks may have formed the structure by chance and not because he understands how to make them stay. Another may have the correct idea, either from the beginning or from his first experience with the material; however, he may be too clumsy to put his plan into effect. He may give up or persist, depending on his emotional attitude. The clinician must be able to differentiate carefully among physical, intellectual, and emotional factors that influence the outcome. Therefore, she must observe the child's working process, his trials and hesitations, as well as the end product. As in many other test situations, the end product may yield an objective score which ranks the child among his peers, but the process leading to the result may explain how it came about and, therefore, may be more informative.

3—Putting Blocks in Box

Produce a box to fit the blocks. Say, "Let us put them away so we can play with something else." E may start to put one or two blocks into the box, and the child may enter into this activity spontaneously or upon invitation.

Note: Does the child want to "help," or take the lead, or do it completely by himself? Does he "take turns" spontaneously? Some children may throw the blocks into the box and enjoy most of all the noise they produce. Others may clear the blocks away haphazardly, interested only in discarding them. Still others may try to fit and to arrange the blocks neatly in the box; they may reveal their comprehension of spatial relationships or their lack of it. They may try to force a block into a space largely occupied by another one (*two-year level*), or learn to separate two blocks enough to fit a third in between (*three-year level*). Other observations may be made when the top of the box is put on. An immature (*eighteen months to two years old*) or tempestuous child may force the top onto the box with no regard for its shape or for any obstructing blocks. An older child (*up to four years old*) may try out the way the top fits best. After that age a child normally considers both the shape of the box and that of the top, and fits them properly without delay.[4]

4—Two Colors

A second set of twelve-inch blocks of a different color may, in some instances, be introduced to replace the first one. A change in color may give some children a needed new start. Occasionally, the second

---

[4] In the Merrill-Palmer Scale, the item "fitting 16 blocks in box" is placed on the two- to two-and-a-half-year level (within 125 seconds) and on the two-and-a-half- to three-year level (within 100 seconds). The directions there call for more supervision and prompting than is generally given in the above procedure. See Rachel Stutsman, *Mental*

set may be held in reserve for use later in the examination if repetition and verification of certain findings appear desirable.

4A—Two different sets of colored blocks may be used simultaneously. If the second set is added to the first, note spontaneous reactions of the child. Does he accept the new material immediately? Does he try to put the first blocks away or integrate the new ones into his previous activities?

4B—Say, "I am making (a bridge) in red. You make one in green," or, "Let us build one green bridge and one red one."

4C—Arrange two-color models. Examples: bridge (see 2) with two green blocks as base, one red block on top; six-cube pyramid with two green and one red blocks as base, two red blocks above, and one green block on top.

Note: Does the child spontaneously pay attention to the color, or must he be reminded? How systematic is he about it? Does he copy the proposed color scheme? Experience shows that only a few children *under five years of age* respond correctly to color in this situation, where more emphasis on building than on color seems inherent.

5—Serial Patterns

5A—ALTERNATING ROW. With both sets of blocks in loose order before the child, say, "Let us make something different now. Look, watch me. We will make something pretty"; or, "I will take a green one, and a red one, a green one, and a red one, and a . . . which one do you think comes next? Yes, a green one. We will make it 'a red one, a green one' all the way to the end of the table." If the child does not pick up the next block correctly, point to the right one and help place it. If a wrong one has been placed, keep saying, "That is fine, but let us put a green one in between so that it is always one green one and one red one in between." Help in correcting errors two or three times. After this, leave the child to do as he chooses.

Note: Does he pay attention to what is proposed to him? Is he interested only in lining up blocks? Does he seem to understand the inherent rule of the pattern, but not carry through to the end? Does he understand immediately, or does he learn gradually? How does he accept help and intervention?

5B—TWO-AND-ONE ROW. Use pattern of two green, one red,

Measurement of Preschool Children, with a Guide for the Administration of the Merrill-Palmer Scale of Mental Tests (Yonkers, New York: World Book Company, 1931), p. 208.

two green, one red, in the same way as above. With older children use 5b following 5a, or omit 5a.

Note: As above. Also, does the child find it easy enough to adapt to a new pattern, or does he persist in a previous one?

This procedure is an adaptation of other commonly used techniques. The Revised Stanford-Binet Scale, Form L, at age VI uses an alternating pattern of beads to be repeated from memory.[5] The Revised Stanford-Binet Scale, Form M, at age VI uses a two-one-two-one bead pattern to be copied.[6] Successful completion of these tasks requires comprehension of an inherent rule and ability to continue in a given mental set without being distracted by any other stimulations offered by the material. The use of blocks instead of beads reduces the need for fine motor control. The use of color instead of form material precludes failure which might be caused by lack of form discrimination alone. A child who in other tests shows that he is able to discriminate color but fails completely in this task probably does so because he lacks comprehension of the rule. He may be unable to perceive the parts of the whole in their relationships, even though he may be able to distinguish properly some isolated parts.

In general, normal *three-year-olds* are capable of understanding how to alternate the colors in a row (5a). However, they are not always able to keep it up until all the blocks are used. At about *three-and-a-half years of age* the majority of normal children complete the task satisfactorily. Between *five and six years of age,* the two-one pattern (5b) is understood and accomplished.

One may vary the test with a somewhat more difficult three-color pattern (green, red, yellow, green, red, yellow), repeating the series until all blocks are used. Experience shows that ascending-descending patterns (green, red, yellow, red, green, red, yellow, red, green) seem to be much more difficult (*seven to eight years of age*).

6—SORTING COLORS

6A—SORTING/MATCHING. Use two identical plastic boxes of a neutral color like white. Place before the child and say, "Let us put the blocks away. The green ones go in one box, the red ones in the other." Wait for a response. If none is forthcoming, or if the child continues to play with the blocks in other ways, put one block in each

---

[5] Terman and Merrill, *op. cit.,* pp. 95, 222.
[6] *Ibid.,* pp. 154, 348.

box and say, "This is going to be the green box, and this is going to be the red one." Repeat if necessary. Then watch the child proceed. Should it become clear that the child does not follow directions but puts blocks into the boxes without attention to color, one may start to teach him in various ways. One may remove unobtrusively each wrong block as soon as it has been placed, or one may say each time, "I do not think that this one goes there. It goes in the other one." Or one may wait to the end and then pick out the wrong blocks and say, "Let us find a better place for these." In this situation the child learns most easily if his errors are corrected immediately. If one allows several wrong blocks to accumulate in a box, it becomes more difficult for the child to discriminate between those that belong and those that do not. Similarly, a box becomes more definitely the "red" or "green" box as more and more blocks of the correct color accumulate in it.

Note: Does the child initially follow verbal directions? Does he follow directions after demonstration, immediately or after delay? Does he notice E's corrections? How does he react to them? Does he accept her interference, or is he annoyed at it? Does he realize why she is changing his placements? Does he seem to learn? Does he carry through to the end, or does he forget in between? Note his method of putting away (see also 3).

This procedure is adapted from other commonly used techniques. In the Revised Stanford-Binet Scale, Form M, a sorting test using twenty-two black and white buttons is placed on the III 6-year level.[7] The Merrill-Palmer Scale[8] includes a color-matching test. Both are described in Chapter VI. In comparison with either one of these techniques, the use of blocks as described reduces demands on fine motor skills. It varies also in other features—in the color of the boxes, for instance, and in the number of colors and units to be sorted (see VI:1,2).

The test procedure described above is one in which normal *three- to three-and-a-half-year-old* children are successful. Many children at *two-and-a-half* come to understand the principle but are easily distracted and cannot complete the test without error.

6B—TRUE SORTING. Sorting without matching can be arranged if high containers (no. 2 cans of a neutral color) are used instead of flat boxes. Thus, the containers remain neutral because the blocks which have been sorted disappear from sight and cannot determine the choice

[7] *Ibid.*, pp. 144, 339.
[8] Stutsman, *op. cit.*, p. 175.

of container. Using this method, sorting colors becomes considerably more difficult. Elements of memory and learning enter in and may add interest for the clinician.

Blocks may be useful in studying number concepts of young children. They may serve as a first gauge of the level of number comprehension with older children whose learning ability is under question.

7—Counting Blocks

Blocks may be spread out in front of the child. Say, "Will you see how many we have? Let us count them." Use all blocks at first, then proceed to isolate smaller groups.

Note: Does the child count the blocks, or does he only recite numbers in their correct order, or incorrect order? Does he coordinate what he says with what he does? Does he point to blocks one by one, or touch one after another? Does he skip any, count some twice? Does he know that the final number is the correct answer to the question "how many?" or has he only understood that he should "count"? Does he run out of either blocks to point to or numbers to recite?

Often young children are able to count verbally before they know how to count a number of objects, or they may be able to count a few objects but not know how to respond to "How many?" Gesell finds that *four-year-old* children in our culture usually can count up to ten but cannot count more than three objects with correct pointing. *Five-year-olds* can recite up to thirteen or more, but can count only ten objects with correct pointing. *Six-year-olds* count thirteen objects without error.[9] Similar standards are presented in the Revised Stanford-Binet Scale.[10]

8—Isolating Small Quantities from Larger Ones

8a—With all blocks in front of the child, E may open her hand and ask, "Please give me three blocks (or two, seven, etc.)."

Note: How does the child go about it? Does he count the proper number first and then hand them out? Is he interested in the social action of give-and-take only, or does he also count the blocks he is handing out? Is he able to perform equally well with larger or smaller units?

8b—As above, say, "Please give me two green blocks and

---

[9] Gesell, *op. cit.*, p. 172.
[10] Terman and Merrill, *op. cit.*, pp. 93, 221, 155, 350.

three red ones," or "four green ones and two red ones," etc. Or say, "Give me five blocks in all, but give me three red ones and two green ones."

These last tasks require more comprehension than do the earlier ones (8a). Quantitative and qualitative elements are combined. The child may easily be diverted by one or another aspect of the request. For instance, he may pay attention only to the demand for red or green blocks, or simply to that for five objects. Similar procedures involving two conceptual areas simultaneously are described in several of the commonly used scales: Gesell finds that the normal *three-year-old* is usually able to give "just two" objects out of ten; the *four-and-a-half-year-old* is able to give "just three" correctly.[11] The Revised Stanford-Binet Scale, Form M, on the V-year level includes one such test item. Within a test of number concept of "three's" the child is asked to give "two blocks and one bead."[12] Here block and bead take the place of the two colors featured in the tasks described above (8b). Gesell lists another similar but more complex procedure: in a test of "drawing bubbles," the child is asked to draw from one to four circles representing soap bubbles "under" or "above" or "in front" or "in back" of the figure of a boy. Drawing the circles and placing them correctly are combined here with the task of reproducing the exact number of circles. Gesell finds that in general *five-year-olds* succeed in these tasks, though occasionally some fail to draw exactly four circles. *Six-year-olds* have no difficulty with these tasks.[13]

9—COMPARING CONCRETE QUANTITIES

9A—Arrange six blocks in a row, allowing one inch of space between each. Ask the child to take the same number of blocks for himself.

Note: Does he begin by counting the blocks in the row? Does he start arranging a new row for himself? How does this row compare in length with the first one? Is each of his blocks arranged opposite one in the first row? Does he end up with an equal number of blocks? Do these blocks have an arrangement of their own, or are they just in a heap?

Various interesting studies about the development of number concepts

[11] Gesell, *op. cit.*, p. 174.
[12] Terman and Merrill, *op. cit.*, pp. 151, 346.
[13] Gesell, *op. cit.*, p. 173.

have yielded interesting findings which can easily be duplicated in these test situations.[14] After *six to six-and-a-half years of age,* most children start by counting the number of blocks in the first row and then proceed to put an equal number of blocks in a separate heap. Less mature and younger children may proceed in either of two ways: they may make a new row and arrange to make it as long as the first one without trying to use the same number of blocks, or they may reach a correct solution by concretely matching each block, one by one. This latter is a frequent solution at *five years of age.*

9ʙ—Arrange four blocks in a square. Ask the child to do the same. Then ask him to count his blocks. If he does this correctly, cover the first square and ask him, "Guess how many I have." Many children up to *five years of age* find it impossible to answer this question without being given a chance to count the blocks in the first square. They do not understand that there must be the same number of blocks in both arrangements since the second copied the first exactly and was made of identical units.

Many of the test situations using blocks help in the study of a child's nonverbal comprehension. If necessary, most of them can be used without verbal directions but with demonstration substituting for words. In most of these situations the child can, in one way or another, reveal his comprehension of the material even if he does not have the necessary motor skill to handle it properly. With severely handicapped children, one may use a proxy method. The child may be invited to direct E how to proceed by whatever way his particular handicap permits. This method requires some adjustments in arrangement of material.

For instance, in serial patterns (5a) one may leave all colored blocks in their respective boxes and place the boxes far apart from each other. Even a child handicapped by a severe motor impairment and lack of speech still may be able to indicate by his glances, his head motions, or other traces of movements which box contains the block he wants to choose. In sorting colors (6) the empty boxes may be set far apart from each other. A child able to grasp a block but unable to drop it into the box properly, may still show which one he is aiming for. Or, if he is unable to grasp the blocks at all, E may hold one block

[14] Jean Piaget, *The Child's Conception of Number,* trans. (London: Routledge, 1952), Parts III and IV. Also Alina Szeminska, "Essai d'analyse psychologique du raisonnement mathématique," *Cahiers de pédagogie expérimentale et de psychologie de l'enfant,* Number 7 (Geneva: Institut des Sciences de l'Education, 1935).

after another up to him and each time ask to be shown where it should go. After a while several blocks of the same color may be picked up together, to avoid fatigue. In blockbuilding tests (2 and 4) E may place the model in front of the child and construct several copies for the child to choose from. One copy may be identical with the model, while others may show slight variations. The child given this multiple choice who refuses all but the correct copy shows better comprehension and discrimination than one who does not seem to see any difference between a straight and an oblique bridge (2), or a building with a green base and one with a yellow base (4).

T:I.   Most suitable procedures for various age ranges

Procedure	Age
1a, 2a, 3	Up to two years
1–9	Two to six years
5, 7–9	Six to ten years

II

Pictures

PICTURE BOOK

Use a picture book showing a few single, clearly outlined common objects on each page.[1] To facilitate grasping, for children with motor impairment, mount the pages on cardboards held together by rings. A picture book may be useful at any time during the examination of children *between fifteen months and four years of age.* Since most young children are accustomed to "looking at pictures," the sight of a book may tend to reassure an apprehensive child or to relax an overexcited one. Sometimes, if a child has strayed away from the examining table, a book proves a lure to get him back to it. A child who has previously said little may start to talk when he sees a book. Sometimes a book offers the child a welcome opportunity to approach his mother again when he may feel that he has abandoned her to play with E. A few children reject the picture book, a fact which in itself may be significant. Often this happens when families have persistently urged the child to say and/or repeat things and have used picture books in this connection.

1—Spontaneous Activity

Place the book on the table and watch the child's response to it. If none is forthcoming, open the book with, "Let us see the book."

Note: Does the child approach the book? Does he grasp it like an object to be manipulated? Does he push it or drag it, as *twelve-month-olds* are apt to do? Or does he seem to treat it appropriately? Does he seem to notice pictures as color spots to be patted (*fifteen months*)? Does

[1] *What Baby Sees* (Platt and Munk, Inc., No. 742) has been found to be satisfactory for the purpose. It is made of resistant material and is available at many good toy stores.

302

he look at pictures "selectively" (*eighteen months*)? Does he turn several pages at once (*eighteen months*)? Or one at a time (*twenty-four months*)? Does he, on his own, point to and name any of the pictures (*eighteen to twenty-one months*)?[2] Does he vocalize at all? Does he look for an audience and use the book as an opportunity to be social, or does he "read" silently?

2—NAMING

Use with the youngest children only. Try to elicit vocal responses by pointing to some picture, saying, "Look, what is that?" Select a picture for which the child is likely to have a name, as dog, shoe, car. Select at the beginning only one picture on each page, because most young children like to turn pages. When they are very young, frequently they perceive only one dominant picture on each page. This first procedure invites the child to give a name to a familiar object, although it may be pictured in an unfamiliar way; the test is not intended to evaluate how he differentiates among several pictures on the same page—such an attempt would be of a higher order of difficulty.

Note: Does the child seem to respond to the question, or does he continue to name spontaneously what he sees and knows? Does he name the objects with discrimination, or does he keep on using the same word persistently? Does he voluntarily go on to new pictures on the same or a new page? Does he use gestures *with* his words or *instead* of them?

3—POINTING

Use with the youngest children only. Study the child's responses to questions like "Where is the dog?" (or house, or shoe, or kitty). Turn to the proper page or fold the book so that a single page is before the child.

Note: Does the child differentiate between cat and dog, lamb and horse, car and wagon, shoe and sock, apple and orange? Does he point out objects he has not been asked for?

Among children of the same age there is considerable variation in responses to such tasks. For some children, it is simpler to point toward a picture than to name it. Pointing on request involves the ability to scan all the possibilities which the page offers and to resist the attractions of everything but the requested picture. In order to differentiate

[2] Arnold Gesell, *The First Five Years of Life* (New York, Harper, 1940), p. 211.

between similar objects, the child needs powers of observation and of discrimination. However, much also depends on what the child may have seen or been taught at home. At *two to two-and-a-half years of age* many children who have had the normal opportunities are able to point correctly to a considerable number of different pictured objects and to discriminate between similar ones.

4—DIFFERENTIAL POINTING

Study the child's comprehension of subtler differentiations and descriptions.

4A—Ask, "Show me the mouth of the doll," or "the eyes of the teddybear," or "the tail of the horse."

4B—Ask, "Where is the tail of the lamb?" or "Where are the wheels of the automobile?" For these questions choose places in the book that show on the same page both a train and a wagon (or a horse and a lamb).

Note: Does the child respond correctly immediately or only after the request has been repeated? Does he point only to the eyes of the doll or to the whole doll (4a)? Does he show the wheels or the automobile; if he shows the wheels, does he point just to the automobile wheels or to all wheels on the page?

Correct response demands verbal comprehension of the whole question and ability to structure perceptions accordingly; any response stimulated by only a part of the question must be inhibited. In general, *three-year-olds* are capable of responding adequately to this type of question. At higher age levels, failure in these tasks may show a lack of reasoning ability or of ability to concentrate, or it may suggest a lack of auditory acuity. Hearing difficulties which are not immediately obvious may often be suspected if an otherwise responsive child fails these tests even though he succeeds in 3.

5—PICTURE IDENTIFICATION

5A—BY USE. Ask questions about usage: "Which one goes on our feet?" or "on our hands?" "Which one do we eat with?" or "drink from?" Choose pages showing both shoes and mittens, or both cup and spoon. Choose a page with pictures of hairbrush, comb, toothbrush[3] and ask, "Which one do we fix our hair with?" or "Which one do we brush (or comb) our hair with?" Note whether the child responds to the first

[3] *What Baby Sees.*

question as well as to the second, or whether he misses the first but responds correctly to the second because the word "comb" or "brush" directly suggests the respective pictures.

One may expect most normal children at *two-and-a-half to three years of age* to respond correctly to such questions. These norms, which have been derived from experience only, seem to agree with those established in scales such as the Revised Stanford-Binet in situations differing somewhat from those described above. Similar questions are asked with regard to objects in the Revised Stanford-Binet Scale, Form M, on the II 6- and III-year levels, and in Form L on the II 6- and III 6-year levels. Similar questions are also asked regarding black and white pictures in the Revised Stanford-Binet Scale, Forms M and L, on the IV- and IV 6-year levels.[4] (See II:9.)

5B—BY SIMPLE GROUPS. Say, "Let us find all things to eat" or "all animals" or "all toys." For each question go through every page of the book.

Note: Does the child go through the book page by page, looking over each one to find only the relevant pictures? Does he scan the pages silently, or does he verbally discard (with "Not this one") those pictures not applicable? Does he find several pictures on the same page or only one on each? Does he go through the book systematically, or does he become distracted by other pictures and forget what he started out to do? Is he always certain which ones to choose? Does he know that the fish is an animal, or does he have doubts? Does he choose edibles only, or include eating utensils too?

The task demands verbal comprehension, ability to discriminate, to choose, and to discard. It requires background information and sustained attention. Experience shows this is within the range of most normal *three-and-a-half- to four-year-olds,* though there may be some individual variations.

5C—BY COMMON USE GROUPS. Ask such questions as, "Which ones do we eat for breakfast?" or "With which ones do we play outside?" or "Which one makes juice (or applesauce)?" (Common-sense questions of this nature will be discussed in Chapter X.) This type of question must be scrutinized carefully and revised from time to time; for instance, the "orange juice" or "applesauce" questions have become more or less obsolete in this age of frozen and canned foods.

---

[4] Lewis M. Terman and Maud A. Merrill, *Measuring Intelligence* (Boston: Houghton Mifflin, 1937), pp. 78, 84, 137, 140, 198, and 87, 91, 146.

BLACK AND WHITE PICTURES

6—Picture Description

Use the following picture material from the Revised Stanford-Binet Scale, Forms M and L, III 6- and VI-year levels: (Form M) Grandmother's Story, Birthday Party, Washday; (Form L) Dutch Home, River Scene, Post Office.[5]

 6a—standard presentation. Present and evaluate as directed.

 6b—questions. Add questions ranging from a neutral, "And . . . ?" or "What else . . . ?" to more direct questions, such as, "What are they doing?" or "What do they (he) think?" or "What would they (he) like to do?"

Note: Does the child notice relationships and meanings at once, or does he name isolated items, seeing the relationship among them only after delay? Does he spontaneously, or only after suggestion, mention the more important items (people, fire on the stove), or does he concentrate on details (leaves, flowers)? Does he show more interest in people and their activities and interactions ("She is talking to them") or in objects and furnishings ("things cooking")? Are there any interesting emotional tones, such as, "She is mad at them" or "They would rather play outside"? Do E's questions seem to change his responses, and if so, in what direction? Does his tendency to enumerate pictures seem to be a customary routine with him? Is he able also to give interpretations when asked for them?

The test situations here (6a, 6b) may be used to evaluate vocabulary, fluency of speech, sentence combinations, perceptions, and comprehension of situations as well. A child may not initially give many good responses, but may produce more when he is asked. However, unless the child is at a stage near immediate comprehension, he is not likely to function on a higher level of comprehension as a result of questioning.

 6c—simple problems of reasoning. On Birthday Party: Ask, "Could you guess how old the child is going to be? The one that has a birthday?"

Note: Some children may at once count the candles on the birthday cake which is visible in the window (*five- to six-year level*). Others,

---

[5] *Ibid.*, pp. 84, 204, 143, 155, 335.

without looking at the picture, may smilingly declare, "Four years"; but when these latter children are asked "Why?" or "How did you know?" they may reply, "Because I am four—I know," or "My sister is five." One may receive responses somewhere in between the two described here. A child may not yet have learned how to find the right answer, and yet may no longer rely on his own immediate experience for it. Previously learned replies to "How old?" no longer help him to solve another similar question. When he declares that he does not know, E may introduce a series of graded suggestions: "Look at the cake—how old is the child?" "Look at the candles—how old is the child?" "Count the candles—how old is the child?" "How many candles does he have on his birthday cake? How old is he?" (The question "How old is the child?" should be added after a proper interval during which the child has had time to consider the suggestion.)

On Grandmother's Story: Ask, "What are they cooking?" or "What is cooking on the stove?"

Note: Some children may study the picture and point out that there is a teakettle with boiling water on the stove and a pot of boiling soup spilling over on the floor (*approximately six years and over*). Others may hardly look at the picture, but enumerate any items they can think of, as, milk, chicken soup, "their supper." Some children look at the pictured stove but do not study it carefully enough; they may say, "Water or soup or something," but not notice the difference between the steaming kettle and the dripping pot.

On Washday: Ask, "What did he take?" The most observant *five-year-olds* may respond, "A shirt" or "A blouse." Younger ones may say, "His pants," "A sweater," or, indiscriminatingly, "Mother's clothes."

6D—HABITS AND EMOTIONAL SET. Some more specific questions may elicit information about the child's home life and emotional attitudes.

On Washday: Ask, "Why did he take the clothes away?"

Note: Answers may vary from, "He wanted to have fun" or "to play" to, "He wanted to be bad" and, "He wanted to run away." Continue asking questions, such as "Why?" or "And then?" or "What happened?" or "How does he feel?" Answers may be similar to, "She is chasing him. He is running away. He is going to get a spanking. He will never do it again"; or "He will do it over again right away"; or "He does not want to be bad anymore. His mother is mad at him. She sits him in a chair."

All situations described under 6b to 6d are given simply as samples, to show the type of psychological information obtainable with any appropriate picture material. There seem to be certain advantages in using the material from the Revised Stanford-Binet Scale for the various purposes described and not only in standard fashion. It appears natural for most children to keep talking about the pictures they have been shown. Also, it may often be advisable not to change sets of material more frequently than necessary, but rather to exploit each one as thoroughly as the child's interest span permits.

7—PICTURE VOCABULARY

Use either of the following series of black and white pictures representing simple objects, from Revised Stanford-Binet Scale:[6] (Form L) shoe, clock, chair, bed, scissors, house, table, hand, fork, basket, glasses, gun, tree, cup, umbrella, pocketknife, stool, leaf; or (Form M) automobile, hat, telephone, key, airplane, ball, knife, soldier hat, block, flag, horse, foot, coat, boat, can, pitcher, arm.

7A—STANDARD PRESENTATION. Present and score as directed. The original "purpose of this test is to determine whether the sight of a familiar object in a picture provokes recognition and calls up the appropriate name."

7B—STUDY OF RESPONSES. Use this material to study any response provoked by the sight of a familiar object in a picture. Any response that has to be scored minus by scoring standards may have significance. It may reveal the quality and special character of a child's perceptions and associations, his experiences, and his ability to remember. It may show his special modes of expressing himself.

Note all responses obtained. Does the child find some responses for every picture, or is he apt to say, "I do not know?" Does he try to find a new word for each picture, or does he use the same word several times, successively or at intervals? Does he seem to grope for the correct word, or does he seem to say the first word that comes to his lips? Do his errors show associations easily recognizable as such (spoon for fork) or meaningful to those around him ("Daddy go" for airplane)? Does his naming show that he tends to perceive pictures in a primitive, diffuse,

[6] *Ibid.*, pp. 77, 195, 136, 328.

global way, paying attention to "qualities of the whole" rather than fine details (stick for knife)?[7]

Are his errors the result of a carryover from a previous picture or from other familiar verbal patterns? Carefully observe the child's enunciation; note which of the consonants may be missing or defective. Watch for dropped consonants (coa- for coat, fla- for flag). For children with very poor articulation, note and check with the mother on nuances in sound productions which may mean different words to the child even if only barely perceptible to outsiders. Observe gestures and whether they accompany or replace verbal responses. Are they relevant and meaningful or only incidental? If they are the child's only form of response, do they indicate that he is, or is not, familiar with the picture?

7C—GESTURES. The same picture material may be used to study more specifically a child's ability to express himself without words. Show a knife (or airplane, ball, spoon) and ask, "Show me what it does" or "Show me what we do with it." For children who do not seem to understand language, show by a sample what is wanted of him.

Note: Does the child use varied appropriate gestures, or does he tend to use the same gestures with all pictures? Are his means of expression mostly manual, facial, or both? Is there any sign that he indicates objects of the same category in similar ways? Does he, for instance, describe animals by their sounds and movements, tools by their use? or does he point to a chair in the room to indicate a stool or chair? Observation of a child's use of gestures can be of considerable diagnostic significance with respect to development of communication.[8]

7D—ALTERNATE NAMING. If the child has designated an object either in words or through gestures, E may ask, "What else could it be?" The child may or may not find a second response, produce a synonym, a better word, or a better gesture.

7E—POINTING. This picture material may also be used to investigate comprehension of language. Use all cards of a series at one time, or use them in groups of four to six. Present the material by asking, "Where is the spoon?" etc. (as in 3). The child can indicate by pointing or nodding at the pictures, or in any other way he chooses. For a

---

[7] Heinz Werner, *Comparative Psychology of Mental Development* (New York: Harper, 1940), p. 116.

[8] Helmer R. Myklebust, *Auditory Disorders in Children* (New York: Grune and Stratton, 1954), Part 3, Chapter VII, "Aphasia."

severely handicapped child who is unable to point accurately or to turn his head freely, the pictures may be spread far enough apart to avoid equivocal responses, yet near enough so that they all remain in the line of vision.

Note whether the child scans the field for the proper picture or responds haphazardly, pointing first to one, then to another? Does he point to the correct picture only? Does he know at least the general area in which it belongs? (Does he point to a fork when asked for a knife, for instance?) Does he seem to see all the pictures correctly, or does he make unexpected errors? Are they possibly due to sensory difficulties? Check whether a wrong picture is pointed to because of poor perception, eyesight, or hearing. Does he not *understand* or does he not *see* (or *hear*) the difference in the looks of gun and knife, or the words house and horse?

This procedure is on a higher level of difficulty than that described under 3. The pictures are more complex and more differentiated than those of the picture book; they are also black and white, and small. Experience shows that, in general, normal children are able to point out all pictures adequately before or at least at the same age they can find names for them (see 7a). Often one may find children who can point correctly to something long before they are able to name it. It may often be important for the clinician to discover whether a child understands more language than he is able to express. The procedure is therefore of considerable value in all cases of speech retardation, as well as in those where sensory difficulties are suspected.

8—MEMORY FOR PICTURES

Use either series of the picture vocabulary material described under 7, but avoid introducing this procedure if 7 has preceded. Choose three (or four or five) pictures; avoid those that may create the more obvious kind of association. For example, use hat, horse, and ball in the same series, but not airplane *and* automobile, or hat *and* coat.

8A—NAMING MISSING ONE OF THREE (OR FOUR OR FIVE). Say, "Let us play a guessing game. First I will show you pictures." Present the first picture. Say, "This is a . . . ," waiting for the child's response. Accept and repeat any name he gives. Supply a name if the child does not produce one. Place the picture in front of the child and present the second and third pictures in the same manner, placing all pictures in a horizontal row. Say, "Let us look at them," and repeat,

"This is a . . . , this is a . . . , and this is a. . . ." Again supply the words if the child does not do it on his own. Use the same word name as before. Repeat as above, but shift the positions of the pictures in the row in order to change the auditory and visual sequence. For example, change "hat, horse, ball" to "horse, ball, hat."

Say, "Now let us play the guessing game. You close your eyes tight so you can't see them. And while you're not looking, I'm going to take one away, and then you open your eyes and guess which one I took away." Some children are too active to listen to the complete directions. Then say only, "Now close your eyes tight." Some children may be apprehensive and may not like to close their eyes. Instead, say to them, "You look at Mommy," or "Look out of the window so you cannot see the pictures." Put up a screen or shield the pictures in some other way. Remove one of the pictures. Keep it face down but visible on the table; close the gap between the remaining pictures and say, "Now you may look. Which one did I take away?"

Note: Does the child look at the remaining pictures and conclude from them which of the pictures has been taken away? Or does he point to the face-down picture and say, "That is the one." Does he want to see the picture again, or try to wrest it away from E? If he knows that he may find the answer by looking at the remaining pictures on the table, does he try to remember what was there before, and does he or does he not come up with the right response? On the other hand, does he name in a haphazard fashion any of the pictures which he sees still lying on the table and thereby reveal his lack of comprehension of the problem?

If the correct solution has been found, proceed to the next series (four or five new pictures) and present in the same way. If the correct solution has not been reached with the first series, present the same three pictures once more in the same way, but remove a different picture from the one used before.

Note behavior in all repetitions. Does the child use the same method in all presentations, or does he learn from experience? Does he learn better ways as time passes, or does he try to find the answer in a more primitive way as soon as he is faced with a longer series of pictures? Note also whether the child is elated and excited or anxious and uncertain. Does he become stimulated and amused by the social situation involved, or does he become angry and aggressive?

Successful performance of these tasks requires attention, learning, and reasoning ability. The pictures in each series have to be separately remembered, and each series must be so manipulated that the sight of the remaining pictures helps in finding the solution, yet is not itself the solution.

Accurate age norms are not available for the procedure in the form in which it is presented here. Comparison with similar items in other scales and with the norms available for these helps to evaluate performances in children with marked deviations in attention, comprehension, etc. In a similar test, Kuhlmann uses three pictures at the three-year level and four pictures at the four-year level.[9] The Revised Stanford-Binet Scale, Form L, includes on the IV-year level a similar memory task, with small objects presented in a series of three, but covered rather than taken away.[10]

8B—NAMING COVERED-UP ONE OF THREE (OR FOUR OR FIVE). A simpler procedure may be used with children for whom the removal of the pictures and the special give-and-take involved proves overstimulating and confusing.

Present pictures as above. Do not remove any picture, but place a hand over one and ask, "Guess what picture I am covering." Note behavior as before.

9—PICTORIAL IDENTIFICATION

Use material from the Revised Stanford-Binet Scale, either Form L, IV-year level, or Form M, IV 6-year level.[11]

9A—STANDARD PRESENTATION. Present and evaluate as directed. Ask questions such as: "Which one do we cook on?" "Which one do we carry when it is raining?" (from Form L) and "Which one can fly?" "Which one swims in the water?" (from Form M).

9B—ADDED QUESTIONS. Ask, "Which one says meow?" (See 5a.) "Which one hops?" Note all the child's responses, whether they are correct or not. Does he name the object and point to it spontaneously or after he has been asked to do so? Does he seem to have a verbal answer all ready without looking at the picture? Or does his answer come after he has scanned the page and found the proper picture? What are his errors? Does he point to a specific picture and mean it, or does

[9] Frederick Kuhlmann, *A Handbook of Mental Tests* (Baltimore: Warwick and York, 1922), pp. 157, 160. See also Florence L. Goodenough *et al., The Minnesota Preschool Scale* (Minneapolis: Educational Test Bureau, 1932).
[10] Terman and Merrill, *op. cit.,* pp. 86, 209.
[11] *Ibid.,* pp. 87, 146, 210.

he seem to point haphazardly at any one? What, if any, is the relationship between the picture he chooses and the question? Did he misunderstand or reply only to some aspect of it (to "Which one gives us milk?" he might show "the cat").

9C—IDENTIFICATION BY GROUPS. Use same material. Say, "Show me all the animals" or "Show me all the things that we can eat."

Note as above (see also 5b).

9D—IDENTIFICATION IN REVERSE. Present following 9a and use same material. Say, "Now it is your turn. Ask me one. Make me guess."

Note: Does the child understand immediately and formulate a new question? Is his question exclusive or could it apply to several of the pictures ("Which one is in the tree?" Does he mean the apple or the bird?). Does he repeat a question which has previously been asked of him? Does he point to a picture and ask, "This one?" or "What is this one?" or does he lead to the picture he wants to have guessed by asking, for example, "Where is the fish?" or "What do we cook on the stove?" or "Which bird says peep?"

This technique requires more maturity of reasoning than does 9a. The child has to think in terms of another person's point of view. He must formulate a question. He must manipulate the relationship between picture, word, and action, but resist reacting himself to these relationships as they present themselves to him. It is an often observed fact that a child may act properly in a given situation long before he is able to understand or describe this action. Children of *five-and-a-half to six years of age* in general respond adequately to this task. The younger they are the more often they themselves respond to the stimulus, either by pointing to the picture or by asking for it by name. At an in-between stage they may invent an elaborate and well-reasoned question, yet not abstain from incorporating the name of the object in their question. Again, they may formulate a correct question, yet at the same time keep pointing to the corresponding picture.

9E—SUGGESTIONS. Try several explanations for children who do not understand spontaneously. Say, "You make it too easy for me. You are showing me (or telling me). I made it harder for you. I only talked about the fish and you guessed right away, but I never showed it to you. Try again but do not tell me which. Just tell about it."

For some of the older children, this may be explanation enough and may help to produce the correct response. Younger ones may thus be induced to refrain from pointing or naming directly, although they still may resort to any other of the above described primitive forms of behavior.

10—ANIMAL PICTURES

Use material from the Revised Stanford-Binet Scale, Form M, III 6-, IV-, and IV 6-year levels.[12]

10A—STANDARD PRESENTATION. Present as directed. Say, "Find me another one just like this one." Evaluate as directed.

10B—"FIND ANOTHER (RABBIT)." Present as above. Say, "Find me another (rabbit) just like this one." Naming the animal seems to make the task easier, probably because it gives a firmer structure to the task.

10C—"THIS IS MY (RABBIT), WHERE IS YOURS?" Present as above and say, "See this one here in the window. This is *my* rabbit. Where is *yours*?" or "See, this one here is *my* rabbit. Look around and find one for yourself. Where is *your* rabbit?" This procedure is easier than 10a or 10b. It creates a social atmosphere which seems to motivate most children better than either one of the previous tasks.

10D—NONVERBAL MATCHING. For deaf children or others who do not seem to understand language, the situation may be presented without the use of words. E, by pointing, may explain what is to be done. Put one finger on each of a pair of animals simultaneously. This may help the child to understand that there are two pictures to be matched.

Note in 10a through 10d all choices, whether correct or not. Note whether the child succeeds immediately in 10a or whether his performance improves with the facilitated presentations, 10b and 10c. Does he understand what is asked of him in 10b and try to find a picture matching the one shown to him? Or does he seem simply to be looking for *any* rabbit picture? How does he react to the social or competitive note in 10c? What may be the basis for his errors, if any? Are they determined by primitive perceptual qualities, such as the upright position (cat—squirrel), or four-legged squatness (bear—pig), or long-leggedness (goat—giraffe)? Or are they determined by meaningful associations (cat—mouse)? Are his errors in the choice of those pictures which are more difficult to differentiate (deer—goat), or do they involve also pictures that seem to be easily distinguishable be-

[12] *Ibid.,* pp. 143, 148, 335.

cause of size, posture, etc. (elephant—mouse)? Does his performance get better or worse? As the task proceeds does he catch on to it, or do his interest and attention fade?

11—ANIMAL PICTURES

Use the same materials (Revised Stanford-Binet Scale, Form M, III 6-year level). Use bottom card only.

11A—NAMING. Introduce this task either after 10a, or without it. Do not have it precede 10a.

Say, "Look, you know all these animals. Let us tell who they are, as fast as you can." Point to the picture (cat) in the upper left corner, and start, "This is a. . . ." If the child hesitates in giving a response, add "cat." Then point to the next, with "This is a. . . ."

Note: Does the child seem at ease, or is he hesitant and insecure? Does he seem hurried or challenged, or does his desire to be fast help to keep him from wondering if he might be wrong? Note his enunciation, manner of speech, etc. (as in 7). Does he use infantile expressions, such as "bow-wow" or "billy goat"? Does he have a different name for each animal, or does he repeat the same one frequently or invariably? Does he distinguish properly between animals that may have similar size and posture (see above), or do his errors indicate that he still has diffuse concepts that may embrace varied objects which are vaguely similar only in some global perceptual quality? Does he remember and use names used before in 10b or 10c?

Experience shows that the task of naming these animals is well within the limits of ability of normal *six-year-old* children. Most of them can correctly name all the twelve animals pictured on the card except the deer. The younger children may not find names for goat, bear, and squirrel.

11B—POINTING. Ask child to show the (squirrel, giraffe, etc.).

Frequently, a child who is not yet able to think of or produce the proper name may know how to point correctly when asked. This variation of the procedure allows E to differentiate between those children who do not know the animal at all and those who are not yet able to say its name. In some cases this distinction may be of some importance especially with children whose speech retardation calls for qualitative analysis.

11C—IDENTIFICATION. Say, "Let us play a guessing game." Ask: "Which one says meow? Which one gives us milk? Which one eats cheese? Which one eats nuts? Which one brings Easter eggs? Which one do we see in the circus?"

11D—IDENTIFICATION IN REVERSE. Say, "Now it is your turn. Ask me one. Make me guess."

Note all responses (as in 9a to 9d). Note (as in 9d) how the child puts his questions. Does he find original ones that reveal richness of information ("Which one can go in the desert without water?"), or are they repetitive ("Which one says bow-wow?"), or commonplace ("Which one hops?")? Are his questions so formulated that they can mean only one specific animal ("Which one squirts water with his trunk?"), or could they apply to several ("Which one makes noise?")?

Experience shows that above questions (11c) are answered satisfactorily by most normal *five- to six-year-old* children. Both questions and material seem to be more difficult than those described under 5 and 9a. The pictures here are more nearly identical than in either of the other tasks, and the questions involve more specific knowledge.

11E—IDENTIFICATION BY DIFFERENTIAL QUESTIONS. Say: "Show me the one that has the longest nose; show me the one that has a curly tail. Show me the one that has a bushy tail. Show me the one that has pointed ears. Show me the one that has a very long, thin tail. Show me the one that is pictured sitting."

These questions are solved by children *six years of age and older*. They test scope and comprehension of vocabulary. This task also may be suited to children with speech difficulty who use a restricted vocabulary but may or may not understand more language than they produce. The task may also be useful with children who appear fluent in their everyday conversation but may not always know exactly what the words they use mean. It may show a lack of comprehension which is hardly noticeable in everyday life. (See also Chapters X and XI.)

T:II. Most suitable procedures for various age ranges

Procedure	Age
1–4	Up to two years
1–11	Two to six years
6–8, 9d, 11	Six to ten years

III

Paper and Pencil

1—Spontaneous Drawing

Use plain, medium-sized sheets of paper. Use crayons with children up to three or four years of age and medium-sized pencils with blunted points for older ones. (Over- or under-sized sheets of paper and long or extra-sharp pencils are awkward to handle.) An ample supply of paper and pencils assures the child that there is no restriction on his use of paper and no necessity to worry about breaking pencil points.

Note: Does he seem to have experience with paper and pencil; does he like to use them, or do they make him apprehensive? Does he grasp the pencil (or crayon) immediately with the proper grasp? Does he apply it to the paper? Does he use the proper strength, or is his stroke too weak or too strong, unsteady or irregular? Does he consistently use the same hand, and which one is it? Does he begin to draw something, or does he wait for instructions? Does he seem to have a subject in mind, or does one develop while he is working? Does he stick to his plan, or does he change it? Does he begin to scribble to try his pencil or for lack of an idea, or does he scribble when his attempts prove frustrating? Are his productions recognizable? If they are not, is this caused by motor disability or immature perception or both? Is his drawing planned in relation to the size of the paper? Is it over-sized and does it not fit the available space, or is it noticeably small and condensed at the bottom of the page or in one corner?

Spontaneous drawings of children of all ages have been of interest to many investigators who have studied them from various angles.

It is, for instance, well known that very young children (from *eighteen months on*) are apt to scribble only, until they gradually (at about *three years of age*) come to name their productions spontaneously, or later (at *five years of age*) name a project before starting. In between (at about *four years of age*) they may have a plan but alter it during their work to fit the production.[1] With advancing age, more and more depending on individual differences, a child *older than six* may prefer to follow a plan of his own or to draw a subject chosen for him. With advancing age, most children become more critical of their lack of skill and more reluctant to display it. After *ten years of age* it is often difficult to obtain any uncoerced free drawing except from children who like to draw and are used to it. Cramped, small-sized drawings are more often made by anxious, inhibited children than by exuberant ones. Occasionally, however, such a drawing may be produced by some child mainly because of poor motor coordination or because he has been taught to save paper. Over-sized drawings are supposed to be characteristic of outgoing, optimistic personalities. Often, such overexpansion may also point to lack of foresight and planning. Overmeticulous, carefully pencilled drawings may indicate compulsiveness. Overemphasis on detail at the expense of the whole is seen in schizophrenic as well as in brain-injured patients. It seems that brain-injured children are more apt to dwell on decorative details (flowers on a dress, stripes on socks), whereas children with schizophrenic tendencies stress less obvious or even hidden functional details (bricks of a house, stamens in a flower, bony structures in animals). Exaggerated dissociations of details, so-called "piecemeal" productions, and lack of organization (a head with the mouth and eyes next to and unrelated to it) are most frequently seen in the drawings by brain-injured children. Similar dissociations, however, are also found in those of schizophrenic patients.[2] It is important to remember that normal children at young age levels also frequently show a tendency to juxtaposition or to global, "syncretic," over-all impressions. They are apt to show both tendencies in their various drawings; at the youngest age level, single subjects are frequently represented globally, but with progressing age are represented in a more differentiated way. Complex scenes or simultaneous events

---

[1] Arnold Gesell, *The First Five Years of Life* (New York: Harper, 1940), pp. 140ff.
[2] Lauretta Bender, *Child Psychiatric Techniques* (Springfield, Illinois: Thomas, 1952), p. 306.

often are pictured side by side in primitive juxtaposition by younger children but in more coordinated relationships by older ones.

Drastically changing a project while drawing is normal for a young child because mental organization still allows optimum fluidity. In older children, however, it may be a sign of something else. It may be due to abnormal flightiness in some, for instance, or, on the contrary, be an alibi to cover up imperfections in the more critical ones.

Many kinds of considerations too numerous to mention must enter into the evaluation of an individual child's spontaneous drawings. E must have had ample experience with drawings by normal children at various ages, or else refrain from elaborate interpretations which cannot be justified or verified. When judged with caution, drawing is a useful clinical technique which can, in many cases, offer an easy approach to the child and a tentative first impression of his motor, intellectual, and emotional condition.

2—SUBJECT DRAWING

Propose a special subject to the child. Ask him to draw "a lady walking in the rain."[3]

2A—DRAWING A LADY WALKING IN THE RAIN. Allow not more than ten minutes. If necessary emphasize the fact that the picture need not be beautiful but that the child should try to include everything needed to show the scene. See scoring directions below.

Note the child's manner of work, his motor characteristics, and the way he arranges the drawing on the page (as in 1). Note his attitude toward the task, the speed with which he begins or proceeds. Does he keep to the directions or make counterproposals? Does he voluntarily elaborate on the theme? Does he follow a plan or haphazardly add one feature to the next? Does he start with the main figure or with some detail? Which details attract him most? Does he constantly remember the

---

[3] This procedure was originated by Fay and published first in 1924. It was later revised and newly standardized by Wintsch. The latest standardization, on 1,300 Swiss children, published by Rey in 1947, combines a scoring system adapted from Goodenough with that of earlier authors. See H. M. Fay, "Le dépistage des arriérés à l'école," *La médecine scolaire*, pp. 282–290, December 1924; *L'intelligence et le caractère* (Paris: Foyer Central d'Hygiène, 1934), pp. 69–76. Also J. Wintsch, "Le dessin comme témoin du développement mental," *Zeitschrift für Kinderpsychiatrie* 2:33, June; 2:69, August 1935. Also André Rey, "Epreuves de dessin témoins du développement mental," *Archives de psychologie* 31:369–380, December 1946; 32:145–149, February 1947; *Monographies de psychologie appliquée,* Number 1 (Paris: Delachaux et Niestlé, 1947). Also Florence L. Goodenough, *Measurement of Intelligence by Drawings* (Chicago: World Book Company, 1926).

T:III:2a.   Wintsch's scoring system for "une dame se promène et il pleut"

Item	Points
a. A lady	1
A human figure without feminine attributes	½
b. Walking indicated (by position of feet)	1
c. Outside, indication of landscape	1
A line instead of landscape	½
d. Rain	1
Rain poorly indicated, not down to ground or around person	½
e. Rain protection	1
Umbrella folded or not over head	½
f. Interesting details (pocketbook, heels, dog on leash, etc.), in all	½
Adapted from Wintsch, *op. cit.*	

T:III:2a.   Wintsch's age norms for "une dame se promène et il pleut"

Age (years)	Points
7	1
8 to 9	2
10 to 11	2½
12	3
Adapted from Wintsch, *op. cit.*	

theme, or does he, while working, forget some important point (rain, motion)? Does he correct, erase, and try to improve his work, or leave it as it is? Listen to his remarks while he is drawing; note especially all features (in the lady or the scene) which may point toward a child's emotional situation.

In normal children up to *ten or twelve years of age* the procedure described here is designed to measure the level of intellectual maturity. The young child draws what he knows rather than what he is able to draw properly. Before the age of ten he rarely finds any theme technically too difficult to do. He tries to represent the scene as best he can. After the age of ten many normal children become more conscious of the difficulties which might be involved. Because of their frequent reluctance to try, the test procedure tends to lose its usefulness as a measure of maturity for children older than twelve. Up to this age, normal children become more and more able to see the necessary details in their proper relationships. Even those children who do not draw well can show how they mean to arrange the various details of the scene. They then combine these in a total picture which is meant to describe what they set out to draw. As they advance in maturity, they no longer produce

T:III:2a. Rey's age norms, based on sum of points, for "une dame se promène et il pleut"

Age (years)	Percentile				
	0	25	50	75	100
4 to 5	0	5	9	11	20
5 to 6	3	10	13	15	24
6 to 7	5	13	17	20	29
7 to 8	6	15	19	24	31
8 to 9	9	18	22	25	34
9 to 10	9	20	23	26	35
10 to 11	13	21	26	29	35
11 to 12	14	23	26	30	40
12 to 13	15	26	29	32	40
13 to 14	16	25	28	31	41
14 to 15	16	27	29	32	42
15 and over	17	30	33	37	43

Adapted from Rey, *Monographies de psychologie appliquée.*

a sexless human figure standing, but a lady in walking posture. They properly indicate how rain is falling and no longer find it enough to jot down somewhere on the paper some symbolic marks for raindrops. They may even add puddles and resist conventions which might tempt them to add a sun to their landscape. They also may show an umbrella, a raincoat, or the like, to protect the lady from getting wet. The norms based on genetic studies show that children's performances in this procedure improve steadily up to *twelve years of age* and that their drawings become increasingly richer in details and better organized.

The test proves to be a useful tool for a clinician. It appeals to children either because it involves drawing *per se* or because the particular scene seems amusing to them. The test provides a simple way to get a first impression of a child's mental maturity. The Rey scoring system may be more complicated than the older Wintsch scores; however, since it is more detailed, it allows finer differentiations and therefore is often more satisfactory than the shorter form. While these scoring systems are based on both quantitative and qualitative criteria, the clinician can add qualitative observations of her own, as in any other test procedure. The results can be significant in many ways: in this test a child may show good reasoning ability as well as skill, but because of emotional, educational, or other problems, the same child may do poorly in tests of a more academic nature. Another child may draw poorly because of inadequate motor coordination but show clearly that he means to represent correct relationships (the umbrella covering the person, or her feet touching the ground). Still another child may haphazardly place a drop

T:III:2a.   Rey's scoring system for "une dame se promène et il pleut"

Item	Points
1. Human form (head with legs)	1
2. Body distinct from arms and legs	1
3. Some clothing (buttons, scribbles on body)	1
4. A female figure	1
5. Profile: head and at least one other part of body in profile (body, feet, arms)	1
6. Motion indicated (gait, posture)	1
7. Rain roughly indicated	1
8. Rain properly indicated (touching ground, regularly distributed, raindrops on umbrella and lower parts of picture)	1

For drawing featuring umbrella

Item	Points
9. Umbrella roughly indicated	1
10. Umbrella in two lines (round, oblong, top, handle)	1
11. Umbrella clearly shown (ribs, points, scallops)	1
12. Umbrella dimensions 1/3 to 2/3 of body length	1
13. Umbrella positioned to cover at least half of body	1
14. Umbrella attached to hand at end of arm	1
15. Position of arm adequate	1

For drawing featuring raincoat, raincape, hood, without umbrella

Item	Points
16. Hood indicated (if there is a hood and an umbrella count only point 42—clothing)	1
17. Head well covered by hood	1
18. Raincoat or raincape	1
19. Shoulders, arms covered by coat or cape, hands showing only	1
20. Arms fully covered by cape, with shoulders clearly indicated	1
21. Shoulders not shown, but asked, "where are the arms?" child answers, "under coat."	1
22. Eyes shown (one line, dot)	1
23. Eyes in double lines, several parts	1
24. Nose shown	1
25. Mouth shown (one line)	1
26. Mouth shown in double lines, lips front or profile	1
27. Ears shown	1
28. Chin shown (front or profile)	1
29. Hair or headgear (except hood)	1
30. Neck or collar shown clearly	1

If the lady's face is covered by umbrella or if her back is turned, give credit for nose, mouth, eyes, etc. Credit 2 points if the quality of the picture suggests the more mature form of these details.

Item	Points
31. Hands (credit one point if hands are in pocket)	1
32. Arms shown (one line)	1
33. Arms in double lines	1
34. Arms attached to body at shoulder level	1
35. Arms in proportion to body or slightly longer	1
36. Legs shown (one line)	1
37. Legs in double lines	1
38. Legs properly attached	1

T:III:2a.   Rey's scoring system for "une dame se promène et il pleut" (cont.)

Item	Points
39. Legs in proportion to body	1
40. Feet shown	1
41. Shoes shown clearly	1
42. Clothing: 2 articles (skirt and blouse, jacket and skirt; if the hood goes with an open umbrella, it is considered clothing)	1
43. No transparency, if such could be possible	1
For a picture that shows a definite artistic trend or technique (silhouette, etching, skilled schematization), credit total number of points possible up to here: 37 points.	
For landscape	
44. A baseline, a road, a path, in one line or dots	1
45. Figure clearly positioned on baseline or road	1
46. Road or path shown	1
47. Pavement or gravel shown	1
48. Flower border, tree, doorway, house shown	1
49. Special details showing imagination	1

Maximum 43 points

Adapted from Rey, *Monographies de psychologie appliquée.*

of rain here, a sun there, and an umbrella somewhere in the sky, and not realize that the scene is incongruous because the details do not fit together. Lack of cohesion between various features may point to attention difficulties and to difficulties in reasoning of the kind often seen in retarded children and especially in children who have brain injuries.

Many children like to draw small details like flowers on the walk or decorations on the lady's dress. Some may add these as an embellishment after having finished the main picture satisfactorily. Others are carried away by details and forget to draw important parts of the scene. This may often be the case with flighty, poorly organized children or emotionally disturbed children. The diagnostician has to consider what kinds of details are being overstressed by the child. Again, the brain-injured child may become involved with flowers on a dress or feathers on a hat, whereas the disturbed child may be concerned with somber, less obvious details, such as cracks in a wall, threads in dress material.

Many of the productions may throw light on a child's body image and its distortions. This is frequently of interest, especially in the development of brain-injured children.[4] When used with due regard

[4] Zelda Klapper and Heinz Werner, "Developmental Deviations in Brain-Injured (Cerebral-Palsied) Members of Pairs of Identical Twins," *Quarterly Journal of Child Behavior* 2:288–313, July 1950. Also Lauretta Bender and Archie Silver, "Body Image Problems in the Brain Damaged Child," *Journal of Social Issues* 4:84–89, 1948.

for normal developmental characteristics, additional interpretations in line with Machover's "draw a person" test may add width to the evaluation of a drawing.[5]

With children who are unable to draw because of motor impairment one may try to use this test procedure in the proxy form described with other techniques. The child then may indicate by any means at his disposal what E should draw and where to place it. In "dictating" the picture, he may be able to give some impression of how he understands the task and what in it seems important to him.

The test can be used with deaf children. If the child is able to read, E writes the subject of the picture on a paper. Through his drawing the child may be able to express comprehension, observation, and reasoning, and this may help E to appraise a deaf child's intellectual potentialities.

2B—TELLING A STORY ABOUT HER. When the picture is done, ask the child to "tell a story about her." If the child does not start to tell a story, encourage him by saying, "Let us together make up a story about her. Who is she? Where is she going? Where does she live? Who is at home?" The child frequently produces material which is revealing in many respects and which may be used like other projective material. Conversation about his picture may surprise one child and seem natural to another; it frequently amuses and stimulates a previously untalkative child and opens the way to further conversations.

2C—WRITING NAME. One may ask the child to write or print his name on the picture, "So I know it was you who made it."

2D—WRITING TITLE. One may also ask him to write the title of the picture, "lady walking in the rain." Both 2c and 2d allow E a first impression of ability in academic matters (see also XI:9). If the child declares that he cannot spell one or another word (as "lady," "walking"), one may tell him the necessary letters and find out how he writes single letters on dictation. Normal children with ordinary school experience print their first names at least by the *age of six* and often younger. By the time they have reached the third grade, they generally are able to write the title of the picture (2d) with not more than one or two mistakes. During their second school year they may produce letters on dictation but occasionally confuse printing and writing if they are just learning in school how to distinguish between them.

---

[5] Karen Machover, *Personality Projection in the Drawing of the Human Figure* (Springfield, Illinois: Thomas, 1948).

3—SUBJECT DRAWING

3A—SPONTANEOUS DRAWING OF A MAN. Frequently, this subject is chosen spontaneously by the child (1) or proposed by him instead of the "lady" (see 2). Most children have had some experience with this subject. Often they may have "made a man" spontaneously, but more often they may have been shown and encouraged by others. Almost invariably, adults in our culture choose this theme to amuse children at one time or another. The child's spontaneous productions, therefore, frequently carry at least an element of learning; various studies in this country and abroad show, however, that in spite of individual differences and variations in skill or opportunity, drawings of the human figure, as the child grows older, show progressively more details and better organization. The *three-year-old* may draw nothing but one or two vertical lines, some circles, or, at best, a circle with some appendages which may be interpreted as legs. The *four-year-old* may be variable in his productions, but he makes obvious attempts to furnish a representative drawing, frequently a circle with eyes or nose or both, and legs attached to it. *Between five and six* a trunk and frequently arms and legs are shown. Two-dimensional legs begin to appear at this age, but become more common from *six years of age on.*[6]

3B—DRAWING A MAN. Ask the child to draw a picture of a man.[7] Goodenough's scoring rules and norms to measure intelligence in the young child by careful analysis of his picture of a man may be used to evaluate his attempts to draw a man. However, great caution is necessary in applying these norms. Goodenough's original norms are based on drawings by children who, in groups in schools, were given the following specific instructions: "On these papers I want you to make a picture of a man. Make the very best picture that you can. Take your time and work very carefully. I want to see whether the boys in [this] school can do as well as those in other schools. Try very hard and see what good pictures you can make."

When working with the individual child, E should try to come close to these directions by emphasizing that the "very best picture" is being asked for. The element of competition of the original instructions is not easily simulated and hardly enhances the examination of an individual child. Still, the Goodenough scores can be useful if it is clear that the child has tried to do a good job. However, the setting in which

---

[6] Gesell, *op. cit.,* p. 148.
[7] This test is adapted from Goodenough, *op. cit.,* pp. 90ff.

T:III:3b.   Goodenough's scoring system for all drawings recognizable as
attempts to represent the human figure*

---

1.   Head present
2.   Legs present
3.   Arms present
4a.   Trunk present
4b.   Length of trunk greater than breadth
4c.   Shoulder indicated
5a.   Both arms and legs attached to trunk
5b.   Legs attached to trunk; arms attached to trunk at the correct point
6a.   Neck present
6b.   Outline of neck continuous with that of head, of trunk, or of both
7a.   Eyes present
7b.   Nose present
7c.   Mouth present
7d.   Both nose and mouth shown in two dimensions; two lips shown
8a.   Hair shown
8b.   Hair present on more than the circumference of the head, and nontransparent. Method of representation better than scribble
9a.   Clothing present
9b.   Two articles of clothing nontransparent
9c.   Entire drawing free from transparencies when both sleeves and trousers are shown
9d.   Four or more articles of clothing clearly indicated
9e.   Costume complete without incongruities
10a.   Fingers shown
10b.   Correct number of fingers shown
10c.   Fingers shown in two dimensions, length greater than breadth, and the angle subtended by them not greater than 180°
10d.   Opposition of thumb shown
10e.   Hand shown as distinct from fingers or arms
11a.   Arm joint shown—either elbow, shoulder, or both
11b.   Leg joint shown—either knee, hip, or both
12a.   Head in proportion
12b.   Arms in proportion
12c.   Legs in proportion
12d.   Feet in proportion
12e.   Both arms and legs shown in two dimensions
13.   Heel shown
14a.   Motor coordination. Lines reasonably firm and mostly joined
14b.   Motor coordination. Lines all firm and correctly joined
14c.   Motor coordination. Head outline
14d.   Motor coordination. Trunk outline
14e.   Motor coordination. Outline of arms and legs
14f.   Motor coordination. Features
15a.   Ears present
15b.   Ears present in correct position and proportion
16a.   Eye detail; brow or lashes shown
16b.   Eye detail; pupil shown
16c.   Eye detail; proportion
16d.   Eye detail; glance directed to front in profile drawing
17a.   Both chin and forehead shown
17b.   Projection of chin shown
18a.   Profile with not more than one error
18b.   Correct profile

* A credit of one point is allowed for each item scored plus.
  Adapted from Goodenough, *op. cit.* For more detailed scoring criteria consult original text.

T:III:3b.   Goodenough's age norms, based on sum of points, for all
drawings recognizable as attempts to represent the human figure

Age (years)	Points
3	2
4	6
5	10
6	14
7	18
8	22
9	26
10	30
11	34
12	38
13	42

Adapted from Goodenough, *op. cit.*

a child spontaneously offers to "draw a man" (3a), or is casually asked
to "draw a man" (3b) is not necessarily one in which he makes the
best possible effort. He may have finished only a casual symbolic representation which does not necessarily contain all he knows about the
human figure. For this particular situation he may omit features which
are not important to him at the moment.[8] The Goodenough scores
applied to such productions can help E to form only an initial and
rough impression of the child's maturity level; they frequently give a
rating that is several points below what it should be. E may try to
compensate for this error by adding questions ("Is that the best man you
can do? What else does he need? Can you think of something more
he should have?"). Such questions are hardly apt to change radically
the original structure of the drawing. They may, however, result in the
addition of a few details and therefore better the performance. The
Goodenough scores used with caution may then help E at least to
judge the range within which the child might have functioned if properly motivated.

Added questions, such as, "What else would you have liked to do?"
or, "What else should he have?" may help to establish what a child
might have wished to do if he had known how. In the Goodenough
test (as in 2a) children may produce less than their best once they
have reached the stage of development at which they become critical of
their own work because they are able to recognize the difficulties in-

[8] The multiple functions which drawings may fulfill for young children have been
discussed by many authors in varied ways. See, amongst many others, George Henri
Luquet, *Les dessins d'un enfant* (Paris: Alcan, 1913); Günther Mühle, *Entwicklungs-
psychologie des zeichnerischen Gestaltens* (Munich: J. A. Barth, 1955).

volved. The influence of emotional attitudes on results in Goodenough drawings has been discussed by Goodenough herself and also by various other authors.[9]

3C—DRAWING OTHER SUBJECTS. Give the child other subjects to draw. Ask him to draw a cat or a dog, or "his cat" or "his dog." Ask him to draw his house, his kitchen, his bedroom, garden, school.

Note whether he tries to show individual differences stressing special dominant and characteristic features or whether he represents all animals (or houses or gardens) in similar or identical ways.

Schematic, nonindividualistic drawings are characteristic of younger age levels. Their gradual disappearance with advancing age (probably at least up to the age of school entrance) seems to parallel other significant trends in the mental development of young children.[10]

With children who like to stress some individual features, such picture making may easily lead to topics of conversation that are interesting to the clinical investigator.

4—IMITATION

4A—SIMPLE FORMS. Take the child's crayon or pencil and produce on the paper before him a circle, a cross, a line. Hand the crayon back to him and ask, "Can you make one just like that?"

Note: Does he like to do what is proposed to him, or does he dislike to have his spontaneous use of the crayon interfered with? Does he wait and seem interested in seeing the finished product, or is he intent only on getting the crayon back? Does he watch the movement of the crayon in E's hand? Does he put his own mark near the one on the paper? Does he try to keep it approximately the same size, or is it bigger or smaller? Does he try to do what he has been shown? Does it result in a similar product, or does he intentionally or unintentionally achieve something different? Note whether he is satisfied, nonchalant, or critical about his own drawing. Does he seem to differentiate among the different models he has been shown, or does he each time respond with the same scribble, circle, etc.?

It is easier for children to imitate what has been drawn for

---

[9] Goodenough, *op. cit.*, p. 56. See also Wally Reichenberg-Hackett, "Changes in Goodenough Drawings after a Gratifying Experience," *American Journal of Orthopsychiatry* 23:501–517, July 1953.

[10] Heinz Werner, *Comparative Psychology of Mental Development* (New York: Harper, 1940), p. 21.

them while they watched than it is to copy a ready-made model. Often the child comes to imitate the motion producing the drawing, rather than the drawing itself. The child of *eighteen months* is, in general, capable of imitating a vertical line and keeping it in the same direction as the model. At *two years of age* he can imitate a circle properly; at the same age he may put down two marks in imitation of the straight cross, but does not necessarily make his lines meet in an angle; at *three years of age* he imitates the straight cross properly.[11] At *three-and-a-half,* he imitates a diagonal cross.[12]

4B—DIFFERENTIATION OF DIRECTIONS. Produce a vertical scribble on the paper; while doing it say, "Up and down, up and down," and then, "Can you make one like that?" On the same paper, but not crossing the previous scribble, do the same in a horizontal direction, saying, "This way and this way, this way and this way," and then, "Now you can make one like that." Later, take a new sheet and scribble in circular direction, saying, "Round about and round about," and then, "You make one like that."

Draw a straight cross on the paper (4a). Have the child imitate it, then draw a diagonal cross and ask him to reproduce it. Repeat both if necessary.

Draw a square, as above; then a tilted square of the same size.

Note: How does the child differentiate directions? Does his end product clearly show the difference in directions, or does he try to show different directions but does not succeed in producing them? Does he seem to remain unaware of the difference of the two strokes, or of that of the crosses or squares?

These tasks help E to study a young child's comprehension of simple spatial relationships. Normal children at *two-and-a-half years of age* are capable of differentiating between horizontal and vertical strokes when they are presented successively on different sheets of paper.[13] In the above described task, the same sheet of paper is used with verbal re-enforcement added; probably this is somewhat easier. *Between three and four years of age,* normal children come to distinguish a straight cross from a diagonal cross in their drawings; about *a year later* they may recognize the difference between the straight square and the tilted square and try to represent it.

[11] Gesell, *op. cit.,* pp. 158ff.
[12] Terman and Merrill, *op. cit.,* pp. 85, 207.
[13] Gesell, *op. cit.,* p. 169.

Some children, especially handicapped ones, may perceive and understand differences in directions before they are technically equipped to show these in their finished products. Their unsuccessful attempts, their dissatisfactions and verbal comments show their intentions, which the examiner must take into consideration. Even if a child's finished product does not show any clear evidence of spatial differentiation, it is important to determine whether or not the difference between the two models has been noticed by the child. If he has perceived it but is unable to reproduce it, he may be on a higher level of mental maturity than a child who by a fortunate chance position of his pencil produces a suggestion of differentiation of directions without meaning to do so.

The above tests prove useful in determining a child's readiness for various school subjects. It is generally accepted that children who, visually at least, discriminate spatial relationships at the proper age have less difficulty in learning how to read than those who do not. For writing and printing, however, they may need not only the ability to discriminate between directions but also the skill to reproduce them with paper and pencil.

5—COPYING

5A—SIMPLE FORMS VARIOUSLY ORIENTED. Show a ready-made model, drawn in pencil on a separate paper or printed on individual cards.[14] Ask the child to "draw (or make) one just like that" on a piece of paper before him. Present successively: circle, cross, square, triangle, diagonal cross, tilted square, star, British flag (rectangle with diagonal, horizontal, and vertical mid-lines), horizontal diamond, and vertical diamond (see Figure 2).

Note the child's motor characteristics, working habits, behavior, approach to the task, interest in his product, etc., as before. Note also how he uses the model. Does he recognize or name the form? Does he study it? trace it in the air (especially crosses, diagonals)? approve it or reject it? Does he, after a brief initial look, work from a mental image? Does he arrange his drawings in a row or haphazardly distribute them over the paper? Does he try to fit the size of his next drawing to the still available space? Does he ask for a new sheet of paper, or does he disregard his previous product and have his drawings overlap? If he does the latter, is he surprised or disturbed, and does he admit not having planned correctly, or is he unconcerned and no longer interested

[14] *Ibid.,* p. 357.

FIGURE 2. Simple geometric forms (2/3 original size)

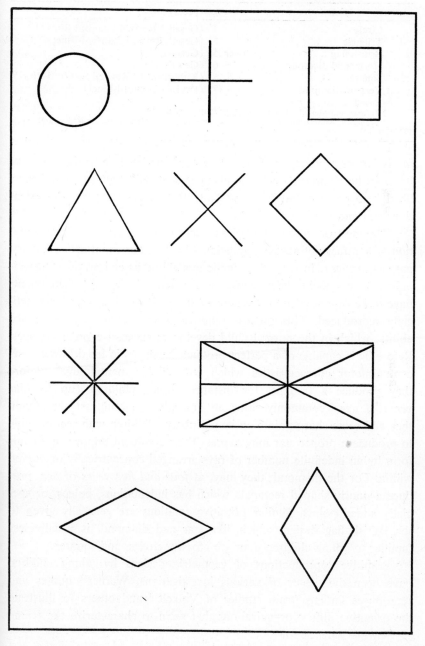

T:III:5.   Age norms for correct and objective copy of geometric forms

Form	Age (years)
Circle	3 (Gesell,* Revised Stanford-Binet†)
Triangle	5 (Gesell, Revised Stanford-Binet)
British flag	over 5 (Gesell)
Horizontal diamond	6 (Gesell)
Square	5 (Kuhlmann,** Revised Stanford-Binet)
Vertical diamond	7 (Revised Stanford-Binet)

* Gesell, *op. cit.*, p. 169.
† Terman and Merrill, *op. cit.*, pp. 82, 92, 201, 219, 98, 230.
** Frederick Kuhlmann, *A Handbook of Mental Tests* (Baltimore: Warwick and York, 1922), p. 102.

in his former product, or anxious to cover it up because he does not like it? Does he comment on his drawing and explain how he would have liked it to come out differently? Note the discrepancy between intentions and end product (as in 4).

Copying from a model involves a more complex process than imitation (4), a fact not always appreciated by amateur examiners (doctors, parents, uncles). Instead of a kinetic model and its end product, there is only a static model to be perceived as a structured whole. Its components have to be organized into a system of successive actions and kinesthetically reproduced. This process requires perceptual as well as motor ability, which in the normal child develop in successive orderly stages. Before he is capable of a perfect product, he shows in his drawings perceptuo-motor characteristics which indicate his mental level. Before they produce a triangle, for instance, young children (up to *four years of age*) commonly draw an amorphous circular stroke. Often they add some sharp points on its periphery. Children who seem unable to produce a proper star may express their dominant impression of this form by an indefinite number of rays arranged concentrically or curved within. For the diamond, they may, at *four and five years of age,* produce a poorly shaped rectangle which has indentations, bulges, or specially added points. Similar primitive solutions are generally given to the British flag design, which, like star and diamond, is usually less familiar to young children than are crosses, circles, and squares.

Primitive reproductions of geometric designs by young children have been the center of various investigations. Werner[15] quotes and reproduces findings from studies of Volkelt[16] and others to illustrate the primitive diffuse organizations that seem to characterize the young

[15] Werner, *op. cit.*, p. 118.
[16] Hans Volkelt, "Primitive Komplexqualitäten in Kinderzeichnungen," *Bericht über den VIII Kongress für experimentelle Psychologie* (Jena: Fisher, 1924).

child's perceptuo-motor activities. It is generally agreed that such solutions are not caused by motor incapacity alone. When a child is questioned by an adult on what the various parts of his drawings represent, he may show the pointed marks on his triangular form and say that they mean the "points" of the triangle. For Piaget, the characteristic reproductions of geometric forms by children led to his interesting theoretical discussions on the development of spatial comprehension.[17]

5B—OTHER FIGURES. Other tests dealing with the copying of figures are listed and discussed in Chapter VII.

6—MEMORY

All forms shown above can obviously be used as memory-for-form tests. Expose each form for a brief period, then ask the child to draw what he remembers.

6A—SIMPLE FORMS. The British flag design seems well suited to serve as a memory test on age levels for which other memory-for-design tests are still too difficult. Experience shows that normal six-year-old children usually are able to reproduce this design correctly from memory; occasionally they may still omit one of the mid-lines. This task can also be useful as an introduction to the more difficult designs.

6B—OTHER FIGURES. All other memory-for-design tests are listed and discussed under VII:1–6.

7—CODING[18]

7A—Use material from the Wechsler Intelligence Scale for Children.[19] Present and score as directed.

Note motor habits: how does he use his pencil and how is his stroke, etc. Is he slow, fast, careful, or hasty? Note the shape of his marks: are they well done, just recognizable, or wrong? Does his score penalize him for lack of speed or for inaccuracy? Does he understand the task, does he have technical difficulties, does he seem to fail because of inadequate form perception, poor attention? Does he proceed properly, does he check each figure with the samples, or does he try to remember

[17] Jean Piaget and Bärbel Inhelder, *The Child's Conception of Space,* trans. (London: Routledge, 1956), Chapter II.

[18] The listing of this type of test under Paper and Pencil may seem arbitrary. The procedure uses the test blank rather than an ordinary paper. It could as well fit into VII: Designs, or VIII: Learning and Memory, but no one of these would seem to be more appropriate than any other.

[19] David Wechsler, *Wechsler Intelligence Scale for Children* (New York: Psychological Corporation, 1949), pp. 85–86 and test blank.

what to do? Does he start to pick out one type only and skip others? Does he start and continue properly, or does he get confused as he goes along? Does he understand and proceed correctly after explanations have been repeated?

7B—Use digit symbol material from the Wechsler-Bellevue Intelligence Scale.[20] Present and score as directed.

Note as above. Note also types and frequency of distortions. Do they occur with one figure only, occasionally or each time it appears, or are there distortions interspersed without any apparent regularity among correct markings?

For children, the procedure seems to be demanding in more ways than similar tasks are for the normal adult.[21] Success depends not only on comprehension of the task with proper matching of the respective symbols, but also on a person's experience and skill with pencil and paper. This may vary in children of all ages more than in adults. Depending on some of their motor characteristics, it seems to be more difficult for some children to mark the small areas prescribed 'than it is for others. Also, the somewhat painstaking task appears frequently to be more difficult for the alert, creative, and intuitive normal child than it is for the more pedantic, passive, and slower moving one.

Comparative normative genetic studies with a qualitative viewpoint have not been published, to our knowledge, but might be of interest and value.

Experience shows that the procedure is probably more useful for older children than it is for younger ones. Often it may be of special interest because it affords an opportunity for study of a child's working habits. Distortions of forms, if persistent, may in some cases point toward difficulties in perceptual functioning of the kind seen in children with certain brain injuries. However, because of the complex character of the task and especially because of the purely motor factors involved, suspected symptoms of this kind need careful counterchecking with other

---

[20] David Wechsler, *The Measurement of Adult Intelligence* (Baltimore: Williams and Wilkins, 1944), p. 94 and test blank. This procedure is included in the WAIS. It should be pointed out here that since the completion of this manuscript in 1958, the Wechsler-Bellevue Intelligence Scale (W-B 1) has been superseded by the Wechsler Adult Intelligence Scale (WAIS). Wechsler's *Measurement of Adult Intelligence* has been replaced by his *Measurement and Appraisal of Adult Intelligence,* fourth edition (Baltimore: Williams and Wilkins, 1958). In the earlier editions directions for administering and scoring the tests were incorporated in the book; in the new edition these appear in a separate manual. The new standardization covers ages sixteen to seventy-five, but does not provide measurements for ages ten through fifteen, as do the earlier editions.

[21] *Ibid.*

methods. In some cases the procedure is helpful in the study of attention, especially where difficulties in this area are suspected on the basis of recent injury to a previously able child.

T:III.   Most suitable procedures for various age ranges

Procedure	Age
1, (4a)	Up to two years
1, 3, 4, (5), (6a)	Two to six years
1–3, 5–7a	Six to ten years
2, 6, 7	Over ten years

Parentheses around number indicate that the procedure is suitable only for the older children in the age group.

IV

Fitting and Assembling

1—WALLIN PEGBOARD A

The materials of this test consist of a board with six round holes and six wooden pegs to fit the holes. A board with larger holes (one inch in diameter) and larger, sturdier pegs than those provided with the original material proves useful with children who have difficulties in fine motor coordination.

This procedure was described by its author as a test of psychomotor capacity.[1] As such, it is used in various test scales, such as the Merrill-Palmer[2] and the Cattell.[3] In the procedures described below (as in all others in this chapter) emphasis is on comprehension of spatial relationships, attention, learning ability, social attitude, etc., rather than on motor ability.

1A—ROUND PEGS. Set the board before the child and hand him the six round pegs one by one. Wait to see if he places pegs spontaneously or suggest, "Put these little sticks in the holes." If the child does not proceed or if he starts to play with the pegs in other ways, show him how to place the first peg.

Note his attitude and interest. Does he understand immediately, or after demonstration? Does he finish the task or place only a few pegs? Which hand does he use? How does he use it? Is it easy or hard for him to keep the peg erect and steady?

---

[1] J. E. W. Wallin, "The Peg Form Boards," *Psychological Clinic* 12:40–53, 1918.
[2] Rachel Stutsman, *Mental Measurement of Preschool Children, with a Guide for the Administration of the Merrill-Palmer Scale of Mental Tests* (Yonkers, New York: World Book Company, 1931).
[3] Psyche Cattell, *Measurement of Intelligence of Infants and Young Children* (New York: Psychological Corporation, 1940).

Normal children of *eighteen to twenty-one months of age* are, in general, able to complete the pegboard.[4] Occasionally the younger ones do so, but only with some urging. Experience shows that children of *fifteen months of age* may place one or two pegs adequately but that they usually do not complete the task. Children around *twelve months old* are, in general, not able to hold the peg steady enough, but they may bang it near and around the hole, thus showing that they perceive some relationship between peg and hole.

In the Merrill-Palmer Scale and in the Cattell Infant Intelligence Scale, the pegboard is first presented with all pegs in place. This may render the task somewhat easier, since relationship between peg and hole has been established and can be perceived by the child.

1B—ROUND AND SQUARE PEGS. Present pegboard A to the child; offer him a round and a square peg together. Repeat, presenting him with two pegs to choose from, each time interchanging them in position.

Note: Does the child choose the round peg immediately? Does he do so with all following pegs? Does he try a square peg in a round hole but once and discard it on his own or after E suggests it ("It is no good, put it aside here"). Does he after this disregard any other square peg, or does he try others again in other holes? Does he turn the peg if it does not fit, to try the other end? Is he content to test a square peg in only one of the holes, or is he apt to try it in all or several of the remaining round holes?

Normal children of about *two years of age,* and some younger, reject square pegs either immediately or after a very few trials. They quickly learn to generalize that if one square peg does not fit in one round hole, no other square peg will fit in any round hole. In examinations of normal children one may find with this task some of the earliest manifestations of concrete concept formation: the child recognizes easily that all square or all round pegs are alike and knows that what goes for one also goes for another. The ability for this mental process is significantly lacking in many children with brain injuries. The test procedure described here may, therefore, be useful for the early detection of perceptual distortions, sensory and reasoning difficulties, and resulting disabilities in learning. Elizabeth Lord especially discusses the diffi-

---

[4] These norms correspond to those given by Stutsman. She presented the board with all pegs in place, removed them in full view of the child, and asked him to put them back. Stutsman, *op. cit.,* p. 206. The same method is used in the Cattell Infant Intelligence Scale.

culty that some brain-injured children have in tactile-sensory recognition (astereognosis), which may show up in this procedure.[5]

One may test further the child's ability to learn by repeating the same procedure several times and watching for improvement in the performance, or one may proceed to 2.

1c—ALL PEGS. Use this test instead of 1a or 1b. Present pegboard A and place the box containing round and square pegs near the child. Have him choose for himself the proper pegs for A.

Note as above.

2—WALLIN PEGBOARDS B AND C

2A—SQUARE PEGS WITH B. Use pegboard B, which has six square holes, and provide six square pegs to fit. If 1b has just preceded, show the child that the previously discarded square pegs will now fit. If 1b or 1c has been omitted, present the six square pegs without explanation.

2B—ALL PEGS WITH B. Use the same board. Present, as in 1c, the box containing all the pegs.

Note as before. Also watch how the child fits the square peg into the hole. Does he adjust the peg to the hole by turning it correctly before inserting it? Does he screw it into the hole gradually or try to hammer it in without giving it the proper rotation? Does he gradually learn to adjust the pegs properly? Does his difficulty seem due to lack of comprehension of spatial relationships, or does it appear to be primarily caused by motor inability to manipulate the pegs as he wishes to? If the task follows 1b, note whether he shifts easily to the new setting, or whether he continues to mistrust the square pegs.

Normal children of *two to two-and-a-half years of age* are able to complete pegboard B successfully.[6]

2C—THREE ROUND AND THREE SQUARE PEGS WITH C. Present pegboard C, which has three round and three square holes, to the child together with three round and three square pegs. Let him proceed on his own. If he seems about to discard a square peg because it does not fit a round hole (as in 1b), say, "Try another hole." Eventually help him by removing a round peg which he has placed in a square hole before.

---

[5] Elizabeth Lord, *Children Handicapped by Cerebral Palsy* (New York: The Commonwealth Fund, 1937), p. 38. Out of print.

[6] These norms correspond to those given by Stutsman. She used pegboard B immediately following pegboard A, presenting it as before without intermediate tasks. Stutsman, *op. cit.,* p. 207.

Do this unobtrusively, or point to the misplaced peg and say, "That one does not fit. Why don't you try to take it out and see?"

Repeat without suggestions or other aids. Occasionally the pegs may seem to have been placed correctly with proper comprehension, when in reality they were so placed only by chance. Renewed mistakes may show that comprehension of spatial relationship is still lacking.

Note as before.

Normal children of *two-and-a-half years of age* learn to adjust the pegs properly in this task. At about *three years of age* some few children may still make a mistake, but generally they proceed without trials and errors.

3—NESTED BOXES

Use a set of four or five hollow boxes which fit into each other. Present the assembled set to the child; ask him to take the boxes apart and later to put them back together again. If necessary, separate the boxes while the child is looking on. Arrange them in a loose order. If the child does not start, show him how to fit two of the boxes, then separate them and let him proceed.

Note behavior and manipulations of the child. Note especially how he goes about dealing with the task. Does he start by grasping two of the boxes (one in each hand) and trying to assemble them, or is he interested in exploring the boxes, looking into them, banging them, turning them over. If he starts to fit one into another, is he trying to find the correct ones or is he content with putting any one into any other? Does he try to fit larger boxes into smaller ones? Does he try to pile a third box into the space occupied by the second one? Does he try to correct his errors by changing boxes, removing those that do not fit? Does he try to force boxes into each other even though they do not fit, or does he give up? If he experiments with the boxes, does he seem to learn from experience, or does he repeat the same kinds of mistakes? Does he finally succeed in assembling all boxes in one nest, or is he left with a group of two or three boxes side by side?

This procedure involves comprehension of spatial relationships such as young children are apt to acquire early in life.[7] They gradually learn that a space occupied by one object cannot be occupied by another; they learn that a small object can fit into a larger one, but that a large

---

[7] Jean Piaget, *The Construction of Reality in the Child,* trans. (New York: Basic Books, 1954), Chapters I and II.

object will not fit into a smaller one. Through their manipulation of objects they learn to appreciate gradations in sizes (which at a later age they may perceive without experimentation).

In a study of spatial comprehension of normal preschool children a set of nested boxes of triangular shape was used with fifty-eight children ranging in age from eighteen months to five-and-a-half years.[8] It was found that until the age of *two-and-a-half to three years* a child does not seem to show any appreciation of the sizes and forms of objects which he wants to assemble. He handles the boxes for the sheer pleasure of handling and putting them together. He may or may not happen to succeed, but he neither knows nor learns why some fit and others do not. Up to the *age of four* a child learns as he plays with the material. He may not know beforehand which boxes will fit, but he learns through his trials and errors; he is not apt to repeat the same kind of mistake, and he succeeds soon. From *four to four-and-a-half years* onward, children seem to know right away how to go about fitting the boxes. Before they begin they may look the situation over and pick boxes of the right size. They do comprehend the form relations involved and no longer need trials and errors.

Similar nested box material is used in various scales.[9] In the Merrill-Palmer Scale the material consists of four hollow cubes.[10] The method of assembling them is first demonstrated to the child. This, and the shape of the boxes, may make this procedure easier for the child. This test is placed on a *two- to two-and-a-half-year level,* with 240 seconds allowed for its successful accomplishment, whereas the *two-and-a-half- to three-year-old* group is allowed 220 seconds to perform the same task.

4—MONTESSORI CYLINDERS

The material for this test consists of a set of ten wooden cylinders, graded both in height and diameter, which fit into holes in a solid wooden base.[11]

Remove the cylinders from their holes while the child is watching.

[8] Edith Meyer, "The Comprehension of Spatial Relations in Preschool Children," *Journal of Genetic Psychology* 57:119–151, 1940.

[9] Charlotte Bühler and Hildegard Hetzer, *Testing Children's Development* (New York: Farrar and Rinehart, 1935).

[10] Stutsman, *op. cit.,* p. 212.

[11] This is the second (B) of the original three boards described and standardized in terms of time required for successful test performance. See Helen T. Woolley and Elizabeth Cleveland, "Performance Tests for Three-, Four-, and Five-Year-Old Children," *Journal of Experimental Psychology* 6:58–68, 1923. Also, Bird T. Baldwin and Lorle I. Stecher, *The Psychology of the Preschool Child* (New York: Appleton, 1927).

Say, "See how these come out of their holes. Now see how they fit—the biggest one in the biggest hole, and here the smallest one in the very small hole." Again remove all the cylinders and place them beside the base, well mixed up. Ask the child to put them back, "Each one in the hole in which it belongs."

Note how the child proceeds. Does he understand the task, does he pick up any cylinder, or does he look for the largest or the smallest one? Once he has grasped it, does he look for the proper hole, or does he try it in the nearest one? Does he have any preconceived idea of where it might fit? Does he try the smaller cylinder in holes that are only slightly larger, or does he also try holes that are obviously too small? Does he avoid holes which he on one try found too small, or does he try them with the same cylinder, or with another larger or smaller one? Does he seem to notice that the holes become larger on the right and smaller on the left? Does he remove a cylinder which fits well enough when he comes upon one better suited to the hole, or is he not inclined to correct any previous placement? Does he notice gross size differences only, or also finer ones? Does he learn from experience, or does he repeat the same kind of error over and over again? Help the child if necessary.

Repeat the procedure whether or not he received help. Note any changes in method, speed, etc.

It is normal for children approximately *three years old* to go about this task sensibly and to learn from their experiences. On a second trial, most three-year-olds make no mistakes, or only tentative ones. Children younger than this may proceed by trial and error and usually do not succeed completely; they are not apt to learn much from experience. Around *two years of age,* one may find children who try a large cylinder in a hole obviously too small. In spite of this they keep persisting by banging the form against the wrong hole. Their attempts to force it in seem to show their disregard for spatial properties and their inability to realize that a space occupied by one body cannot be occupied by another one. Children *over four years of age* who continue to have difficulty in the task may have poor attention spans, difficulties in size discrimination, and poor comprehension of spatial relationships. This may often be a sign of difficulties in reasoning and learning of the type associated with certain kinds of brain injury.

In general, the procedure is not well suited to children with serious motor difficulties. However, occasionally E may want to use it with the proxy method to study gross size discrimination in an older child where severe retardation is suspected. One may show a very small or a very large cylinder and observe if the patient turns to or otherwise indicates the right kind of hole, or whether he seems to make gross errors.

5—THREE-FIGURE FORMBOARD

Use material from Gesell.[12] This consists of a board measuring 36 x 16 cm. and painted green. There are three holes cut to fit three white wooden forms (circle, triangle, square), each 2 cm. thick.

5A—STANDARD PRESENTATION (GESELL). Present the board with the three blocks placed in front of their respective holes. Say, "Put them where they go."

Note as in 1a and 2a. Also, does the child first try each block in the correct hole, or in any hole? Does he hold the blocks (triangle and square) poised in correct position for insertion? Or does he try to force them into their holes? Or does he, by trial and error, find out which way they can fit? If he tries the wrong hole, does he soon realize that the block does not fit? Or does he persist in banging and try to force it in? Does he learn from experience and repetition?

Normal children *eighteen months of age* are apt to pile the three blocks, without placing them. From then on, they may start to place one or another block correctly. At *twenty-four months of age,* they generally place all blocks correctly without much hesitation.[13]

5B—PILED PRESENTATION. Present blocks in a pile. Note whether this arrangement changes the child's performances. This task seems to be more difficult, probably because there is not as direct and immediate a perceptual attraction between, for instance, the round block and the round hole.

5C—ROTATED STANDARD PRESENTATION. Use only after successful repetition of 5a.

Rotate the board 180 degrees. Be sure child is watching. Leave blocks as before (round block facing square hole, as directed by Gesell).

Note: Does the child try each block first in the hole nearest to it, or does he shift to the correct hole immediately or after one quick trial that proves wrong? Note as in 5a.

[12] Arnold Gesell, *The First Five Years of Life* (New York: Harper, 1940), pp. 130–133.
[13] *Ibid.,* p. 133.

Normal children of *two to two-and-a-half years of age* learn to adapt to the rotation of the board gradually and with increasing speed. *Three-year-olds* adapt within a short time without repeating any errors.[14]

5D—ROTATED PILED PRESENTATION. Rotate the board as in 5c, but remove blocks and present them in a pile. The task is then easier than 5c. Only one block at a time has to be decided upon. The child does not have to break up the fixed perceptual arrangement of the three blocks.

5E—STANDARD PRESENTATION (REVISED STANFORD-BINET). Use the material from the Revised Stanford-Binet Scale, Forms L and M, II- and III-year level.[15] This board is smaller than the Gesell board. Three red blocks (circle, square, triangle) fit into recesses which are painted the same dark green color of the board.

Present and score as directed. One success out of two trials (direct presentation as in 5a) receives credit on the *two-year level;* two successes in two trials (rotated presentation as in 5c) receive credit on *three-year level.*

Note as before. From the perceptual point of view, this task seems more difficult than the larger Gesell board. The forms seem less clearly outlined on this board because of the dark recesses. This difference may be of importance, especially in examinations of brain-injured children. Also, for other children with handicaps in fine motor coordination, the smaller insets may be more difficult to handle than the sturdier Gesell blocks.

6—SEGUIN FORMBOARD

This is a large wooden board with insets to fit ten forms level with the board; the forms are circle, oval, square, lozenge, elongated hexagon, rectangle, star, half-disk, triangle, and cross. It is used in the Pintner-Paterson[16] and Merrill-Palmer[17] scales. The Goddard board used by Gesell[18] is essentially similar; however, the board is dark brown, the forms are heavier and thicker than the board and do not fit level with it. This latter board may occasionally be more suitable than the Seguin board for children with motor handicaps.

[14] *Ibid.*

[15] Lewis M. Terman and Maud A. Merrill, *Measuring Intelligence* (Boston: Houghton Mifflin, 1937), pp. 75, 136, 193.

[16] Rudolf Pintner and Donald G. Paterson, *A Scale of Performance Tests* (New York: Appleton, 1923).

[17] Stutsman, *op. cit.,* p. 187.

[18] *Op. cit.,* pp. 133–134.

6A—FIRST PRESENTATION. The board with all forms fitted is presented briefly to the child. Say, "How would you like to play with this puzzle?" Remove forms by turning the board upside down.[19] (With a child who might be easily startled or frightened by unexpected sounds, one may warn, "This is a noisy game. It will make a big clang." Or watch the child's reactions to the sudden noise of blocks dropping on the table.) Arrange the blocks loosely in three piles with the round form on top nearby, or leave the forms lying around the board, but avoid leaving any form adjacent to its hole. Say, "Now you put them back where they go." Unless the child starts at once, hand him the round block first and say, "Where does this one go?" Point out the place, if necessary, "See, that fits well here. Now let us find places for the other ones." Some children may continue on their own, others may wait to have one block after another handed to them. Select blocks whose places on the boards are not adjacent. Try to have the child proceed without help, but assist if he gets frustrated. For children who have serious difficulty, one may place difficult pieces (lozenge or hexagon) or remove a wrongly placed form. Assure in every way possible that the child is comfortable, well disposed, and eager to continue.

This task is used frequently near the beginning of the examination. The material is appealing and invites active participation without requiring verbal exchange. It may be useful with children as old as seven and eight years of age. It may help to reassure an anxious child and to provide E with a first general impression.

Note the child's attitude and motor habits, as before. Note work methods, as in 4 and 5. Does he first study the board, or pick up some block to find a place for it? Does he see some relationship between the form he holds and a hole he sees, or does he start haphazardly to fit the block into any nearby hole? Does he try the same form in different holes? Does he persist in unsuccessful trials by pounding and hoping to force the block into the hole, or does he keep trying the same block in the same hole, turning it different ways? Does he use a similar work method with all forms or with some difficult ones only? Does he keep changing his attack throughout? Does he seem impulsive or more careful at first or as time goes on? How does he accept and use

---

[19] This form of presentation varies from that recommended in other scales. In other scales the child is shown the board only after the insets have been removed and have been arranged on the table.

help if it is offered to him? Does he appreciate it, ask for it, or resist it? Does he make use of it or repeat the same mistakes?

6B—VARIATIONS. (1) Repeat the same presentation to see how the child learns and remembers; or (2) remove only those forms which were most difficult for him, and ask him to replace them (for children who have difficulty with some shapes only); or (3) leave the most difficult forms in the board and remove some of the simple ones only (for children who have difficulty with all shapes); or (4) repeat only one of the above presentations, asking the child to use "the other hand." Note how he obeys. If he does but soon forgets again gently take hold of the hand he used before in order to remind him to use the other one, and note whether or not he is able to heed the request when the favorite hand is again released. Note as above.

The Seguin formboard is interesting in various respects. In the form presented here it is particularly useful for the study of perceptual ability and comprehension of spatial relationships in young children. Besides this, it shows a child's learning ability in these areas, his work habits, reaction to success, frustration, social interaction, etc. Normal children *three years of age* use the trial and error method.[20] They are usually able to finish, though slowly. When starting, they commonly have no preconceived idea of where a certain block might go; as they grow older, they continue in trial and error fashion, but may prefer to try the blocks first in places that seem vaguely familiar because of certain dominant characteristics. At about *four years of age* this tendency becomes more marked; children are apt to pick up one or another block and then visually peruse the board. For their first trials they choose places which have characteristics seen also in the block which they hold ("roundness" common to oval and semicircle, "lengthiness" common to oval and hexagon, "multi-angularity" seen in star and cross). However, *four-year-olds* complete the board with very little or no help. *Five-year-old* children work quickly with no errors, or only a few made in haste. They either first choose a place and then look for a block to fit it, or hold a block poised until they find the proper place for it.

7—FIVE-FIGURE FORMBOARD

Use material from the Pintner-Paterson Performance Scale.[21] This consists of a wooden board with five recesses (square, oval, round, hexagon,

---

[20] Stutsman, *op. cit.*, p. 191.
[21] Pintner and Paterson, *op. cit.*

and cross) and eleven wooden insets to fit into the recesses, two for each except three for the cross.

7A—FIRST PRESENTATION. Introduce the task as another "puzzle." If given after 6, prepare the child for the fact that it is a more "difficult" one. Remove pieces while child is watching; arrange them loosely, separating pieces that would fit together. Say, "You put them back where they go." If he hesitates, tell him to try, but assure him that he will get help if he needs it. Let the child proceed on his own. If it becomes clear that he is not apt to find a solution on his own, systematically introduce some suggestions. First place one half of the oval, then encourage the child to proceed. If he completes the oval, but fails to learn from this suggestion that the other forms are also divided in several pieces, place either the larger part of the round form or one of the pieces of the cross. Frequently, no help is needed until the child fumbles with square or hexagon or both. Occasionally the suggestion, "Turn it," may be all that is needed to help him succeed.

7B—VARIATIONS. Repeat as above, or remove the most difficult forms only, or the easiest forms only (see 6b:2 and 3).

Note the child's attitude, motor ability, work methods, and learning ability, as in 6. Note also whether an erroneously placed piece is speedily removed by the child, whether he understands why it does not fit, and whether he repeats the same error twice. Note which pieces seem difficult and apt to produce errors. Are the errors mainly due to inattention and haste? Are they due to confusion of similar looking pieces (square and hexagon) or to inability to turn the piece the right way (hexagon)? Or are gross errors of perception noticeable in his trials (circle in oval, rectangle in square)? Does the child immediately recognize which two pieces go together and join them before placing them, or does he find out only by trying which pieces may constitute a whole form?

This procedure, like other formboard tasks, may fill many purposes in the clinical examination.[22] The above presentation may be useful

[22] The original norms published for most formboard tests are in terms of number of moves and time required. However, the authors of these and similar tests were well aware of their qualitative aspects and emphasized the need for minute observations to complement the scores. With the growing stress on rigid statistical measurements, it has been easy to forget that study of attitudes and work processes were meant to be an integral part of these procedures. See Walter F. Dearborn, E. A. Shaw, and Edward A. Lincoln, *Series of Form Board and Performance Tests of Intelligence.* Harvard Monographs in Education, Series 1, Number 4: Studies in Educational Psychology and Educational Measurement (Cambridge: Graduate School of Education, Harvard University, 1923). Also R. E. Leaming, "Children Applying for Working Certificates," *Psychological Clinic* 14:163–179, 1922.

for the appraisal of perceptual ability, form comprehension, spatial orientation, learning ability, etc. It requires all these, as well as imagery, to recognize how the form segments belong together and how they fit in their respective recesses. Experience shows that normal children between *five and six years of age* complete three to four forms without help. They may immediately recognize and join the pieces of the oval or the square. They may proceed by trial and error in the relative arrangements of the pieces of the cross. They may find only after delay the proper position for the small segment of the circle. Many children at this age level still have trouble, at least initially, in differentiating parts of the square from those of the hexagon. At *six years* and slightly above, some difficulties with the hexagon only are still common. Even if a child at this age has placed these segments correctly once simply by chance, he may not be able to fit them properly when he tries again. Children who at *eight years of age* or over still cannot distinguish at a glance which pieces belong to the square and which ones to the hexagon, and who cannot easily place them in their respective recesses, must be considered weak in comprehension of spatial and perceptual relationships. This applies even more to those who at these age levels have difficulty with the cross or circle.

8—Casuist Formboard

Use material from the Pintner-Paterson Performance Scale.[23] This consists of a board with four recesses (three circles of varying sizes and one oblongated oval) with twelve pieces to fit (three each to the two larger circles, two to the smaller circle, four to the oval).

Present board as in 6 and 7. Have the child proceed on his own. If he has difficulty, give systematic suggestions by placing first one of the circle segments, and later, if necessary, other pieces. Give assistance as in 7.

Note as before. Also note how the child discriminates among the sizes of the circle segments. Does he recognize immediately the difference in sizes? Or does he notice it after some delay? Or does he have to look for the proper size each time through trial and error? If he places two of the three circle segments in one circle, does he place them so that they leave space to add a third one, or does he leave them so that only two small spaces are left between them on each side? Does he see how to remedy the situation? Does he place semicircles in the

---

[23] Pintner and Paterson, *op. cit.*

ends of the oval where they do not belong but then notice his errors, or does he rigidly persist and is he unable to remedy this arrangement which superficially seems at first satisfactory enough?

The interest of this test procedure seems to be in the direction discussed in 6 and 7. This board is more difficult because it is more complex. It seems to require more judgement, more flexibility and readiness to revise one's first impulses. Some pieces (semicircles) seem to fit where they do not belong, some others (segments) look alike at first sight, but are not. Some of the perceptual organizations must be broken up in order to get a total and satisfactory solution.

Normal children of *eight to nine years of age* usually complete the task successfully.

9—LINCOLN HOLLOW SQUARE FORMBOARD

A board with a 4½-inch square cut out to fit combinations of three and four of eleven pieces of wood which exactly fill the square hole. The pieces are rectangles, triangles, a square, and several other odd shapes (see Figure 3). These pieces are inconspicuously numbered. E has formulas for each of eight combinations handy to help her present smoothly one task after another. The tasks vary in difficulty, the first one being the easiest and the last the hardest. (The true comparative difficulty of some of the intermediate tasks has not been definitely determined.)

The procedure has been tentatively standardized.[24] So far, systematic attempts to establish norms have been directed only toward evaluating the amount of time needed by the subject to successfully complete the task. Qualitative norms have not yet been developed, but would seem well worth while. Pending more normative studies, the diagnostician may find this procedure most useful in observing comprehension of spatial relationships, persistence, attention, learning ability, etc.

The test situation appeals to children up to *ten years of age*. Since eight problems have to be solved, the factor of chance appears to be diminished in comparison with other formboard tasks (described in 7 and 8). Experience shows that normal *nine-year-olds* are frequently able to solve without difficulty at least seven out of the eight problems.

All test procedures described under 1 through 9 may be adapted

[24] Edward A. Lincoln, "Tentative Standards for the Lincoln Hollow Square Form Board," *Journal of Applied Psychology* 11:264–267, 1927. Also Dearborn, Shaw, and Lincoln, *op. cit.*

FIGURE 3.   Lincoln hollow square formboard

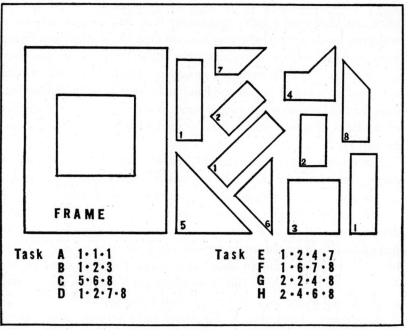

Task	A	1·1·1		Task	E	1·2·4·7
	B	1·2·3			F	1·6·7·8
	C	5·6·8			G	2·2·4·8
	D	1·2·7·8			H	2·4·6·8

From Augusta F. Bronner, William Healy, Gladys M. Lowe, and Myra E. Shimberg, *A Manual of Individual Mental Tests and Testing,* Judge Baker Foundation Publication Number 4 (Boston: Little, Brown, 1927), p. 159

for use with handicapped children. All test situations are well suited to the study of children with whom it is difficult or impossible to establish verbal communication. All procedures demand a minimum of verbal instruction, and gestures can be substituted for words if necessary. When dealing with children with motor handicaps, it may be important to distinguish errors due to motor disability from those due to lack of comprehension. Qualitative observations of the kind described above are therefore more satisfactory than evaluations based on speed or skill. Children with motor handicaps must be carefully observed; the level and character of their form comprehension may show in their intentions and trials rather than in their actual performances. For those with handicaps serious enough to preclude the actual handling of material, the proxy method described in connection with other techniques may be in order. For instance, in test procedure 6 (Seguin formboard), E may hold up one form after another and have the child indicate as best he can where each should go. The sequence of blocks must be selected so that ambiguity is avoided as much as possible. Formboards described under 7 and 8 lend themselves to the same adjustments. The proxy method often may yield more reliable information than the fumbling of children with poor motor control, who may move or drop insets where they do not want them. With other procedures other adjustments may be necessary and effective. With the pegboard procedures (1, 2), for instance, one may hold up a square peg in one hand and a round one in another and have the child choose which peg he wants to see placed in one or another of the holes. Similar methods may be used with the three-figure form-board (5).

Experience shows that even children who have had no chance of gaining experience by their own motions or manipulations will gradually acquire correct notions about form and spatial relationships if they have the intellectual potentialities to do so. Allowing for some delay because of lack of sensory-motor experience, the clinician may find evaluation of spatial comprehension one of the most reliable methods by which to judge a child's ability to understand the relationships between objects around him. This is especially so for children whose delay in speech and motor skill renders other methods difficult.[25]

Experience shows that in the above tasks severely handicapped children of *four years of age* whose later development proves them to be mentally intact choose correct forms at least as well as normal *three-year-olds,* and frequently do better. *Eight-year-old* handicapped children may do at least as well as normal *six-year-olds,* and frequently better. Rules of thumb which develop from such experiences may seem vague and arbitrary; however, they help the clinician at least to avoid being either much too pessimistic or too optimistic.

10—CONVENTIONAL MANIKIN

Use material from the Wechsler-Bellevue,[26] Pintner-Paterson,[27] and Merrill-Palmer[28] scales. This consists of six pieces representing a conventional figure of a man. In the original version of this test and also in the early editions of the Wechsler series, wood was used instead of the cardboard that is commonly used now. Wooden pieces seem more suitable for use with young or handicapped children.

[25] See similar discussion in Chapter V.

[26] David Wechsler, *The Measurement of Adult Intelligence* (Baltimore: Williams and Wilkins, 1944), p. 96; *The Measurement and Appraisal of Adult Intelligence* (Baltimore: Williams and Wilkins, 1958), p. 82. Manikin is included in the WAIS.

[27] Pintner and Paterson, *op. cit.*

[28] Stutsman, *op. cit.,* pp. 196–198.

T:IV:10.   Pintner-Paterson scoring system for manikin

	Points
Perfect performance	5
One or both arms up or out, *i.e.,* not exactly fitting in joints	4
One reversal, *i.e,* right arm for left arm and *vice versa,* or right leg for left leg	3
Two reversals, *i.e,* both arms and both legs reversed	2
Legs or arms interchanged or arms at sides or any other results that look like a man	1
Failure to see that it is a man	0

Adapted from Pintner and Paterson, *op. cit.*

T:IV:10.   Pintner-Paterson age norms, based on sum of points, for manikin

Age (years)	Percentile		
	75	50	25
4	2	1.5	0
5	4	3	2
6	5	4	3

Adapted from Pintner and Paterson, *op. cit.*

10A—STANDARD PRESENTATION. Set pieces before the child. Place body of manikin in center, arms and legs on either side, and head on extreme right; place leg with rectangular end at opposite side of body from where it fits, and place the other leg and the two arms in similar relationship. Present and score as directed by Pintner and Paterson, by saying, "Put this together as quickly as you can," or present and score as directed by Wechsler, by saying, "If these pieces are put together correctly they will form something. Go ahead and put them together as quickly as you can."

Note: Does the child recognize immediately what the figure represents and join head and trunk and later legs and arms, or does he handle the pieces as if they were just so many pieces of wood to be banged on the table, joined in a row, or piled indiscriminately? Or does he study the situation and discover what the figure will be while experimenting with the joining of edge to edge? Is his idea of a "man" only global and rough, so that either of the long pieces can stand for arms or legs without discrimination, or does he know how to distinguish between arms and legs and to fit them carefully in their respective places? Does he discover their rectangular and round fittings after delay, or not at all?

This test demands some constructive ability besides perceptual skills. The child has to assimilate the single pieces in an internal scheme of the conventional figure of a "man." Unless he is able to do so, he most likely will use at least some of the pieces inappropriately. Only occasionally may one find a child who arrives at a perfect performance by carefully fitting edge to edge without realizing until he has finished what the figure represents. Younger children often recognize the figure early in the procedure, but are content with fitting head to body, or head, body, and some appendages (not unlike what they do in their drawings of a "man," see III:3).

The Pintner-Paterson scoring system is simple and useful for a quick appraisal of a child's maturity level.

10b—VARIATIONS. One may omit saying that the child should be quick. One may use various suggestions if the child does not seem to recognize the figure, or if help seems indicated for some other reason. For example, one may first place the head and trunk in the proper relationship; then the head, trunk, and a leg; then the head, trunk, leg, and arm. Wait after each suggestion to see whether the child gets the idea.

One may arrange the pieces as in 10a and suggest, "It's going to be a man."

Vary the original presentation, for example by (a) scattering the pieces on the table or by (b) arranging them in various structures (as body in the center, legs diagonally above body, head on top, arms loosely at each side of body). Normally the child finds it more difficult to break up and rearrange the pieces (b) than to construct the figure after the parts have been presented in standard manner or scattered as in (a).

11—WISC Manikin

Use as directed the manikin from the Wechsler Intelligence Scale for Children.[29] This material does not seem to lend itself to as many interesting observations as that described under 10. When dealing with children handicapped by motor deficiencies, both manikins have to be used with caution because of possible emotional reactions to the mutilated human figures. The WISC material, with its shortened leg, seems especially suggestive in this respect, apparently more so than the schematic, conventional figure of 10.

[29] David Wechsler, *Wechsler Intelligence Scale for Children* (New York: Psychological Corporation, 1949), pp. 80–81.

12—OTHER OBJECT ASSEMBLY TESTS

Use the profile and hand from the Wechsler-Bellevue Intelligence Scale[30] and/or the horse, face, and automobile from the Wechsler Intelligence Scale for Children.[31]

12A—STANDARD PRESENTATION. Present and score as directed.

12B—VARIATIONS. Say, "Put these together as they go." (Omit mentioning that it is a horse, hand, profile, face, or automobile.) Present pieces as directed. Say, "Can you guess what it is going to be?"

Note: Does the child immediately have an idea, or does he prefer to manipulate the pieces first? Is his idea correct, or does he have notions that may make it difficult for him to reach the correct solution? If it becomes clear that he will not arrive at a solution, introduce systematic suggestions by placing some significant part (a finger of the hand, the head of the horse) and by gradually adding more. Or make verbal suggestions, for instance, "It is an animal" (or a horse, or part of a man, or a hand, face).

All the object assembly tests described (10 through 12) can be used with handicapped individuals in ways described before. These procedures are, in general, most useful with individuals who lack speech because of hearing difficulties and the like. For those handicapped by motor impairment, they may be less effective.

13—MARE AND FOAL PICTURE BOARD

Use the material from the Pintner-Paterson[32] and the Merrill-Palmer[33] scales. The picture represents in color a mare and foal in a field with two sheep lying down and three chickens in the foreground. In the background are seen two houses. Seven pieces have been cut out (head of mare, head of foal, a lamb, a chicken, front legs of mare, front leg of foal, piece of meadow).

13A—FIRST PRESENTATION. Briefly show the board to the child. If other formboard tasks have preceded, one may say that "this puzzle is somewhat different." Remove the pieces and scatter them right side up around the board. Say, "Put these back where they go."

---

[30] Wechsler, *The Measurement of Adult Intelligence*, pp. 96–98, 181–183; *The Measurement and Appraisal of Adult Intelligence*, p. 82. These are included in the WAIS.

[31] Wechsler, *Wechsler Intelligence Scale for Children*, pp. 82–84.

[32] Pintner and Paterson, *op. cit.*

[33] Stutsman, *op. cit.*, pp. 194–196.

Note, as in other formboard tasks (6 to 9), trials and errors. Does the child first try to find the correct piece for a specific hole, or a hole for a specific piece? Or rather does he pick up any piece and try it in any hole? Does he try longitudinal pieces in similarly shaped recesses, or does he try pieces without regard for their general shapes? Does he seem to go by the shapes of inset and hole only, or does he try to go by content (horse needs a head, chicken goes with other chicken)? Does he try to fit the piece into its correct position, or does he try to force it in by pounding and banging on it? Does he turn it after experimenting? (See also 2, 3, 4, 6.) Does he realize when he has a piece face down, and does he try to adjust it?

Successful completion of this test procedure requires skills similar to those needed with other formboards. The fact that each piece can fit into one spot only makes it somewhat more difficult than other formboards where each one of the cutouts is one entire piece which can fit in various ways (Seguin). However, besides form perception, color as well as content may be used to solve the puzzle. Normal children between *three-and-a-half and four-and-a-half years of age* are, in general, able to complete the board, though the youngest ones take a long time and proceed largely by trial and error.[34] They may try small pieces in larger holes or be unable to turn the pieces as they should. From *four-and-a-half years of age* on, the board can be completed more easily with fewer trials and quicker adjustments. The Merrill-Palmer Scale, which evaluates the performance by time alone, gives credit on the *four- to four-and-a-half-year level* for success within 150 seconds, and on the *five-to five-and-a-half-year level* for success within 86 seconds.

13B—VARIATIONS. The procedure may be modified by varied systematic suggestions. If it seems indicated, one may place one or another piece for the child or remove a piece that was poorly placed. One may turn one or another piece to a position which may suggest how it should be fitted; or one may help by proposing that it should be turned or that "it goes the other way" or that "it is too big."

13C—QUESTIONS. In certain cases the same test material offers an opportunity for E to get a first impression of a child's language and stock of information. A child who has been uncommunicative during preceding tasks may become willing to enter into a casual conversation about the picture. Once he has finished the board, one may ask him to name or point out certain objects or animals, or to show "all

[34] *Ibid.*, pp. 196, 228.

animals," or "white animals, brown animals" (see II:2–4,5b), or to name other animals, or to answer "What do we get from chickens, lambs, cows?" (See Chapter XI.)

14—ASSEMBLING CUT-UP PICTURES

Use material from the Wechsler Intelligence Scale for Children, "Picture Arrangement," A to C (pictures of dog, mother, and train).[35] Present and score as directed.

Note: Regarding train, does the child notice that the train consists of separate units with two pieces belonging to the engine? Does he see to it that the engine is followed by a tender and coal car, or does he match individual parts like wheels, or does he mostly seem to fit line to line? Note at what point the child seems to recognize what the puzzle represents.

Normal *six-year-olds* usually put the train together, though they may do so with some initial errors.

Similar simple puzzles are used in various other test scales. In the Revised Stanford-Binet Scale, Form M, III 6-, IV 6-, and V-year levels[36] the materials are a block disk, a pig (each cut vertically), and a rectangle cut diagonally.

T:IV.   Most suitable procedures for various age ranges

Procedure	Age
1, (2), (3), 5	Up to two years
1–6, (7), (9), (10), (13), (14)	Two to six years
6–12, 14	Six to ten years
8, 9, 12	Over ten years

Parentheses around number indicate that the procedure is suitable only for the older children in the age group.

---

[35] Wechsler, *Wechsler Intelligence Scale for Children*, p. 74.
[36] Terman and Merrill, *op. cit.*, pp. 142, 334.

V

Following, Finding, Retrieving

In his behavior with people and objects a young child may show how much he understands of what is going on around him. In many of the manifestations of the first two years, motor, emotional, and intellectual factors are intimately linked. Therefore, the clinician who wants to use her observations on babies as a basis for evaluation must take notice of any minute symptoms of behavior. These may help show what the child can understand, as opposed to what he is able to do or what he wants to do—either just then or at any time.

In all test procedures described below, note a baby's motor pattern. Note his general behavior and his awareness of objects, people, and events in his environment. Observe whether he is interested, cheerful, smiling, and enterprising, or aloof, anxious, unresponsive, and lethargic. Note whether he is observant and attentive, or dull and remote. Is he lively and agile, or slow and clumsy? Does he seem able to do all he wants to, or is his motor equipment inappropriate to his needs?

Use colorful or otherwise attractive objects as lures (rattles,[1] colored rings, jingle bells, sets of measuring spoons, keyrings) unless other specific objects are mentioned in the description of procedures. Maintain the child's interest and cooperation. Make sure he keeps on being attracted by what is shown to him. For some children a variety of objects may be needed. Others may like one special toy and want to keep on with it. Some may even prefer their own toys to the strange ones proffered by E. With older children, and especially with severely handicapped ones, the clinician has to consider the child's apparent level of com-

---

[1] As described by Arnold Gesell, *The First Five Years of Life* (New York: Harper, 1940), p. 76.

prehension when choosing a lure. Even if, for good reason, E uses infant procedures for such children, she should not pick a rattle to test loco-motion or persistence in a child of late preschool age. The child may feel that the rattle is not worth the effort of reaching; yet he might be more eager to try reaching for some, to him, more attractive and interesting toy.

1—NOTICING AND REACHING FOR OBJECT

Hold the object directly in the baby's line of vision; move it slowly in front of him. Later touch it to each hand and place it in his hand unless it has been grasped spontaneously.

Normal babies, in general, notice an object in their line of vision by the time they are *four to six weeks old*. By *eight weeks* the sight of the object increases their general activity. They regard the object con-sistently at *three to four months of age,* approach it with both hands at about *five months,* or with just one hand at *seven to eight months.* By *three months* they may begin to hold on to the object which is placed in their hand. They may notice its loss by *four months* and show some attempt to re-secure it by *six to seven months.*[2]

2—FOLLOWING AND FINDING MOVING OBJECT

Move object sideways, first slowly, then rapidly. Later move it rapidly in all directions.

Normal babies of *three to four months of age* can usually follow the slowly moving object,[3] but may not be able until about *nine months* to find an object visually again after it has been momentarily lost from sight.[4]

3—REACHING FOR DISTANT GOAL

Place an object or person within sight but out-of-reach of the baby, with no obstacles in between.

To reach the desired object, normal babies in this situation change their body position as follows: they may turn from back to side by *six to seven months,* may draw up legs or assume a creeping position

[2] For similar norms see Arnold Gesell and C. S. Amatruda, *Developmental Diag-nosis* (New York: Harper, 1941), "Developmental Schedules."

[3] *Ibid.*

[4] Jean Piaget, *Construction of Reality in the Child,* trans. (New York: Basic Books, 1954), Chapters I and II. Note that here, as in all following references to Piaget's writings on infants, the age levels mentioned are those given for the three children whom Piaget observed. These are not statistical norms derived from large numbers of subjects. The interest is in the sequence of developmental stages rather than in exact age norms.

by *ten to eleven months,* or, when slightly older, pivot on belly or start to creep.[5]

4—RETRIEVING HIDDEN OBJECTS[6]

4A—FROM ONE PLACE. Place an object in which prolonged interest has been shown under a nearby cloth (or edge of pillow) while the child is watching.

Note whether the baby pursues the object and tries to uncover it as normal children of *eight to nine months of age* may do, whether he no longer pays attention to it and has forgotten it, or whether he still wants the object but does not know how to get it back.

4B—FROM A SECOND PLACE. Once the object has been retrieved several times from the same place (4a), hide it under another cloth (or pillow) nearby while the child is looking on.

Note whether the child goes immediately for the object in the new spot or whether he, like a normal child up to *ten or twelve months of age,* turns again to the spot in which he found the object before. Note whether he gradually learns to find the object in either place, as seems normal at this age.

4C—FROM A THIRD PLACE. Once the child has learned to retrieve the object from either hiding place, hide it in a third spot in the same manner.

Note whether the child can find it right away, or whether he first looks in either of the previous places but gradually learns where to find it. To solve 4c normal children may have to be a *month or two older* than to solve 4b.

5—RETRIEVING HIDDEN OBJECTS AFTER DELAY

Use material from the Revised Stanford-Binet Scale, Form M, II-year level.[7] This consists of three boxes and a toy cat.

5A—STANDARD PRESENTATION. Present as directed. Say, "I'm going to hide the kitty and see whether you can find it again." Hide the kitten under one of the boxes which are lined up in a row. Screen the boxes and count aloud from one to ten. Then reveal the boxes and say, "Now, can you find it?" Repeat three times, hiding the toy each time under a different box (first center, then right, then left).

---

[5] Gesell, *op. cit.*

[6] The following procedures are adapted from Piaget, *op. cit.*

[7] Lewis M. Terman and Maud A. Merrill, *Measuring Intelligence* (Boston: Houghton Mifflin, 1937), "Delayed Response," pp. 135, 327.

Score as directed; two successes are required for passing at *two-year* level.

5B—VARIATIONS. Vary the above procedure. Omit counting, but say (while the boxes are screened), "Can you find it?" Uncover the boxes. Say, "Now, where is the kitty?" Lengthen the intervals between screening and uncovering in the second trial by adding patter such as, "Are you sure you can find it? You think you can?" and more of the same in the third trial.

Note success and failure. Note whether, in the second and third trial, the child tries to find the kitten where he found it before, whether he modifies his search correctly in response to the change, or whether he searches haphazardly anywhere. Note whether he is interested in finding the kitten each time, or whether he gradually becomes carried away only by the pleasure of uncovering the boxes or the enjoyment of repeating, "There it is," regardless of whether he has found it.

This procedure seems to be a more social and meaningful situation for the child than 5a. It seems less artificial to fill the pause between hiding and uncovering with E's chatter than with counting. Since the child's interest and expectation are deliberately kept alive, his span of attention rather than his memory is being evaluated in this version. This may be helpful for early detection of attention difficulties that are often characteristic for children with certain types of brain injury.

6—INTERMEDIARIES

6A—OBJECT NEARBY. Use a ring with a string,[8] or a similar object with a string of similar length. Place in front of the child; the end of the string should be within reach of the child, but the ring should not.

Note whether the child strains directly for the ring (as is normal for children about *seven months of age*) or whether he, although wanting the ring, gets interested in the string, pulls it, and seems surprised when the ring approaches (*ten months*). Note whether he wants the ring but immediately structures the situation adequately and pulls the string, and shows by his constant gazing at the approaching ring that he knows it is coming (*ten to twelve months*).

6B—OBJECT FARTHER AWAY. Place the object, with a longer

[8] Arnold Gesell, Helen Thompson, and C. S. Amatruda, *Psychology of Early Growth* (New York: Macmillan, 1938) pp. 39ff. The "dangling ring" used by Gesell consisted of a wooden embroidery ring 11 cm. in diameter and painted red, suspended on a string 25 cm. long.

string, farther away from the child behind some barrier (crib-rail, chairback). Place the string within his reach.[9]

Note (as in 6a) whether the child pulls the string without anticipating the approach of the object, or whether he uses the string to get the object nearer to him. This task is frequently more difficult than 6a. A loop in the string, or the barrier itself, may interfere with direct perception; the child must act on what he knows about such situations rather than on what he perceives. Also, he has to act upon an object which is outside of his immediate realm. Occasionally, children, especially those with motor handicaps, are not accustomed to this.

6c—OBJECT HIGH UP. An object (ball, bell) is placed out of reach of the child in a high place while the child is watching.

Note whether he tries to reach it directly by straining toward it, standing on his toes with arm extended, as children of *eighteen months* are apt to do, or whether he uses a nearby chair or a handy stick, as is common in *two-year-olds,* or gets a chair or something else to climb up on, as normally enterprising children from *two-and-a-half years* on may do.

7—DISAPPEARING OBJECTS[10]

7A—OBJECT TEMPORARILY OUT-OF-SIGHT. A moving toy is moved so that it disappears temporarily behind a screen or in a tunnel.

Note whether the child watches for the toy at the spot where it vanished, as a child *up to ten months of age or older* may do, or whether he correctly watches for it to come out at the other end of the screen. Note whether, after several repetitions, the child learns to expect reappearance of the object in the proper spot (*twelve to fourteen months*).

7B—OBJECT LOST OUT-OF-SIGHT. A ball may roll out-of-sight under the sofa or some other large piece of furniture.

Note whether the child goes for it at all, whether he tries to follow the track of the ball directly (*eighteen months*). Note whether he keeps straining for the ball even when it seems clear that he cannot reach it this way. Note whether he gives up or whether he realizes that he might retrieve it by reaching it by a detour (around the sofa, etc.). Experience shows that children of *two years and older* may be able to do so.[11]

---

[9] Adapted from Charlotte Bühler and Hildegard Hetzer, *Testing Children's Development* (New York: Farrar and Rinehart, 1935).

[10] Adapted from Piaget, *op. cit.*

[11] See similar situations described in Piaget, *op. cit.;* Edith Meyer, "The Comprehen-

8—Objects and Containers

8a—removing pellet from bottle. Use small glass bottle and pellet. Present pellet to the child. Have him manipulate it for a while. Then introduce the bottle.[12]

Note how the child handles the pellet. Does he grasp it with two fingers (*nine to ten months*)? Does he retain it (*eleven months*)? Does he combine it with the bottle, hold it over the bottle, or release it (*twelve months*)? Or does he drop it inadvertently somewhere on the table as soon as he gets hold of it (*under eight months*)? Or after he has retained it for a while? Does he notice that he has dropped the pellet anywhere, or in the bottle? Does he try to re-secure it after he has dropped it?

If pellet was not dropped into the bottle point to the bottle, and say, "Put it here." After this is done, say, "Can you get it out again?"

8b—variation. Omit handling of pellet previous to presentation of bottle. Present bottle and pellet simultaneously and drop pellet into bottle while child is watching. Note spontaneous behavior first, or say, "Get it out again," or, if the child makes no attempt to re-secure the pellet, demonstrate by turning the bottle upside down so that the pellet rolls out. Put pellet back into bottle and hand it to the child.

Note: Does he immediately try to get the pellet, or does he seem to study the situation first? Does he poke at the pellet through the glass or from the top of the bottle (as babies of *eleven to twelve months* are apt to do)? Does he bring the bottle to his mouth (*ten months*)? Or shake and wave it and watch the pellet inside? Does he use these more primitive activities only to explore the situation, but resort immediately afterwards to turning the bottle over? Normal babies of *eighteen months and older* get the pellet by turning the bottle upside down.[13] At about *fifteen months of age* they may learn to do so after one demonstration.

8c—removing object from narrow box. Use a tubular box, 8 inches high and 1½ inches in diameter, with a set of cat bells or a red disk. Drop the bells (or disk) into the box while the child is watching (as in 8b), or have the child first manipulate bells (or disk), as in

---

sion of Spatial Relations in Preschool Children," *Journal of Genetic Psychology* 57:119–151, 1940.

[12] The following procedures are adapted from those described by Gesell and Amatruda, *op. cit.*, p. 389.

[13] *Ibid.*, p. 69.

8a. Invite him to "get it out again" or watch his spontaneous attempts to do so.

Note whether he turns the box upside down immediately, or whether he tries to poke at the desired object from the top, trying to reach it in direct prehension, even though the box opening is too small for his hand. This situation is more difficult than the preceding one, since the box is opaque and therefore the object is no longer visible after it has been dropped into the box. Normal children may not necessarily succeed in this problem as early as they do in 8a and 8b, even though, from an adult point of view, the same principles seem to be involved. Experience shows that only at about *twenty-one to twenty-four months of age* do normal children immediately turn the box over in order to get the object.

Various ones of the test procedures described under 1 through 8 can be adapted for use with children with motor handicaps who may show the degree of their comprehension by the way in which they participate in the situation. Even children who are essentially unable to proceed alone may show through their trials, attempts and frustrations, or even through eye movements alone, what they would like to do or would expect to see. In 2, for instance, a child may follow a moving object with his eyes, and find it again. In 4, 5, and 7a, he may indicate by his persistent gaze toward a distant place that he expects the object to show up there. In 8, either he may seem to anticipate that the object (pellet or the like) will drop out or he may seem surprised to see it fall out when the container is turned over.

In all of the preceding test situations, comprehension of spatial relationships is involved. It has been shown that in the normal child the notion of space develops gradually as interaction of sensory-motor and mental activity enlarges the scope of his experiences.[14] This development is distorted in children who, because of motor handicap, have not the necessary motor patterns by which to gain normal experiences through handling objects and moving around in space. In their case, comprehension of spatial relationships must come from what they see, hear, or otherwise perceive.[15] Their progress in this

[14] Piaget, *op. cit.* and *Origins of Intelligence in Children,* trans. (New York: International Universities Press, 1953).

[15] Similar considerations are discussed by Alfred A. Strauss and Newell C. Kephart, *Psychopathology and Education of the Brain-Injured Child,* Volume II (New York: Grune and Stratton, 1955).

area, therefore, may be delayed; however, such children commonly seem to adjust to these modified conditions of learning if they have enough mental ability to do so. Test situations involving spatial comprehension may therefore prove useful in the evaluation of a child's ability to learn from his contacts with his surroundings. Experience shows that even children with serious physical handicaps and lack of speech, but with potentially adequate mental capacities, will show comprehension in the above test situations by *three to three-and-a-half years of age,* at the latest. An examiner may be justified in expressing doubts about such a child's learning ability if no evidence of such awareness and comprehension can be elicited at about that age or somewhat later.

T:V. Most suitable procedures for various age ranges

Procedure	Age
1–4, (5), 6–8	Up to two years
5, 7b, 8c	Two to six years

Parentheses around number indicate that the procedure is suitable only for the older children in the age group.

VI

Matching, Sorting, Grouping

1—SORTING

1A—BLOCKS BY COLOR. Use two sets of blocks of different colors (see I:6).

1B—BUTTONS BY COLOR. Use material from the Revised Stanford-Binet Scale, Form M, III 6-year level.[1] This consists of ten black and ten white buttons. Present as directed.

1C—STICKS BY SIZE. Use sticks of two, three, or four sizes (see VII:6c).

2—MATCHING AND SORTING FOUR COLORS

Use material from the Merrill-Palmer Scale.[2] This consists of four small boxes, each of a different bright color (red, yellow, green, blue) opening like match boxes. Each contains six disks of the same color as the box.

2A—IN FOUR COLORED BOXES (SPONTANEOUSLY). Open the boxes and remove the disks; spread them before the child and mix them. Place the empty boxes in a row before the child. Their order may be yellow, blue, red, green, or the like, as long as blue and green are separated, since confusion is more likely between these two colors than between others.

While emptying the boxes one may say, "See all these pretty things, and here there are more and more. . . ." Leave the child to con-

---

[1] Lewis M. Terman and Maud A. Merrill, *Measuring Intelligence* (Boston: Houghton Mifflin, 1937), pp. 144, 339.

[2] Rachel Stutsman, *Mental Measurement of Preschool Children, with a Guide for the Administration of the Merrill-Palmer Scale of Mental Tests* (Yonkers, New York: World Book Company, 1931), pp. 175–178.

template the situation and to initiate any activity he chooses. Let him play for a short while.

Note: Does he pile, line up, or roll the disks? Does he pay any attention to their different colors? Does he relate them to the boxes, place them in or on top of the boxes? Does he make artistic arrangements with the various colors? Or does he become intrigued with the boxes themselves?

2B—IN FOUR COLORED BOXES (AFTER DEMONSTRATION). Say, "Let us put them back in the boxes where they belong." Show the child how to place a red disk on top of the red box and slide it into the box, then place a yellow one in the same manner. Say, "This one is a red one. It goes in the red box. This one is a yellow one. It goes in the yellow box." Then hand a blue disk to the child and ask, "Where does this one go?" If he places it correctly, let him proceed alone from here on. If he places it in the wrong box, correct his error, saying, "No, this is a blue one. It goes in the blue box." Correct one or two more successive errors, then let him proceed without interference. Let him pick the disks or hand them to him in mixed order.

Note: Does he seem to follow a system and place all colors without mistake (*three- to three-and-a-half-year level*), or does he correctly place only some and not carry through (*two- to two-and-a-half-year level*)? Does he place all the disks in one box without color discrimination but occasionally assemble a few disks of the same color in one hand (*eighteen-month to two-year level*).[3] Does he start systematically but become distracted, or does he begin without comprehending but learn gradually? Does he begin or end up by being interested only in sliding any disks into boxes? Does he lose interest in the whole situation entirely?

2C—REMOVING WRONG PLACEMENTS. Present as before, but inconspicuously remove wrong disks from boxes as soon as they have been placed. This makes the task easier, since it keeps each box the proper color (see I:6).

2D—TWO BOXES AND TWO COLORS. Use two colors only, removing the two other colors from sight. Present as in 2b.

2E—WITHOUT BOXES. Use all the colored disks without boxes. Show one (red) disk, and ask for "one just like this." If necessary, demonstrate and ask for another (red) one. Ask for all disks of the same color in succession (easy for normal *two- to two-and-a-half-year-olds*) or shift between different colors (somewhat more difficult).

[3] *Ibid.*

2F—TWO BOXES AND FOUR COLORS. Use all colored disks but only two of the colored boxes. Demonstrate as in 2b. This task seems to be more difficult than 2d or 2e, but easier than 2b.

Note all responses as before. Also, does the child seem to learn from the modifications and simplifications described above? How does he use what he has learned when faced again with the more difficult technique 2b? Try to determine what causes his failure—whether it seems to be the multitude of colors, the matching in the boxes, or the length of the task. Does he have difficulty in color discrimination, or might the procedure be too difficult or too absorbing for him because of the motor task involved?

All techniques described under 2b through 2f may be adapted for use with handicapped children. Children who do not understand or respond to language may be shown what to do. If motor disabilities are severe enough to make effective handling of the disks difficult, one may place the boxes far apart so that one may easily see which box the child means; thus one may avoid letting him struggle until he has placed the disks squarely into the boxes. With the most severely handicapped children, one may use the proxy method described before (see Chapter I). E may pick one disk after another and ask the child to indicate where it should go (2b, 2d, 2f), or she may spread all disks on the table and hold the color sample disk (2e) near first one then another color and let him show what it should be.

3—ADDITIONAL USES OF MATERIAL

The same material may lend itself to use with "serial patterns" (see I:5), or to tasks of counting or determining quantities (see I:7–9).

4—DECROLY MATCHING GAME

Use material from the Merrill-Palmer Scale[4] (originally one of the Decroly educative games). This consists of four large cards, each of which contains four silhouette pictures in red, and a set of sixteen smaller cards made by quartering a duplicate set of the larger cards. The sixteen pictures represent star, crescent, cherry, disk or ball, triangle, pear, sailboat, sprinkling can, lamp, square, pitcher, locomotive, apple, basket, flag, and umbrella. (Sailboat and lamp are antiquated designs.)

4A—MODIFIED PRESENTATION. Place the four large cards in

[4] *Ibid.*, pp. 203–205.

a row before the child, the card with the ball farthest to the right. Say, "You see, you get all the big cards and I'll have the small cards and later I will give you the small cards too." Show small card with ball, and say, "See this ball on this card. There is one just like this here (showing the big card). We will put it right on top of it, that is where it goes." Show square (or triangle) next, asking, "Where does this go? Can you find it?" Help the child find the correct place, or correct a wrong placement if he fails. If necessary, help or correct with two or three other cards. Hand out small cards one by one and let the child proceed on his own.

Note: Does he understand immediately, or after delay? Is he interested in choosing the correct place? Does he look all over the field, or make errors? What are his errors? Are they caused by his tendency to fill one card first, or by his haste to fill the cards, or to grab the small cards? Are errors determined by dominant perceptual characteristics rather than by likeness of the whole figure? (For instance, does he place umbrella on flag because they may look somewhat alike in that each has a compact part with an appendage, *e.g.,* handle and pole. Or does he place apple on ball because they have a vaguely similar shape?) Normal children between *four-and-a-half and five years of age* are able to place at least twelve of the sixteen cards without errors. At *three-and-a-half to four-and-a-half* they place some cards correctly, but they often make the kind of perceptual errors described above. The complete task often may be too long for children *under four*.[5]

4B—GIVING A SECOND CHOICE. E may first ascertain on which level the child is functioning when he is working on his own. Later on she may want to add questions about some of the errors and try to understand how they came about. Ask, "Where else could it go?" Such a suggestion may or may not produce the correct choice. If it does immediately, one may often assume that the child might be mentally mature enough to give a perfect solution. His wrong choice may have been due to inattention. He may have chosen on a first impulse too hastily by a superficial impression rather than by accurate comparison. A consistent tendency toward this kind of inaccurate choice may be a significant symptom in some clinical cases.

4C—STANDARD PRESENTATION. In the original directions of the Merrill-Palmer Scale, the small cards are placed in rows below and

[5] These norms correspond to those given by Stutsman for the standard presentation described below (4c).

above the large cards; the child proceeds on his own immediately after one demonstration. E is then only an observer. Occasionally this method may be desirable, for special reasons. For instance, E may be interested in evaluating how well some child can work independently. Or with another child she may feel that he prefers to work without interference by an adult.

For many children, however, the modified form of presentation (4a, 4b) seems better. The large cards on the table by themselves simplify the perceptual situation: the matching of individual shapes becomes the sole concern and is not obscured by the added task of sorting out the loose cards from the solid ones. Also, E can control the sequence of the cards, which has an advantage. From the social-emotional point of view the interaction between E and the child enhances the climate of the test situation.

4D—TWO CARDS ONLY (INSTEAD OF FOUR). For some children it is necessary to reduce the number of large cards from four to one or two. Attention can more easily be focused and maintained on a smaller field. Thus, with children who are much excited and erratic it is still possible to determine whether or not they are able to differentiate some of the pictures. Occasionally, an otherwise ineffective child may surprise the observer by adequate discrimination between two of the more difficult choices (pitcher—sprinkling can, flag—umbrella).

4E—IDENTIFICATION QUESTIONS. Some questions may be added to evaluate simple group concepts (as in II:5). Ask: "Show me the ones we can eat," "Show me the ones that are up in the sky," "Show me the ones that we can carry things in."

Note: Does the child find all the pictures belonging to one concept, as apple, pear, cherry (often called lollypop), ball (occasionally called orange); star, moon, ball (often called moon or sun); or basket (often called pocketbook), pitcher, sprinkling can? Does he stop when he has found all that belong in one group, and does he try to make others do (as calling the triangle candy)? Note such responses as calling the boat a bird, or saying that the flag "is on the roof in the sky."

4F—NAMING AND POINTING. The material may serve for spontaneous or elicited naming (see II:1,2) or pointing (II:3). Since the pictures are all of one color and presented in silhouette, they are somewhat more difficult to distinguish than those in colored picture books. They do not seem to be more difficult than the black and white pictures used in other procedures testing identification (II:9). The smaller number of choices seems to make the group of questions in 4f easier than that described in connection with the picture book (II:5b).

These techniques can be adjusted for handicapped children in various ways. For a child with impaired motor abilities one may space the large cards so that it becomes clear what he means, whether he indicates it by fumbling motions or only by his gaze. In 4a to 4d one may arrange the sequence of cards so that equivocal placements are avoided. With some children one may want to remove the small cards after they have been placed. This avoids confusion and embarrassment that can occur when the child unintentionally upsets cards which have been placed. For those who cannot understand language, one may substitute pantomime for verbal directions where this is feasible.

5—Color–Form Sorting

Use material of the Weigl-Goldstein-Scheerer color–form sorting test.[6] Use two sets. Each consists of square, disk, and triangle in each of four colors (green, red, blue, and yellow).

5a—same color, same form. Place before the child a green triangle, a red disk, a yellow square. Present the second green triangle. Showing it near the first green triangle, say, "See, these are the same. This one is just like this one." Remove the second green triangle, produce the second red disk, and ask, "Which one is like that?" If necessary, demonstrate. Repeat with all forms. If he has learned to choose correctly, proceed to:

5b—choice of form. Place on the table a blue triangle, a blue disk, and a blue square. Present another blue triangle. Ask, "Which one is like that?" When the child has indicated his choice, remove the triangle without giving the child a chance to pile it on top of the first one. Continue with blue disk and then blue square. Repeat.

5c—choice of color. Place on the table a green disk, a red disk, and a yellow disk. Present another green, or red, or yellow disk, as before. Repeat.

Note: Does the child know or learn to choose correctly? Does he hesitate; does he make mistakes? Does he do as well with colors (5c) as forms (5b)?

Experience shows that normal *three-year-olds* choose correctly in

---

[6] Kurt Goldstein and Martin Scheerer, *Abstract and Concrete Behavior.* Psychological Monographs, Volume 53, Number 2 (Evanston, Ill.: American Psychological Association, 1941), p. 110.

the introductory step (5a) as well as in 5b and 5c. Frequently, they pile or fit the blocks also. *Two-and-a-half-year-olds* may choose correctly by color (5c) but be unreliable in choice by form (5b). These norms correspond to those described under 2 and to those described by Gesell with regard to a color–form test consisting of five red forms (disk, half-disk, square, triangle, cross) to be placed on matching red forms of the same size. *Two-year-olds* identify none of these forms, *two-and-a-half-year-olds* place at least one form, and *three-year-olds* place at least three forms.[7]

5D—CHOICE BETWEEN FORM AND COLOR. Present after 5a, or after 5a, 5b, 5c. (A) Place yellow triangle, blue disk, red square. Present red disk, later yellow square, blue triangle. Repeat by placing other combinations such as: (B) blue triangle, green disk, yellow square. Present blue disk, later green square, yellow triangle. Remove each before presenting next one.

Note: Does the child place the red disk with the blue disk or with the red square (A)? Does he hesitate in making his decision, or does he seem to see only one solution? Does he know that there can be no fully satisfactory solution, since, contrary to previous presentations 5a, 5b, 5c, there is no identical object available in 5d? Is the child consistent in his choice? Does he always choose by color, or always by form?

Younger children are generally not bothered by any conflict between choices. They decide on the basis of one quality only and do not seem aware of any other possibility. Awareness of a conflict because of the two possible choices may be shown by children from *four-and-a-half to five years on.* After that age they become puzzled and find it difficult to decide. They may state their dilemma or choose somewhat arbitrarily. The question of whether form or color choice is preferred by normal children of varying ages has been a matter of much discussion.[8]

[7] Arnold Gesell, *The First Five Years of Life* (New York: Harper, 1940), p. 134.

[8] Katz found in his studies on three- to five-year-old children, using material somewhat similar to the above (two shapes and two colors only), that younger children prefer color choices, and older ones prefer form choices. Descoeudres' findings were similar. Both authors found that their younger subjects were undisturbed by any conflict, whereas the older ones seemed to be aware of it. Brian and Goodenough found that children under three may prefer form to color. Heinz Werner, who quotes all these findings, concludes that "the choice of color or form depends on the relevance of the quality. This may change with the age level, with the kind of objects used, and with the experimental situation as a whole." See David Katz and R. Katz, *Gespräche mit Kindern, Untersuchungen zur Sozialpsychologie und Pädagogik* (Berlin: Springer, 1928). Also Alice Descoeudres, "Couleur, forme ou nombre?" *Archives de psychologie* 14:305–341, 1914. Also C. R. Brian and Florence Goodenough, "The Relative

For the clinician it may be interesting to see whether children after the age of six continue unperturbedly to choose one or the other solution without any sign of conflict. This may be in some cases a sign of inattention or impulsiveness, or may point toward a lack of perceptual discrimination. One may find that children suffering from brain injuries that impair their perceptual ability tend to sort by color alone well beyond the age at which this occurs with normal children.

5E—"WHAT GOES TOGETHER." Use one set of the material of the Weigl-Goldstein-Scheerer color–form sorting test, as directed.[9] Spread out on the table and say, "See all these things. Put together what goes together" (A). When the child has finished his arrangement, say, "This is fine. Now let us arrange them some other way. How could they go together some other way?" (B).

Note: Does the child study the material at first and decide how to arrange it? Does he start immediately to handle some of the pieces and get them organized as he goes along? Does he sort and leave loose heaps, or does he arrange carefully, spacing, fitting, and visually balancing the pieces? Does he end up with distinct groups (of four colors or three shapes), or with one, two, or more arrangements each of which combines several colors and several shapes? Does he build neat towers or patterns, fitting surface on surface or edge to edge?

At all age levels the test material has considerable play value. Whereas normal grown-ups can usually resist the temptation to build and arrange patterns, older children frequently may sort by proper classes but still pay attention to the arrangement of the blocks. Younger children almost invariably use the blocks for the arrangement of patterns or buildings only. The request to change to a different arrangement means for them a change in pattern but not a change in sorting principle. A shift to a different principle is rare in children up to *eight years of age.*

The original intent of this technique was to investigate in the adult brain-damaged patient the ability to apply different categories to the material and to shift from one to another. In normal children the ability to apply various categories to the same material develops gradually with age. This has been pointed out by Werner,[10] Piaget,[11]

Potency of Color and Form Perception at Various Ages," *Journal of Experimental Psychology* 12:197–213, 1929. Also Heinz Werner, *Comparative Psychology of Mental Development* (New York: Harper, 1940), p. 237.

[9] Goldstein and Scheerer, *op. cit.*

[10] Werner, *op. cit.,* p. 238.

[11] Jean Piaget, *Judgement and Reasoning in the Child,* trans. (New York: Harcourt, Brace, 1928), Chapter III.

and others. In a study of concept formation in children, Reichard, Schneider, and Rapaport,[12] using the same Weigl-Goldstein-Scheerer material, confirmed these facts. They also found that only *after eight years of age* 75 percent of their subjects could each group the material both ways. Allowing for individual variations, it would therefore seem that the use of the Weigl-Goldstein-Scheerer test as a diagnostic tool for the detection of brain injury may not be valid *before twelve years of age.* Even then it may best be trusted only in connection with other techniques.

6—MATCHING FORMS

Use material from the Revised Stanford-Binet Scale, Form L, IV-year level.[13] This consists of two cards, each with ten geometric forms; one card is to be cut up so that the forms may be placed on the other card at a point, X.

6A—STANDARD PRESENTATION. Put the larger card before the child, point to the forms on the card, and say, "See all these things. I have others here just like them." Place the cutout circle on X, saying, "See, can you find one just like this on the big card?" If the child does not respond correctly, pass finger around the outline of the cutout circle and repeat, "Find me one just like this." If no correct response follows, point to the circle on the larger card: "See, this one is just like this." Proceed to show all other forms one after another, starting with square or triangle and later in any order that differs from the order of their arrangement on the large card.

6B—VARIATIONS. A somewhat easier and, with children, often more popular presentation, is to first briefly place the cutout circle form on X and then demonstrate its likeness to the circle on the card by placing the two forms on top of each other. Remove after demonstration. Hold up the next form. Ask, "Where does this go?" Let the child place the form on the form of his choice. Repeat with all forms. Remove each form after it has been placed in order to give the child full range for the next choice.

Note all choices, whether correct or not. Do his successes come at the beginning, or after a period of learning? Or are they less frequent toward the end? Are they haphazardly distributed in between

---

[12] S. Reichard, M. Schneider, and D. Rapaport, "The Development of Concept Formation in Children," *American Journal of Orthopsychiatry* 14:156–161, 1944.

[13] Terman and Merrill, *op. cit.*, pp. 88, 212. This test is also described in Gesell, *op. cit.*, p. 136, and Frederick Kuhlmann, *A Handbook of Mental Tests* (Baltimore: Warwick and York, 1922), p. 100.

errors? Does he succeed with easier tasks and fail with difficult ones? Or does he have successes and errors with easy as well as with hard ones? Does he choose carefully, or does he follow his first impulse? Does he spontaneously correct his errors? Does he look for E's approval of his choice?

The discrimination of form that is necessary for this task becomes more accurate with age. A normal *three-year-old* is, in general, able to discriminate four of the forms, the *four-year-old* can find eight of the forms, and the *five-year-old,* all ten.[14] Most children find the circle the easiest shape to identify, whereas an irregular shape and a diamond are among the harder ones and cause errors up to *five years of age.* Young children's choices are frequently guided by primitive, global qualities which for them determine the similarity of the shapes. Hexagon and circle may be frequently confused, perhaps because of their similar size and total impression. The ellipse is matched to the rectangle, perhaps because both are equal in length and similar in width, and are oriented horizontally. The diamond frequently is matched with the square or triangle, perhaps because of its angularity. Such fusions are characteristic of many *four-year-olds* (see also 4 and IV:6).

For normal children this procedure is on approximately the same level of difficulty as the Decroly matching game (see 4). It may be more difficult for abnormally distractible children because the shapes are presented in black and white and are not meaningful as are the silhouettes of objects in the Decroly test. Discrepancy between results in the two tests may be viewed with some interest by the examiner. It often may point toward difficulties that need further explanation. The test procedure described above can be valuable to determine the extent of perceptual distortions in older brain-injured children. For children with severe motor or visual handicaps, larger size cards may be better.[15]

7—DISCRIMINATING AND MATCHING ANIMAL PICTURES

For description and discussion, see II:10.

8—MATCHING AND GROUPING OBJECTS

Use small toy objects similar to those that are provided with the Revised Stanford-Binet material,[16] but use a greater variety and larger numbers of objects. Some of the objects are identical in shape, size, and color;

---

[14] Gesell, *op. cit.,* and Terman and Merrill, *op. cit.*

[15] The cards originally used by Kuhlmann are about twice as large as those of the Revised Stanford-Binet Scale.

[16] Terman and Merrill, *op. cit.,* pp. 75, 135.

others are not. For instance, there are several small green chairs, a red chair, and a yellow stool, several identical green cups, a few blue cups of the same size, larger white cups, blue saucers, small blue spoons, large red spoons and forks. Also among the objects are different animals, musical instruments, a milk bottle, soup cans, bread and other edibles in small, toy imitations. A sizable collection of toy objects provides many opportunities for activities which are psychologically significant. They can be used for evaluation of young, and also older, children. A few samples of test procedures are listed.

8A—SPONTANEOUS GROUPING. Present in succession and leave with the child: a green chair, dog, red spoon, another green chair, cat, green cup.

Note: Watch what the child does with each object. He may immediately name and handle it properly, as stand up the dog or chair, or imitate eating motions with the spoon. He may try to place the dog on the chair or feed the dog with the spoon. Or he may try each object separately but apparently not combine it with another one. He may use all or some of the objects inappropriately and without discrimination, using each one to bang or hammer on the table, to throw in any direction, or at a definite spot, as back at E, or beyond the table, or under his chair.

Most normal *two-year-olds* show that they recognize the objects. They may name them, handle them appropriately, or do both. However, they vary individually in what they do with each object. Beginning at this age, the majority of children like to act out activities (drinking— cup, eating—spoon, cutting—knife, listening—telephone). They may combine several objects (feeding the dog with spoon or cup, placing the cat on the chair, or placing two green chairs together).

Unless the child does not appear to recognize any of the objects in any way, E may proceed to:

8B—SUGGESTED GROUPING. Remove all objects from the table. Then place in two groups.

(A) 1. Green chair with dog beside it; blue dish before dog.
     2. Similar green chair with similar dog. Give a red dish (different shape) to the child.

Note: Does the child place the red dish before the second dog, or does he treat this new object as if it had no relation to the objects standing on the table? If the latter is the case, suggest, "See this is my chair and my dog. He has his dish right here next to him. Now, here is your chair, and your dog, and here is a dish. Where should it go?"

(B) 1. Green chair with dog and red dish with large red spoon.
2. Green chair with cat. Give the child a green cup and a small blue spoon.

Note: Does he react to these groupings? Does he attempt to imitate them or to carry on? Is he able to integrate the new objects in the standing arrangements? Does he initiate new combinations or activities, or does he remain unimpressed by the varied possibilities of the material? Does he handle objects appropriately? Does he become absorbed in each new object, or does he remain interested in all objects?

These procedures have not yet been standardized. Experience shows that in (A) normal children of about *two-and-a-half to three years of age* generally place the feeding dish where it is missing, and thereby act as if they recognized the new dish to be the equivalent of the first one. In (B) the same children are apt to match the dog scene by placing the green cup and the small blue spoon with the cat. From the adult point of view this seems to be a more complex problem than (A). Still it appears that for the child the various objects are not as differentiated by their distinct qualities as they are for the adult: both animals and all feeding utensils seem to go together in a more diffuse total situation of "feeding animals." The child responds perceptually and emotionally to the whole of the situation. He may round it out as he sees fit, or he may make a new meaningful arrangement.

The psychological processes that underlie such activities are the important first steps toward concept formation, though grouping here is still on a practical preconceptual level.[17] Children whose mental development does not proceed in normal orderly sequence may often not be able to respond adequately to these tasks. They may persist in undifferentiated handling of the objects and see no meaning or relationship between, for instance, cup and dish and their respective functions. For them the objects have more primitive values than seems to be normal at their age.

9—MATCHING OBJECTS

Avoid using this technique after 8b. While the child is watching, place objects in three groups as follows: (1) automobiles (a blue, a red, a green); (2) animals (two identical dogs, a cat); (3) dishes (assorted plates, cups, saucers).

Say, "See, here are all these, and all these, and all these" (pointing to one group each time). Give the child a cow, later a yellow automobile,

---

[17] Werner, *op. cit.*, pp. 227ff.

pitcher, spoons, etc. (one at a time). Ask, "Where should it go?" or "Where shall we put it?"

Note: Does the child roll the new automobile to the group of other automobiles, walk the cow to the other animals, or carefully line up automobiles and animals, pile the dishes, etc.? Or does he place the new cow riding in the blue automobile, or feed the cat with the new spoon? Or does he treat the new object independently and place it apart from the others? Does he respond to any added suggestion ("How about putting the cow with the dogs and cat?")? Is such a suggestion effective in leading to other similar groupings?

This procedure has not been standardized. Experience shows that from *three to three-and-a-half years of age* children are apt to place the objects in the groups in which they would belong by adult standards (animals, dishes). But these groupings, for the *three-year-olds,* do not seem determined by logical categories as they would for older children and adults. At the youngest age levels, objects belong together through their similar concrete functional properties (cars can roll or be lined up; cows, cats, and dogs can stand or run).

At the same age and even earlier, objects may be placed in pairs that are meaningful to the child (a cow riding in a car). Around *four years of age* and after, one may find more and more children who favor groupings by kind (animals, vehicles), but even then they still handle and investigate each object separately, place it carefully side by side with another one, or arrange all objects of a group in neat piles or rows; they do not seem to consider their task completed before this is done. When they get older (by *six or seven years of age*) some children may no longer seem to find it important to make concrete arrangements. Now they may assign the new object to the group to which it belongs. They still may also enjoy arranging them, but they do this only later, as a playful afterthought; it no longer seems to them essential for the solution proper. They too sort by category, as would adults who, also, may afterwards be tempted to arrange such objects playfully.

Various genetic studies on sorting have shown similar progression of stages.[18] While the younger children sort by functional qualities and by emotionally attractive properties, they gradually come to sort by form, size, or kind. Even such categories are still for a long time part of concrete actions and probably are not yet the logical categories of the

---

[18] *Ibid.* See also Edith Meyer, "Ordnen und Ordnung bei drei- bis sechsjährigen Kindern," *Neue Psychologische Studien,* Band X, Heft 3 (Munich: Beck, 1934).

adult. Many children go through a stage at which they somehow have double standards: they know how the groups should go (by adult standards), and say so; but they still prefer their individualistic groupings when they have the choice. This fits in with findings showing that normal children understand adults' conceptual groupings before they choose them on their own.[19]

10—MATCHING OBJECTS AND PICTURES

Use picture book (see II:1–5) with such objects as green chair, dog, milk bottle, baby doll, green cup, blue spoon, watch, automobile, trumpet, block (see VI:8). Open the book to the proper page and place the toy dog on the picture of the dog. Say, "See this one. It goes right here. Now see if you can find where the other ones could go."

Note: Does the child understand the task, inspect all the objects, and try to find one to fit on a specific page, or does he pick up one of the objects and then look for a picture to match it? Does he make his choices quickly, with assurance, or does he seem to be puzzled? Does he place the green cup with the green pictured cup, and the naked baby doll on the similar picture only, or does he also place a blue plate with the picture of green dishes, the blue spoon on that of a metal spoon, and the naked baby doll on that of a dressed doll? Or does he place the doll with the chair, the spoon with the cereal, etc.? Does he place an object near or on top of the picture, or does he try to fit the dog lying flat on the picture, or the spoon to cover the pictured one?

This still unstandardized procedure seems well within the abilities of *three-and-a-half- to four-year-old* children. Occasionally a child may hesitate to place a green chair on the picture of a yellow one, but once he sees that E approves of this choice, he may no longer have any doubts about similar placements. Some children may, at this age, take pains also to fit the object form neatly on top of the picture, but most are content to have object and picture correspond in function. Children who at this age and later are unable to combine any object with its pictorial likeness seem to be lacking in some important function. For them the picture may not appear as a graphic symbolization of a three-dimensional object, as it normally should. This may be so even if they do not fail to give the picture the proper object name. Such difficulties

[19] Reichard, Schneider, and Rapaport, *op. cit.*

in pictorial appreciation are occasionally seen in brain-injured children.

11—Matching Objects and Printed Words

11a—choice of objects. Print in large, legible letters in a column, allowing about two inches between words, car, spoon, cat, cup, block, key. Give the child a box containing the corresponding objects, together with a number of other objects. Ask the child to find objects to match the words. Demonstrate if necessary. The child's interest should be on the matching task, rather than on the reading of the words. Do not ask him specifically to read the words; he should not think of this procedure as a reading test.

Note: Does he seem secure and self-sufficient, or is he embarrassed? Does he seem to read the words, study them, or guess them? Is he hesitant with his placements? Does he place correctly, or does he confuse words like cat and car, or cup and cat?

11b—corresponding objects only. The task may be simplified by using those objects only that match the printed words. One may stress the fact that there is one object for each word, or let the child find this out for himself. This procedure is well within the limits of most *seven-year-olds*. Occasionally, one of them may not have "had" one or another word, and immediately recognize the fact. The "game" is enjoyed by many children, even those who otherwise might be reluctant to read during the examination. It may enable the examiner to get an initial impression of a young child's reading comprehension.

11c—for higher reading levels. The task lends itself also for use with children who have higher reading levels. It can be used with more difficult words (automobile, watch, harmonica) and still have the advantage of dealing with objects rather than with the spoken word.

All tasks described here concern functions that are involved in the development of language and communication. Beginnings of concept formation are seen in the earliest groupings of the young child.[20] Putting identical things together is an earlier achievement than seeing equality between an object and its picture. From this point, then, it takes another big step to learn that a printed word may replace either object or picture. The psychological processes that are involved concern

[20] Werner, *op. cit.*, p. 227.

theoreticians whether they are dealing with development of language and thought or of symbols and communication.

The practicing clinician may find the simple tasks helpful, even in their present unstandardized form, since they allow her to observe a child and to estimate his level of comprehension in this area. In some patients with speech retardation, performances in these tests may help to rule out mental defect. In other children whose language development seems delayed, one may find specific difficulties in the comprehension of meaning: they may be interested only in matching object and picture by size and shape (in 10) and may pay no attention to what either picture or object represent. Combined with normal comprehension in other areas (with form material, for instance), such difficulty may suggest aphasoid tendencies. The simple procedures described here seem to prove especially useful in the cases of older children (*over six or seven*) who suffer from acquired aphasia due to a cerebral accident. The tests may help to determine the degree of injury and the rate of recovery. These techniques can without too much difficulty be used with children with serious motor handicaps, whether or not these are combined with delayed speech development. Various adaptations can be made: the proxy methods described before can be used, as can any other arrangement which allows one to see how the child would like to choose.

12—SORTING OBJECTS

Preferably use with children of school age. Use about thirty objects (described in 8). Present all objects in an unsorted pile and ask the child for his assistance in rearranging them. Suggest something to the effect that keeping them all together in one box seems impractical and untidy, and that some new arrangement in packages or boxes is to be planned. Would he have any suggestions about how to organize this best? Many children (*eight years of age and older*) find this a plausible task and seem to go at it with more enthusiasm than when asked only to show "how things go together."

Note carefully all the child does. Does he first inspect the material in order to decide on a plan, or does he seem to find a plan while handling some objects? Does he favor a few large groups, or does he start many small groups? Does he try to make doubtful objects belong in a group in which they hardly go? Does he try to explain? Is he puzzled by, or content with, his decisions? Are his categories obvious (animals, furniture), or plausible (things that go in a kitchen, in a living room), or are they determined by specific personal factors ("toys my sister likes" or "things I need for my doll house")? Are his groups equivalent, or does he have a group of "things that are all green," and "all sorts of dishes" side by side?

Various authors have found the sorting of objects by children to be an interesting manifestation of children's thought processes. Attention may be focused on the criteria which determine for the child "what belongs together," or on the character of the groups themselves, their looseness or narrowness, their relationship to each other. All these aspects are closely related. As the child gets older, criteria as well as organization become more objective and consistent. They come to depend less on a child's immediate actions or emotional relationships to the objects and more on permanent, logical, or abstract qualities; the groups become more distinct and mutually exclusive, and their relationships better defined.

In a study on sorting reported by Reichard, Schneider, and Rapaport it was found that very loose and very narrow groupings are characteristic of the very young. Functional groupings prevailed up to *eight and nine years of age,* conceptual groupings became dominant around *eleven years of age.*[21]

Our test material (described under 12) has not yet been standardized. From her observations of process and of end product, the clinician may nevertheless arrive at some estimate of a child's working habits and level of reasoning. Experience shows that after *eight or nine years of age* it is rare for a normal child to place together all animals and also to include dishes for the animals to eat from. After *seven or eight years of age* children hardly ever use a color group and a functional group simultaneously. At *eight years of age* it is unusual for children to match, for instance, an "animal block"[22] with toy dogs and cats, or a round plate with vehicles "because the plate looks almost like a wheel." Loose groupings of this sort are, however, characteristic of very young children and of those whose reasoning processes are distorted by brain injury and who are at the mercy of their fleeting and stimulus-determined ideas and actions.

The absence of norms demands caution in judging the children's

[21] Reichard, Schneider, and Rapaport, *op. cit.*
[22] Wooden blocks with outline of animals on sides, commercially available under the name of "animal blocks."

choices of categories. The toy-sized objects may be suggestive of concrete and functional categories, even in adults and older children. Up to *ten years of age,* categories such as "kitchen things" or "play-things" prevail. Sometimes they seem to depend on individual preferences rather than on age, except for the very young (*four- and five-year-olds*) who often do not sort at all, but may pick out a few especially attractive objects only and place them in a small (narrow) group without bothering about the rest. Spontaneous sorting by shape (all long, all round), by color, or by material (all wood, all plastic) is, in our experience, so unusual with this material that some significant distortions in thinking may be suspected if it occurs. Such groupings may reveal various types of difficulties. These may be amongst others, in the comprehension of meaning as seen in aphasic patients, or in object relationships as seen in schizophrenic patients.

13—Klapper-Werner Multiple Choice Test

This test consists of eight individual sorting tasks. For each task there are four objects. One of these (the key object) is to be placed by the child with that one of the three others with which it "goes best." The three objects for the first task are: (a) a toy dog made of brown rubber, (b) a yellow cup made of plastic, (c) a glass lens. The fourth (key) object is a toy baby's bottle with a brown rubber nipple.[23]

Note where the child places the key object and ask him why. He may place the bottle with the cup and state that both are for drinking purposes; or he may place it with the glass lens and state that they are made of the same material, or he may place it with the rubber dog and show that the nipple is "like" the dog, or perhaps like the dog's pointed tail.

The other seven tasks are the following:

Key object	Choice objects
(2) Red button	(a) Red lipstick
	(b) Spool of white thread
	(c) Blue poker chip
(3) Small white light bulb	(a) White pingpong ball
	(b) Pink candle
	(c) Wax pear, shaped like bulb

---

[23] Zelda Klapper and Heinz Werner, "Developmental Deviations in Brain-Injured (Cerebral-Palsied) Members of Pairs of Identical Twins," *Quarterly Journal of Child Behavior* 2:288–313, July 1950.

Key object	Choice objects
(4) Metal bottle cover with some	(a) Metal key
red print	(b) Bottle stopper
	(c) Red poker chip
(5) Round ink bottle with red ink	(a) Match cover with red and
	white lines
	(b) Small empty glass bottle
	(c) Sunglass lens—dark
(6) Green toothbrush	(a) Green yo-yo
	(b) Black comb
	(c) Blue pencil
(7) Small black rubber wheel	(a) Black cardboard cover
	(b) Small green wheel
	(c) Lollypop
(8) Pink soap	(a) Pink baby doll sock
	(b) Toy sink
	(c) White soap

In all these tasks note what factor determines the selection. It may be function, color, or form. If it seems to be the latter, it may be that the fact that one object "fits" on top of another or sideways to it is important to the child, but not the shape as abstract category.

In an unpublished study of normal children from *four-and-a-half to ten years of age,* color responses were found to be predominant up to *six years of age.* Some few *nine- to ten-year-olds* gave conceptual responses, and a number of *seven- and some eight-year-olds* chose by inherent property such as material, shape, or size. Brain-injured children were apt to base their choices on color or on some seemingly irrelevant feature, rather than on functional categories, well beyond the age of the normal child.[24] Similar solutions by brain-injured children were reported earlier by the original authors.[25] These findings also agree with a comparable study by Cotton,[26] and are borne out by our clinical experience with similar children. Their choices may be decided by the color of the whole object or of part of an object, by some other minute detail, or by some concrete relationship between two objects. Such choices may be explained in various terms: they may be forced responses to sensory stimuli; they may indicate lack of control, a ten-

[24] Raymond Holden, "An Experimental Investigation of Concept Formation in Children." Term paper, Clark University, Worcester, Massachusetts.

[25] Klapper and Werner, *op. cit.*

[26] C. B. Cotton, "A Study of the Reactions of Spastic Children to Certain Test Situations," *Journal of Genetic Psychology* 58:27–44, 1941.

dency to persevere, or failure to appreciate meaningful wholes. Various authors have pointed to the theoretical and practical significance of distortions of conceptual thinking reflected in such choices. Strauss and Werner[27] discussed them when reporting on the results of sorting tests with children with exogenous and endogenous mental retardation. The above test procedure grew out of these first, now classical, studies. For the observant clinician, the multiple choice test is an interesting and easily handled tool; it is usually much enjoyed by children. Lack of proper standardization is still its greatest deficiency.

T:VI.   Most suitable procedures for various age ranges

Procedure	Age
(8a), (9)	Up to two years
1–10, (11), (12), (13)	Two to six years
(5e), 9, 11–13	Six to ten years
12	Over ten years

Parentheses around number indicate that the procedure is suitable only for the older children in the age group.

[27] Alfred A. Strauss and Heinz Werner, "Disorders of Conceptual Thinking in the Brain-Injured Child," *Journal of Nervous and Mental Diseases* 96:153–172, 1942. Also Alfred A. Strauss and Laura E. Lehtinen, *Psychopathology and Education of the Brain-Injured Child,* Volume I (New York: Grune and Stratton, 1947), Chapter IV. Also William Cruickshank and Jane E. Dolphin, "The Educational Implications of Psychological Studies of Cerebral-Palsied Children," *Exceptional Children* 18:1–18, 1951.

VII

Designs

1—MEMORY FOR DESIGNS

Use designs from the Revised Stanford-Binet Scale, Form M, IX- and XII-year levels, and Form L, IX- and XI-year levels (see Figure 4).[1]

1A—STANDARD PRESENTATION. Present for ten seconds (see Revised Stanford-Binet directions). If the child hesitates, assure him that what he draws is important, not how he draws it. Score as directed.

Note: How does he proceed? Does he study the model in detail or try to take it in at a quick glance? Does he follow outlines with his pencil in the air or try to put down quickly what he has seen? Does he start with simple outstanding structures (squares, etc.) and finish one after the other, or does he work on some isolated lines or small units of the design? Is he self-sufficient and certain, or anxious and hesitant? Does he correct or erase? Is his stroke weak or firm or too strong? If he has difficulties, do they seem due predominantly to insufficient memory of perception or to motor disability? Or to both? As in III:4,5, note his trials, his attempts, and his frustrations in relation to the end result. Question him about his intentions, if necessary. The well-defined task frequently appeals to children better than the request to draw spontaneously (III:1) or to make a picture about a subject (III:2). Those who are uncertain about their ability to draw feel reassured because the test seems to stress memory rather than drawing or good form reproduction. This test situation can be introduced early in an examination. With children of school age, it serves as an initial gauge of graphic skill, fine motor coordination,

[1] Lewis M. Terman and Maud A. Merrill, *Measuring Intelligence* (Boston: Houghton Mifflin, 1937), pp. 104, 108, 248, 250, 160, 169, 362, 386.

FIGURE 4.   Memory for designs models

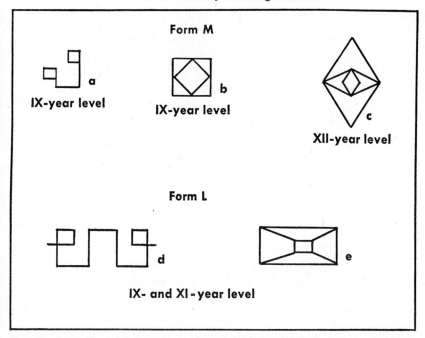

From Lewis M. Terman and Maud A. Merrill, *Measuring Intelligence* (Boston: Houghton Mifflin, 1937), pp. 104, 160, 169.

and perceptuo-motor abilities. Perceptuo-motor difficulties revealed in this test should be neither minimized nor exaggerated. Individuals differ in their proficiency in tasks involving visual memory. They vary equally in their ability to reproduce what they have just seen. Frequently, a person with a motor disability is intent only on overcoming technical drawing difficulties. This may divert attention from the accurate representation of the model. With such variability taken into consideration, this test situation remains a valuable single tool for early detection of perceptuo-motor difficulties as they are seen in children with brain injury. Consistent failure on a ten-year level in a child eleven to twelve years old should warrant further investigation by various methods.

1B—VARIATION. One may repeat the same task or expose the design for copying. Note whether the child shows any tendency to improve his performance. Note whether he can learn to understand the figure better if he is invited to trace the model or to discuss its construction in words.

2—Ellis Visual Designs Test

Use the ten Ellis designs cards (see Figure 5).[2]

2A—FROM MEMORY. Use the designs as a memory-for-design test. Say, "I am going to show you some little designs one at a time. You will see each one just for a little while, and then I shall take it away and ask you to draw it from memory. Look at it carefully so you can make yours just like it; but do not start before I have taken it away." Expose each design for five seconds. Score one point for a good, symmetrical presentation of the figure and one half point for one error or two errors that are symmetrically consistent. For scoring standards see Figure 6, for age norms see tabulation.[3]

Note the child's procedure, manners, working habits, as in 1a.

This test may immediately follow the preceding ones (VII:1). It may help E to reappraise, confirm, or reject findings of those tests. The first Ellis designs are simple and are apt to reassure a child who may have become apprehensive by failure in 1a. Some of the designs (1,2,5,6) seem familiar to many children. They may verbalize this impression by saying, "Oh, just a box" (1), or "two boxes" (5), or "almost a k" (6). The other designs (3,4,7,8,9,10) are unfamiliar to most. Their specific irregularity, imbalance, and intricate configuration have to be perceived, retained, and reproduced.

Normal children improve their performances in this test with age. Brain-injured children frequently have serious difficulty. The test procedure is useful for the detection of perceptuo-motor disturbances when other grossly abnormal findings are absent. Serious deviations from normal are significant symptoms when combined with otherwise normal global ratings. Elizabeth Lord and Louise Wood[4] first showed that children with brain injury frequently show irregularities and very low scores in the Ellis designs test. Such scores are not found in emotionally disturbed children of comparable mental level. It is important to follow Lord and Wood's recommendations when using the test as a diagnostic tool. They propose to consider as diagnostically significant only those scores that fall below the twenty-fifth percentile in the lowest age range. In these terms, children of about *nine years of age* with scores of 3.5 or below may be suspected of having some form of brain injury

[2] Louise Wood and Edyth Shulman, "The Ellis Visual Designs Test," *Journal of Educational Psychology* 31:591–602, 1940.

[3] Samuel Goldenberg proposed a revised and more detailed scoring guide in Alfred A. Strauss and Newell C. Kephart, *Psychopathology and Education of the Brain-Injured Child,* Volume II (New York: Grune and Stratton, 1955), pp. 219ff.

[4] Elizabeth Lord and Louise Wood, "Diagnostic Values in a Visuo-Motor Test," *American Journal of Orthopsychiatry* 12:414–428, 1942.

FIGURE 5. Ellis visual designs

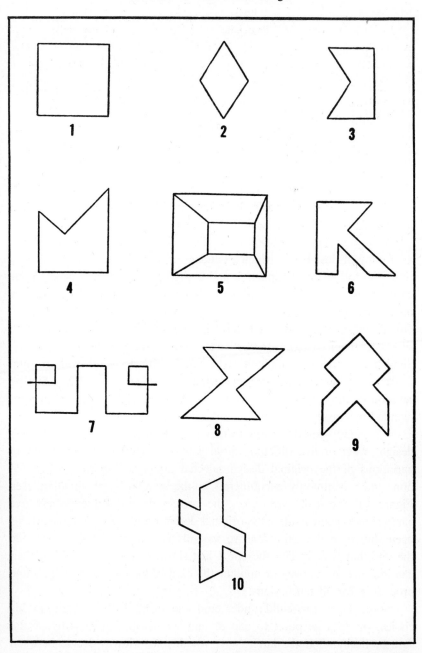

From Louise Wood and Edyth Shulman, "The Ellis Visual Designs Test," *Journal of Educational Psychology* 31:592, 1940.

T:VII:2. Age norms, based on sum of points, for Ellis visual designs test

Age (years)	Boys Percentile			Girls Percentile		
	75	50	25	75	50	25
8/6 to 9/6	6.1	5.1	4.4	6.3	5.2	4.0
9/6 to 10/5	6.7	5.8	4.7	6.5	5.7	4.6
10/6 to 11/5	7.3	6.3	5.2	7.0	6.2	5.2
11/6 to 12/5	7.6	6.6	5.6	7.5	6.7	5.8
12/6 to 13/5	8.0	7.1	5.9	8.0	7.0	6.1
13/6 to 14/5	8.2	7.4	6.2	8.1	7.2	6.3
14/6 to 15/5	8.5	7.7	6.5	8.3	7.3	6.4
15/6 to 16/5	8.7	7.8	6.8	8.3	7.3	6.4
16/6 to 17/5	9.0	7.9	7.0	8.3	7.5	6.6

Adapted from Wood and Shulman, *op. cit.*

which may seriously impair their learning ability and, therefore, their ability to profit from the ordinary academic teaching methods.

2B—BY COPYING. The Ellis designs cards may be presented as a copy-of-design test which excludes the memory factor. This variation may follow 2a or replace it and is preferred in specific cases. Some children become anxious and disturbed by the imminent disappearance of the model in 2a and therefore fail to pay attention to its design. Others become unduly excited by the social interaction with E, who seems to them to tease or challenge them by taking the model away. Significant perceptual difficulties become easily apparent with method 2b, as in other similar copy-of-design tests (see also III:5). Similar revision of the original Ellis-Wood-Shulman technique has been recommended by Cassel.[5]

2C—RECOGNITION (MULTIPLE CHOICE TEST). For each Ellis design, a set of five different cards was developed. Four of them are variations of the original design selected amongst imperfect reproductions most commonly encountered in the standard test situation (see Figure 6); the fifth card shows the correct design. Present these five cards simultaneously after the original design on a separate key card has been shown to the child for five seconds (as in 2a). Ask, "Show me the one that is most like the one I just showed you." The subject then can indicate in one way or another the card of his choice. Use the same procedure for all ten designs.

Note: Does the child understand the task? Is he careful in his choice, or does he point to one or another design haphazardly? Is he sure or hesitant? If the latter, note whether he tries to decide between

[5] Robert H. Cassel, "Relation of Design Reproduction to the Etiology of Mental Deficiency," *Journal of Consulting Psychology* 13:421–428, 1949.

FIGURE 6. Samples of half-point credits on Ellis visual designs test

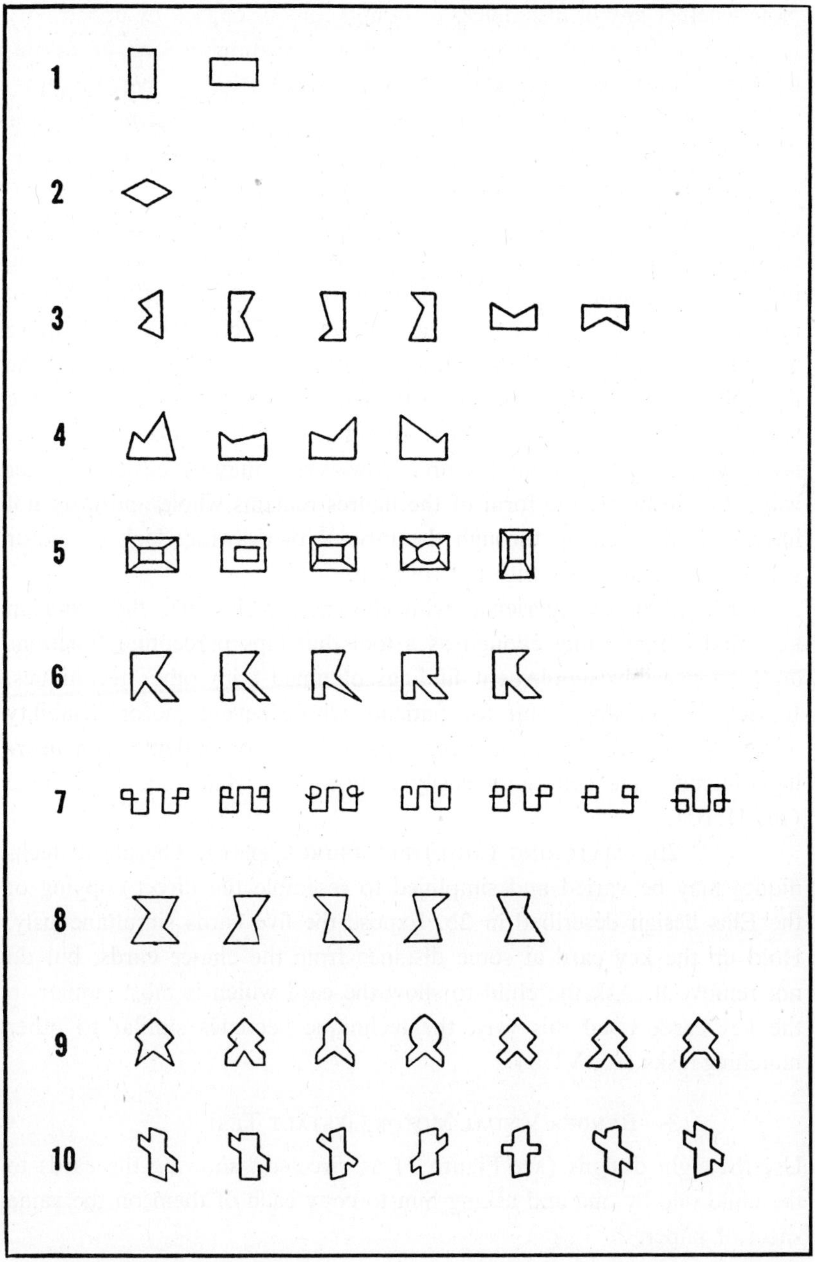

From Louise Wood and Edyth Shulman, "The Ellis Visual Designs Test," *Journal of Educational Psychology* 31:595, 1940.

two reproductions only, or whether he is uncertain about all of them. Note whether any of his choices or doubts may be caused by uncertainty in spatial orientation, or by a lack of appreciation of size or height, or whether there are gross simplifications or distortions of perception.

This multiple choice version of the Ellis visual designs test was developed by this author in collaboration with Kenneth Dinklage. It enables the examiner to distinguish individuals with ability for appreciation of form from those who seem to have a more or less severe lack of it. Before the procedure can be used for finer differentiations among individuals, it will have to be standardized. Also, the psychological processes involved will have to be analyzed and compared with those evaluated by the standard presentation. For instance, it may be that the multiple choice test is more difficult than the original task because the varied choices that are presented simultaneously may obscure the retained image of the original figure. However, it may be easier in other ways. For instance, the form of the figures remains whole and does not have to be broken up through the process of drawing; lack of motor skill does not interfere with the solution.

Pending more experience with this new technique, the clinician may find it interesting enough as a tool that taps perceptual functions and can possibly supplement findings obtained with other techniques. It seems especially useful for patients whose severe motor disability makes the use of paper and pencil impossible. For patients with hearing difficulty one can quite easily demonstrate what should be done (see II:10).

2D—MATCHING (MULTIPLE CHOICE TEST). The above techniques may be varied and simplified to resemble the direct copying of the Ellis design described in 2b. Expose the five cards simultaneously. Hold up the key card at some distance from the choice cards, but do not remove it. Ask the child to show the card which is most similar to the key card. Used this way, the technique becomes similar to other matching tasks (see VI:6).

3—BENDER VISUAL MOTOR GESTALT TEST

Use the eight designs (see Figure 7) as directed,[6] showing the cards to the child one by one and asking him to copy each of them on the same sheet of paper.

[6] Lauretta Bender, *A Visual Motor Gestalt Test and Its Clinical Use* (New York: American Orthopsychiatric Association, 1938), p. 4.

FIGURE 7. Designs from Bender visual motor Gestalt test

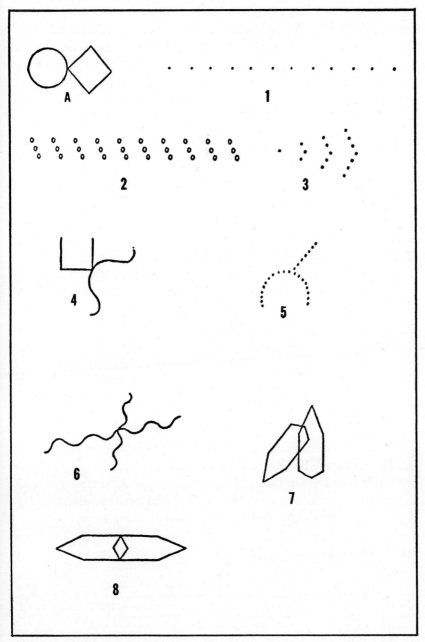

From Lauretta Bender, *A Visual Motor Gestalt Test and Its Clinical Use* (New York: American Orthopsychiatric Association, 1938).

Note as in 1 and 2, and as in Chapter III on drawing. Note working habits, stroke, manner of approach. How does the child proceed, how satisfied is he with the end product? How does he organize his page? Does he try to reproduce the design as a whole, or does he copy its elements one by one? Does he count elements or groups of them; is the form maintained, does the Gestalt become distorted as he goes along, or does it seem to be unessential to him from the start? Watch for gross distortions as well as for left-right or top-bottom confusions. Compare the end result with the standards given.

This procedure is designed to study visuo-motor performance by means of drawings. It is based on the theories of Gestalt psychology that stemmed from studies showing that in normal children the ability to reproduce these designs accurately develops regularly with age. Children who are deficient in mental development produce solutions that may in many ways be similar to those of younger children. However, some of the reproductions of children with abnormal development differ from those of normal children on any age level. The procedure has many merits and is popular with many clinicians. However, the interpretation of specific productions is not always easy, especially not if it becomes important to distinguish with some certainty between children who are retarded and those who have organic brain injury. Since the average normal child is not able to draw the designs with any degree of accuracy before the age of eight, the test seems useful as a diagnostic tool mostly for children over *ten years of age.*

4—BENTON VISUAL RETENTION TEST

Use material as described by Benton for children from eight years of age on. The first seven designs of Forms C and D, respectively, are shown in Figures 8 and 9. On five of these designs there are three forms each arranged in specific sequence, size, and spatial position. Each card is presented for ten seconds and then reproduced from memory.

Use Benton's scoring standards for "correct" and "incorrect."[7] For age norms see Benton (for all ten designs) or tabulation.

[7] Arthur L. Benton, *The Revised Visual Retention Test: Clinical and Experimental Applications* (New York: The Psychological Corporation, 1955); and *A Visual Retention Test for Clinical Use* (New York: The Psychological Corporation, 1946). Also Arthur L. Benton and Nancy Collins, "Visual Retention Test Performance in Children," *Archives of Neurology and Psychiatry* 62:610–617, 1949.

Our experience has been solely with the test published in the older edition. The seven designs of the original Forms A and B, respectively, are included in the revised edition as the first seven (of ten) designs of Forms C and D, respectively.

T:VII:4. Benton's age norms, based on sum of points, for seven designs

Age (years)	Defective	Border-line	Low average	Average	High average	Superior	Very superior
8	0	1	2		3	4	5–7
9	0–1	2	3		4	5	6–7
10	0–1	2	3	4	5	6	7
11	0–2	3	4		5	6	7
12	0–2	3	4	5	6	7	
13–16	0–3	4	5	6	7		

Adapted from Benton, *A Visual Retention Test for Clinical Use.*

Note as in VII:1 and 2, and also note how the child makes use of the model. Does he study it carefully, or only briefly? Is he eager to get going, or does he wait for the model to be removed? Note especially his verbalizations. Does he murmur (concerning C3) for instance, "Two round ones and a little box," or (concerning C4), "A little square, a ball, and a tent?" Does he outline the forms in the air? Does he do this systematically or haphazardly? Does he draw them in succession? Does he try to represent the three figures in their proper relationships, or does he treat them as separate items which may or may not be arranged correctly? Study imperfect reproductions carefully. Are his errors caused by lack of attention to relative size or relative position of the forms? Or by reversals in sequence? Or by omission of some detail? Is a different form substituted for the correct one? Are there perceptual errors in the reproduction of the individual forms? Are these errors gross distortions or reversals only? Is there perseverance from one design to the next?

This memory-for-designs test is in many ways different from those described in 1 and 2. Most of these designs show ordinary shapes (circles, squares, triangles) with some modifications. The forms are arranged in specific sequence, size relationship, and spatial position. The procedure tests predominantly comprehension and retention of such relationships rather than comprehension of the form of any individual element.[8]

After *eight years of age* normal children are familiar with the shapes that are presented. Retention is aided by existing perceptual

[8] The new edition includes designs that seem to be somewhat more complex. This discussion may therefore not apply to the new edition as much as to the old one. For this reason the normative standards for the first seven designs are shown in tabulation. These standards were published as tentative norms in the first edition, which is no longer available. See Benton, *A Visual Retention Test for Clinical Use,* p. 7. In the new edition the author also proposes using the designs as a direct copy-of-design test in addition to the memory-for-design technique.

FIGURE 8.   Designs from Benton visual retention test, Form C

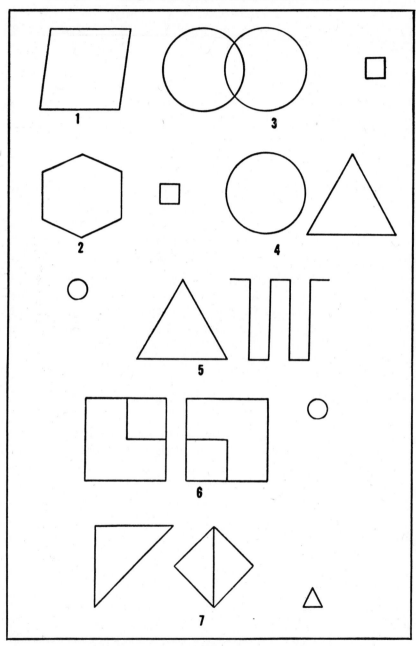

From Arthur L. Benton, *The Revised Visual Retention Test: Clinical and Experimental Applications* (New York: Psychological Corporation, 1955).

FIGURE 9.   Designs from Benton visual retention test, Form D

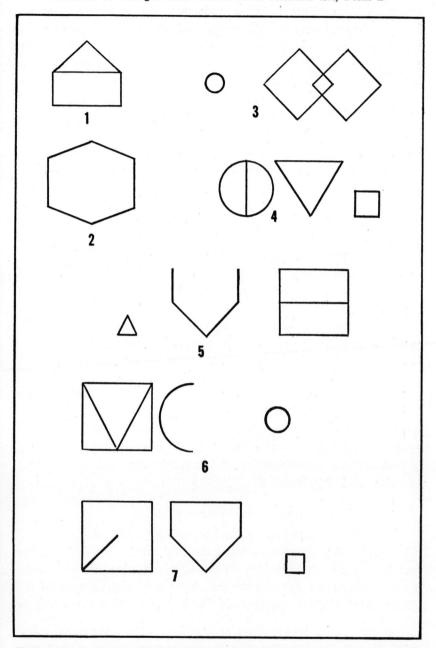

and spatial concepts. Frequently, spontaneous verbalization re-enforces activation, reorganization, and reproduction. For certain children this is easier than memory-for-design tests which require immediate structuring of percepts with no previously acquired schema to fall back on (see Ellis designs 3, 4, 7, 8, 9, 10, or some of the designs from the Revised Stanford-Binet Scale).

It is significant that in clinical experience children who have suffered more or less recent damage to the nervous system (through head injury, encephalitis, etc.) were found to have better scores on the Benton test than they had on the Ellis test. Children with brain injuries of long standing seemed to do equally poorly on both tests. Pending further studies, such findings may suggest the following tentative explanation.

Children with old injuries often show perceptual difficulties from early childhood on. The percepts which they retain are frequently distorted and poorly differentiated. Children who have developed normally up to a certain point before an injury may have retained some well-structured spatial concepts even though they no longer can elaborate new ones with ease. Clinical experiences justify use of the Ellis and the Benton tests together as a diagnostic tool. Flagrant discrepancies between the results of both can be a symptom that needs further explanation and investigation. Good scores on the Benton together with poor ones on the Ellis may suggest, for instance, that the child has a stock of organized visual concepts that must have been acquired in earlier years. This material is still intact and can be used adequately enough. Ability for new organizations, however, is beginning to lag. Good Ellis scores with poor Benton scores, on the contrary, may show good immediate form comprehension, but impulsiveness, lack of sustained attention, and sloppiness.

5—REY-OSTERRIETH COMPLEX FIGURE TEST

Use the design described by Rey and Osterrieth (see Figure 10).[9]

5A—BY COPYING. Present the card bearing the design of the complex figure to the child. Say, "Look at this drawing and try to copy it as well as you can. Try to make sure that you do not forget anything." With an anxious child, one may add that it does not matter how well he

---

[9] Paul A. Osterrieth, "Le test de copie d'une figure complexe," *Archives de psychologie* 30:206–356, 1944. Also André Rey, "L'examen psychologique dans les cas d'encéphalopathie traumatique," *Archives de psychologie* 28:44, 1941.

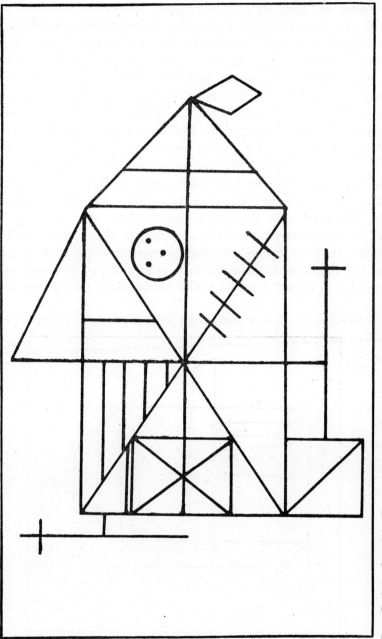

FIGURE 10. Rey-Osterrieth complex figure

From Paul A. Osterrieth, "Le test de copie d'une figure complexe," *Archives de psychologie* 30:206–356, 1944.

draws but that it is essential not to forget any details. If the child still hesitates and finds the task too difficult, sympathize with him, agree with him that the design is complicated, but encourage him to try. If he tries to turn the model card sideways, replace it in its original position. Allow him to turn his own paper as he wishes. Provide a colored pencil without eraser. Invite him to draw with it, and tell him that he will be given a different color later on. (Use of varying colors in a given sequence makes it easy to retrace later the working process used by the child. The examiner introduces a new color whenever she feels that it may help her later to remember how the child proceeded.)

Note: Where and how does the child start? Does he draw distinct units, or does he haphazardly copy isolated lines or details? If he works in large units, does he complete one before getting to the next, or does he change his plan of attack while working? Does he try to get every feature of the design, or is he content with but some? Does he try to reproduce interrelationships between parts, or does he get carried away by some prominent part only and pay no attention to others? Does he realize his mistakes? Does he try to re-

FIGURE 11. Plan of scoring units for Rey-Osterrieth complex figure

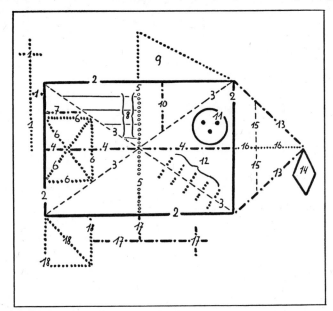

From Paul A. Osterrieth, "Le test de copie d'une figure complexe," *Archives de psychologie* 30:206–356, 1944.

T:VII:5.   Scoring system for Rey-Osterrieth complex figure test (see Figure 11)

Units

1. Cross upper left corner, outside of rectangle
2. Large rectangle
3. Diagonal cross
4. Horizontal midline of 2
5. Vertical midline
6. Small rectangle, within 2 to the left
7. Small segment above 6
8. Four parallel lines within 2, upper left
9. Triangle above 2 upper right
10. Small vertical line within 2, below 9
11. Circle with three dots within 2
12. Five parallel lines with 2 crossing 3, lower right
13. Sides of triangle attached to 2 on right
14. Diamond attached to 13
15. Vertical line within triangle 13 parallel to right vertical of a
16. Horizontal line within 13, continuing 4 to right
17. Cross attached to low center
18. Square attached to 2, lower left

Scoring

Consider each of the eighteen units separately. Appraise accuracy of each unit and relative position within the whole of the design. For each unit count as follows:

Correct	{ placed properly	2 points
	{ placed poorly	1 point
Distorted or incomplete	{ placed properly	1 point
but recognizable	{ placed poorly	½ point
Absent or not recognizable		0 points
Maximum		36 points

Adapted from Osterrieth, *op. cit.*, pp. 221–222.

T:VII:5a.   Age norms, based on sum of points, for copying
Rey-Osterrieth complex figure

	Percentile			
Age (years)	25	50	75	100
4	2	8	10	19
5	11	19	21	31
6	19	23	25	27
7	17	22	27	31
8	27	30	32	35
9	28	30	34	36
10	27	30	32	36
11	30	33	35	36
12	30	32	34	36
13	29	30	34	36
14	30	31	34	35
15	31	32	34	36
Adults	31	32	34	36

Adapted from Osterrieth, *op. cit.*, p. 241.

pair them, or does he ignore them or excuse them? Is he conspicuously slow, careful, and meticulous, or is he impulsive and hastily sloppy? Does he turn his paper sideways occasionally, or frequently? Does this seem to help him or get him confused?

Is his approach, as well as the final product, normal for his age? Evaluate his work as shown below.

Osterrieth investigated from the genetic point of view the productions of 235 Swiss children *from four years of age up*. He studied the drawings from many angles and compared them with those of 60 adults. He found that the youngest children (*four to five years of age*) are apt to produce a design in which some details can easily be recognized, though any global structure is missing. Between *five and ten,* most children either add one detail to another or else produce an undifferentiated global outline of the figure and in it enclose various of the details. The typical adult first constructs a solid, rectangular structure and then gradually adds all necessary details in relation to this rectangle. Aside from such progress with age in the character of the copy, Osterrieth also found that the number of details and the accuracy of their location increases regularly up to *nine years of age*. The norms that were developed in this study are based on a point system which credits separately the quality of each reproduced detail and the manner in which it is placed in relation to other details. This test procedure correlates well with other measures of mental competence.[10] It proves a useful clinical tool for children from *six to seven years of age and older*. Experience has shown its special value for use with brain-injured or emotionally disturbed children. Distorted, primitive, or concretized reproductions are frequently drawn by the first group, whereas compulsively restricted, overmeticulous, regularized, or bizarre arrangements may prevail in the second. More intensive study of test products in well-defined groups of abnormal children would seem interesting and promising.

5B—FROM MEMORY. When the child has finished copying the complex figure (5a), remove his paper together with model and crayons. Ask him, after a rest of three minutes, to reproduce the model from memory on a new sheet of paper with an ordinary pencil. Score the end product as directed.

Note: What is the child's attitude? Is he surprised, challenged, or annoyed about the unexpected repetition? Is he glad to get another

[10] Osterrieth, *op. cit.,* p. 345.

chance at the task, and does he start with more enthusiasm than before? Before starting, does he try to recapitulate what he has to do? Note the character of his work process. Compare it with his previous one. Is he more interested in large units now, or is he more absorbed in some detail? Is the end result better integrated and organized? Are the relations amongst parts more correct than before, or is there now an abnormally high number of missing details?

Since in this test the request for copying from memory comes unexpectedly after the model has been seen and studied for some length of time, for the subject the task is different from other memory-for-design tests (see 1,2,4). Osterrieth found that children from *eight years on* usually reproduce a more compact and better organized design when drawing it this second time. However, in their reproduction from memory, children and adults are apt to omit some of the details which they had in their first copies. It is generally normal that a good rating for the direct copy should accompany an equally high rating for reproduction from memory. If an otherwise willing child (or adult) shows a sharp decline in the second production, one may suspect difficulties in retentive memory. Therefore, it is useful to have the same subject go through both parts of the test (a and b). Comparison of the two performances often may help to elicit an important diagnostic symptom that may help to explain other learning difficulties in various types of cases.

Brain-injured children with impairment of long standing generally do poorly in copying and reproduction from memory because of their difficulties in organizing perceptual material. Children with recent impairment, however, may show greater variability between the two performances.[11] They are occasionally able to reproduce a reasonably good copy by adding carefully line by line. In their second reproduction they may remember a very few features only. Perhaps the difficulty some of these children have with reproduction from memory may be explained by the following factors. They have not yet been able to coordinate the isolated details which they perceived previously. Since they have not organized the details in integrated structures, they cannot recall them easily. It is generally thought to be simpler to remember large single units, whether visually or auditorily, than it is to recall single

---

[11] Similar discrepancy between ability in copying and memory for design has been found by various authors and with varying design materials. See Arthur L. Benton, *The Revised Visual Retention Test,* p. 59.

T:VII:5b.   Age norms, based on sum of points, for reproduction of
Rey-Osterrieth complex figure from memory

Age (years)	Percentile			
	25	50	75	100
4	1	2	5	14
5	4	10	14	23
6	7	13	17	22
7	9	14	18	28
8	16	18	23	29
9	16	19	22	29
10	16	20	22	26
11	17	20	23	27
12	15	18	24	32
13	17	19	23	33
14	19	23	26	32
15	20	22	25	28
Adult	18	22	27	35

Adapted from Osterrieth, *op. cit.*, p. 242.

details (see Chapter VIII). The extra effort this would demand is especially difficult for neurologically impaired children, who are apt to tire easily.

5C—QUESTIONS, SUGGESTIONS, REPETITION. The examiner may want to verify her findings through questions and suggestions. This should be done only when the drawing period is ended (either after 5b, or after 5a if 5b is omitted).

Ask the child who has shown difficulties whether there might be an easier way to reproduce the design than the one he found at first. How would he go about it if he had to do it over again? How would he have to start so that each detail could be fitted easily? Ask him to think about it, and to show (or to draw) the lines that should come first. Rey,[12] who proposes such verification methods, finds that many subjects suddenly find that they should have started with the large rectangle (unit 2) and perhaps with the diagonals (unit 3) or the mid-lines (units 4,5). Others study the design anew when being questioned and gradually find a better solution. Some, however, persist in their first approach or propose an equally primitive alternative. This latter group may have intellectual defects which make it impossible for them to benefit from the new experience. (Such defects are especially common with brain-injured patients.) Those subjects who replace their initial faulty approach quickly by a more mature one may first

[12] Rey, *op. cit.*, p. 48.

have been inattentive and nonchalant, or too hasty or bewildered, so that they performed less well than they could have. The clinician then would have to be concerned with their attitude and working habits rather than with their lack of ability to draw the design.

6—GOLDSTEIN-SCHEERER STICK TEST
(ADAPTED FOR CHILDREN)

Use the stick material from the Goldstein-Scheerer Test[13] or similar sticks in four different sizes (ranging from one to four inches) and one color. To avoid confusion, be seated next to the child, or cornerwise, but not opposite him. Present the sticks to the child. Show him the different sizes. Explain that one can "make" all kinds of things with these sticks and proceed to demonstrate the first design. (It is best not to allow the child to start on any spontaneous play with the material.)

6A—IMITATION. Arrange the first model (square a, see Figure 12). Leave it before the child, point to the pile of sticks, and invite him to "make one just like that."

Note: Does he study the model or look at it briefly? Is he interested only in playing with the sticks on his own? Does he try to imitate the model, or propose another structure? Does he select his sticks carefully beforehand, or pick them up as they come in his hands? Does he pay attention to their size and measure them against the model, or is his structure out of shape because he used wrong-sized sticks?

Correct and explain to the child his errors, if any. Again show the difference in sizes. Then proceed to the next model. If the child plays with the sticks but does not attempt to copy the model, give him the necessary number of sticks of proper size, and ask him to copy the model with them. Children who learn to copy the second model (b) correctly are given the third model (c) to copy also. After this, one may proceed to 6b. With children who have difficulty with the second and third (and other similar models), one may continue to present the series of figures (1–10) to be copied directly (6a) rather than from memory (6b).

6B—FROM MEMORY. Announce that the "game" will be played differently from here on. Say, "I am going to make things for you as secrets. You can't look until I am done. Then you have a good look, and then I'll take it away again before you start yours." Prepare

---

[13] Kurt Goldstein and Martin Scheerer, *Abstract and Concrete Behavior*, Psychological Monographs, Volume 53, Number 2 (Evanston, Illinois: American Psychological Association, 1941), p. 131.

FIGURE 12. Goldstein-Scheerer stick designs (adapted for children)

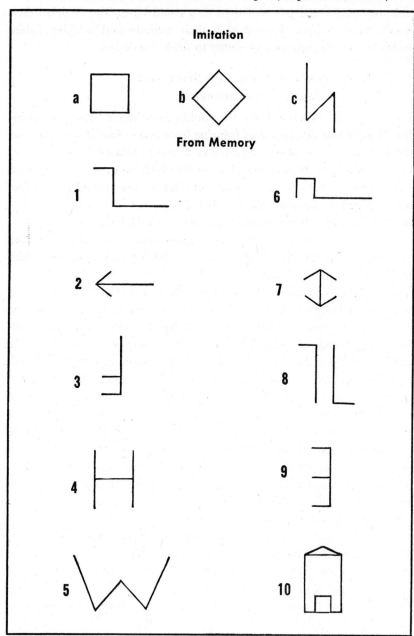

Adapted from Kurt Goldstein and Martin Scheerer, *Abstract and Concrete Behavior,* Psychological Monographs, Volume 53, Number 2 (Evanston, Illinois: American Psychological Association, 1941), p. 132.

each model behind a screen, or have the child close his eyes or turn his back. Produce the models; some of the models present senseless figures (1,6,8); others have more or less specific meanings—house (10), arrows (2,7), letters (4,5), inverted letters (3,9). The examiner may want to vary models or repeat some.

Note as in 6a. Also note carefully other phases of the work process. Note which models are easy for the child and which ones are not. Note those for which he finds names. Does he recognize meanings? Does the child name letters whether or not they are inverted? And does he reproduce the correct spatial orientation of the figures, or does he have a tendency to reversals? Does he overemphasize certain characteristics, for instance, more than three bars in inverted "E" (9)?

Do such primitive productions persist when the model is shown again briefly or when he copies it directly? Does the same kind of error occur with various figures, or only in isolated instances, perhaps owing to diminished attention? This test situation permits study of form comprehension and retention. The material appeals to the child, is easy to handle, and eliminates motor skills necessary for paper and pencil reproductions. Similar techniques were used in early genetic studies of children's productions by Volkelt and other workers in the former Leipzig genetic "Ganzheits" school.[14] These investigators found that young children tend to accentuate primitive perceptual qualities when reproducing two- and three-dimensional figures. The same style of production was shown whether the material was technically difficult to use (drawing, modeling clay) or easy (sticks, preformed shapes).

For Piaget the same primitive solutions (found by him and his co-workers[15] in reproduction of geometric forms with sticks or by drawing) are steps in the development of comprehension of spatial relationships (see also III:5).

Harriet Hyde Sands provisionally standardized the stick test for children (6a, 6b) in an unpublished study of normal children from three to six years of age: she found that gross distortions are common up to *four years of age.* They may consist of simplifications, over-emphasis of one dominant feature (see above). At *five years of age* such gross distortions become rarer. Errors of size predominate at this age and are, in a number of cases, responsible for incorrect proportions

[14] Hans Volkelt, "Fortschritte der experimentellen Kinderpsychologie," *Bericht über den IX Kongress für experimentelle Psychologie* (Jena: Fischer, 1926).
[15] Jean Piaget and Bärbel Inhelder, *The Child's Conception of Space,* trans. (London: Routledge, 1956), Chapter II.

of the reproduced figures. At this age, also, confusion in spatial orientation (reversals in either direction) is still found in some children. By *six years of age* the majority of children reproduce most of the ten figures correctly from memory.

These tentative norms are in general agreement with the findings of other comparable studies. Nevertheless, it would be desirable to obtain more precise norms on larger groups. Then this test procedure could become a valuable tool in determining readiness of *five- to six-year-old* normal children for school. For instance, excessive reversals of figures beyond the normal age may forebode difficulties in reading and printing. Even in its present tentative form the material is useful as a diagnostic aid with children who have suspected or known organic brain injury. Gross distortions in a child of *five,* or persistent reversals at *seven to eight,* must be considered symptoms of perceptual difficulties which have to be verified or disproved by some other procedures.

6C—SORTING STICKS BY SIZE. (See also VI:1c.) This is another good use of the material. Note the child's motor control, work habits, etc. Does the child know how to distinguish all four sizes, or is he certain only about the largest and the smallest, as is the case with very young children? Experience shows that children from *four-and-a-half years up* have no difficulty sorting the four sizes satisfactorily.

6D—NUMBER CONCEPTS. One may have the child count all sticks or certain groups of them. One may use the sticks for concrete arithmetic problems (see XI:11) or for comparisons of concrete quantities (I:7–9).

7—KOHS BLOCK DESIGNS TEST

Use twelve to sixteen blocks with a solid red, white, blue, yellow side, and a white/red and a blue/yellow side each.[16]

7A—STANDARD PRESENTATION. Use the Kohs design cards A, I, II, III, IV, V, and VI (see Figure 13). For older children other cards of that series may be added. Present four blocks to the child. Have him handle and investigate them. Turn two blocks simultaneously to show that "all blocks are alike; each has a yellow (blue, red, etc.) and a

---

[16] S. C. Kohs, *Intelligence Measurement* (New York: Macmillan, 1923). Also Goldstein and Scheerer, *op. cit.,* pp. 32ff. Also David Wechsler, *The Measurement of Adult Intelligence* (Baltimore: Williams and Wilkins, 1944), pp. 91ff; *Wechsler Intelligence Scale for Children* (New York: Psychological Corporation, 1949), p. 77.

FIGURE 13.   Kohs block designs

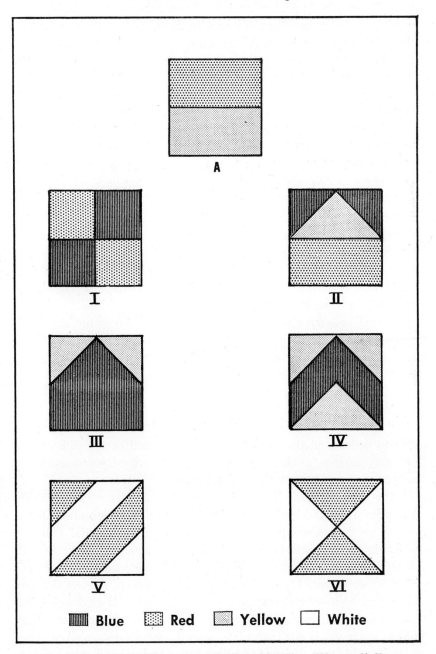

From S. C. Kohs, *Intelligence Measurement* (New York: Macmillan, 1923), pp. 66–67.

yellow/blue and a red/white side." Say, "Let us make something with these." Immediately present card A (demonstration card), saying, "Let us make a design just like this one with these blocks." Wait to see how the child starts, but interrupt any wrong efforts promptly and arrange for him. Let him have a brief look at the complete arrangement, then destroy it and ask him to repeat the same design on his own.

Then proceed to card I, saying, "You try to make this one." If he succeeds, proceed to the next card, etc.

Note: Does the child use the blocks appropriately, or does he start by piling them or lining them up? Does he try to copy the design, pick the right blocks and match their arrangement to that of the card, or does he, at first, copy the color scheme only but later correct wrong positions? Or does he retain only a superficial impression of the design and reproduce it only in a nearly similar arrangement? Does he act differently with designs that require two-color sides? Does he get the two-color sides in correct position? Does he invert them, later correct them, or ignore them? Is he quick or slow, patient, orderly, and over-meticulous, or erratic and superficial? Does he continue in one kind of approach, or does he alter it as need arises?

7B—WITH DEMONSTRATION. If the child does not succeed in producing a design properly, do it for him, then disarrange it and have him repeat the performance.

Note whether he learns from this demonstration. How does he produce the same design? Does he apply what he learned to a following design?

7C—FROM MODEL. If a child fails consistently and seems unable to understand that he is to copy the printed design with blocks, one may arrange a block model for him to copy. Occasionally this method may seem appropriate from the start.

The Kohs block design test investigates a complex variety of skills. The printed designs' intricate relationships must be perceived, analyzed, broken up in a number of squares, transposed to material (blocks) which differs in size, texture, and manipulative qualities. The basic skills involved in this task prove to be of general importance; their lack may often be significant. The numerous valuable aspects of the test situation have been discussed by many authors. The procedure is used with variations in many test scales. Goldstein and Scheerer introduced a method by which, if success is not immediate, graded suggestions are given systematically which are designed to induce better comprehension and a more efficient approach.

The above described procedures combine features of various techniques. The sequence of designs suggested by Kohs has been essentially maintained in 7a. Learning helps proposed by Goldstein are introduced in simplified and abbreviated forms suitable for children (7b,7c). Normal children are able to copy increasingly difficult designs with advancing age. They do so with the help of perceptual habits and experiences with form material which they gradually develop. Allowing for some individual variations in speed and skill, developmental stages may be defined as follows (after Kohs): at *six years of age* children are generally able to do their own arrangement on the checkerboard design (I). At *about seven* they start to use two-color sides properly when contrasted with another solid color (III, blue-yellow/blue). At about *nine to nine-and-a-half* they arrive at an adequate reproduction of designs with four two-color sides arranged with one color for the figure and another for background (IV, blue chevron on yellow ground). By *ten to eleven* a more complex design of similar type no longer presents problems. Normal children who at first have trouble with a design get help from demonstrations (7b and 7c) and learn through them to solve the more difficult next task. Children with perceptual difficulties due to brain injury, however, have considerable difficulty in these tests, as they have in others involving form comprehension and analysis of form relationships. Even the simplest designs may prove hard for some of these children: instead of correct solutions in square formations, they may place isolated blocks either spaced far apart, lined up in a row, or joined at their angles (I). Designs which require two-color sides to be oriented in proper relationships may to them present added difficulties. They may pay attention to the color of the design only. They may have a tendency to reversals. Demonstration often teaches them very little. They may be able to copy from memory what has just been demonstrated to them, but be unable to apply it to the next card. Goldstein described this inability for an "abstract" attitude as typical of adult brain-injured patients also. Experience shows that emotionally disturbed children may produce poor designs showing rigidity or regularization or erratic and impulsive decisions, but that they are not as apt to show the gross distortions and persistent deviations described above.

The procedures described under 7a to 7c are especially suitable for children from six to ten years of age. With few exceptions they enjoy the task and are well motivated to do what they can. Frequently, four to six designs are sufficient. The examiner investigates whether or not the child has adequate ability in perceptuo-motor areas. Difficulty with one or another design, or minor variations from normal, may have various causes and call for restraint and conservatism in interpretation, as does any single failure. However, gross deviations from normal performance which are apparent throughout and interfere with end results, are considered diagnostically significant. An *eight-year-old* child who is unable to get beyond a six-year level has, very likely, perceptual difficulties which call for confirmation and corroboration by other methods. On the contrary, a *six-year-old* who is performing up to age level or better in these tests has, in all probability, no such perceptual disabilities.

Block design methods described under 7 and 8 can be used with handicapped children in various ways. For children who lack speech because of hearing impairment or other conditions, directions can easily be given by pantomime; the procedure then presents no difficulty and has useful results.

For children with motor handicaps, adjustments must depend on type or severity of the condition. A clumsy, awkward child may become tired and discouraged from his physical effort. He must be watched to see whether his production, correct or not, really satisfies him. One may tentatively choose one or another block of his design and propose to put it in another position. One may ask the child whether or not he might prefer this to his original placement. Note whether or not he accepts any wrong position without protest. For severely handicapped children who cannot be expected to arrive at a series of satisfactory reproductions without undue strain, one may use the proxy method. The child is given a choice of turned-up block sides and asked to indicate by word or gesture which blocks he wants the examiner to place and how to do it. For children who are being examined in any other but normal sitting position, a distorted view of the blocks must be avoided to prevent confusion and unexplainable errors. Blocks have to be presented with their tops in the same prominent view as they would be for a person sitting normally. If necessary they may be presented loosely scattered in a large box, so that they can be tipped to suit the child's line of vision. A multiple choice presentation, described below, often serves well as a substitute procedure for the severely handicapped child.

7D—RECOGNITION (MULTIPLE CHOICE TEST). Present three arrangements of four blocks each. Ask the child to choose the one that most resembles the design card shown to him. He has a choice among the correct reproduction, a mildly distorted one, and a grossly distorted one.

For example, for II, present the designs shown in Figure 14. (1) Correct; (2) reversal of both two-color blocks which form a blue instead of a yellow triangle; (3) both two-color sides reversed so that there is no triangle (a), or (if there is reason to believe that the child may have very primitive perceptual habits), one may show a more distorted arrangement (b) using solid colors only without arrangement in a square (yellow center, two blue on top, one red bottom).

For VI, present (1) Correct; (2) both red triangles parallel instead of opposed to each other; (3) one pair of two-color blocks forming a triangle, the other not (a), and four solid color blocks, two red and two white (b).

This procedure proves useful for a more or less rough estimate of a person's skill in analyzing, comparing, and matching perceptual configurations. In many ways it seems to tap the same abilities as do the procedures described under 7a to 7c. It varies from procedures 7a to 7c in other important aspects because several units of blocks, in addition to the design, have to be analyzed instead of one; there is no chance for manipulation and experimentation. The procedure may seem promising and merit more study and standardization. At present, no norms are available. Comparison with Kohs standards may be of some help in evaluating an individual performance, though this must be done with caution.

8—OTHER BLOCK DESIGN TESTS

8A—WECHSLER-BELLEVUE AND WISC, STANDARD PRESENTATION. Use material from the Wechsler-Bellevue Intelligence Scale[17] and the Wechsler Intelligence Scale for Children.[18] Score as directed.

Note as in 7a. Watch work method especially for designs which require more than four blocks. Does the child study the designs first? Does he start with a plan, or does he proceed in small units? Does he construct units of two, three, or four blocks, duplicate these units, and arrange them in proper relationship to each other, or does he seem to work in piecemeal fashion, adding one block to the next and checking with the design at each turn?

[17] Wechsler, *The Measurement of Adult Intelligence*, pp. 183–185.
[18] Wechsler, *Wechsler Intelligence Scale for Children*, pp. 77–79.

FIGURE 14. Kohs blocks multiple choice arrangements

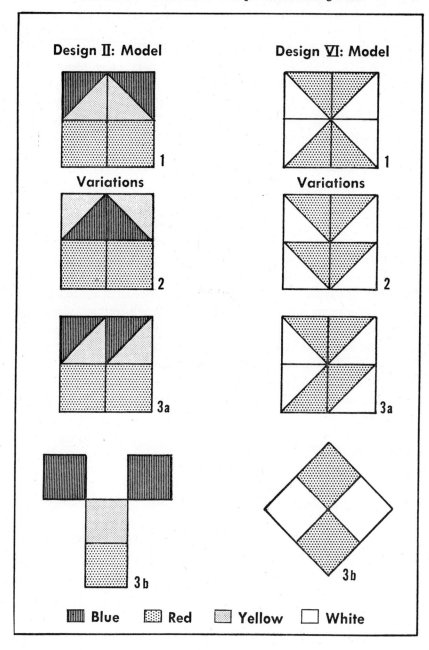

Individuals vary in their work methods with the more complicated designs.[19] Quick global appreciation of the general pattern usually leads to smoother and more efficient performance than does a detailed, slow, piecemeal approach. Children and grown-ups who lack ability for global approach may occasionally earn a reasonably good score by the piecemeal method. This can, at times, obscure the diagnostic picture in a patient whose good scores in the block design tests conceal perceptual difficulties which might be caused by brain injury. Such cases may be more common amongst patients with injuries acquired later in life than amongst those injured from birth or in early infancy.

The examiner may find it helpful to evaluate a child's individual performance in terms of maturity level. Some such estimate can be based on the similarity between some of the Wechsler-Bellevue or WISC designs and those standardized in the Kohs scale.

Wechsler-Bellevue design 1 (red-white)	corresponds to Kohs I (red-blue)
WISC B	corresponds to Kohs I, without dividing lines
Wechsler-Bellevue 2 (red-white)	corresponds to Kohs III (blue-yellow)
Wechsler-Bellevue 4 (red-white)	corresponds to Kohs IV (blue-yellow), 180 degrees inverted
Wechsler-Bellevue 6 (red-white)	corresponds to Kohs V (red-white), four blocks only
WISC 3 (red-white)	corresponds to Kohs VI (red-white) 90 degrees inverted

8B—WECHSLER-BELLEVUE AND WISC, VARIATIONS. Use any of the variations described under 7b to 7d with any of the Wechsler-Bellevue or WISC designs. Where this is done, formal scores should not be rigidly applied or relied upon, since the systematic suggestions offered for one design normally would help the production of another.[20]

8C—GOLDSTEIN-SCHEERER CUBE TEST. Use block design material as directed (12 designs).[21] Graduated aids in six steps are pro-

[19] Goldstein and Scheerer, *op. cit.*, pp. 32–33ff.
[20] *Ibid.*, p. 55.
[21] *Ibid.*, p. 49.

posed with this version of the test. The procedure can be used with older children only; it usually proves to be too long, too cumbersome, and unnecessarily elaborate for children under ten or twelve years of age.

9—RECOGNITION OF FORMS

Use material from the Kuhlmann Scale.[22] This consists of a large card with sixteen figures printed on it (see Figure 15) and a series of small cards each showing a duplication of one of the figures. Show one of the small cards to the child very briefly in inverted position, and say, "I am going to show you this and see if you can find one like it among these." Turn the large card showing the sixteen forms face up for five seconds, then show card 1 of the duplicate set for ten seconds, saying, "Now look at this." Make sure that he keeps looking. After ten seconds remove the small card and turn the large card face up again, saying quickly, "Now show me one just like it among these." Repeat with the other (four or five) cards.

Note whether the child tries to choose, or whether he picks any one to show at random. Note whether or not his correct choices are with the regular closed figures or with the more complicated open figures. If his choices are wrong, are they totally at random, or do they show that he chose by certain dominant features (bars, diagonals, diamonds)? Are his errors mistakes in the spatial orientation of the designs (3 for 15), or failure to see the difference between an open or a closed design (2 for 13)? Does he hesitate between similar ones?

Experience shows that this procedure could have interesting possibilities if age norms with qualitative differentiation could be established. Lacking these the test helps to identify the most serious difficulties of form recognition. It may be used as an additional test to investigate form comprehension, especially with seriously handicapped children who are unable to draw. Some of the duplicate cards of the original Kuhlmann series (Designs 2, 3, 7, 13, 15) are comparatively simple. This may account for the low age range placement of this test in the Kuhlmann scale. Goodenough[23] indicates that the Kuhlmann placement of this test on a *four-year* level (2 successes out of 5 trials) seems low. In clinical experience using duplicates of the more complex designs (6

[22] Frederick Kuhlmann, *A Handbook of Mental Tests* (Baltimore: Warwick and York, 1922).
[23] Florence L. Goodenough, *The Kuhlmann-Binet Tests for Children of Preschool Age* (Minneapolis: University of Minnesota Press, 1928).

FIGURE 15. Kuhlmann recognition of form

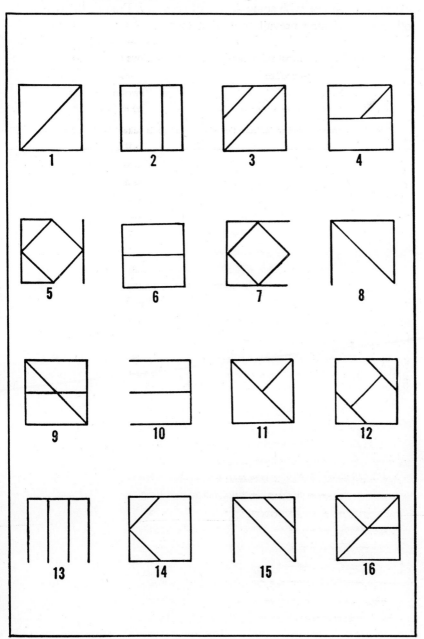

From Frederick Kuhlmann, *A Handbook of Mental Tests* (Baltimore: Warwick and York, 1922).

to 16) it is found that *six- to seven-year-old* children only can be expected to choose with some degree of accuracy. Frequently, one or the other reversal may prevail somewhat longer.

T:VII.   Most suitable procedures for various age ranges

Procedure	Age
(6), (7), 9	Two to six years
(1), (2), (3), (4), 5–9	Six to ten years
1–5, 7–9	Over ten years

Parentheses around number indicate that the procedure is suitable only for the older children in the age group.

VIII

Learning and Memory

1—NONVERBAL (SENSORY-MOTOR) LEARNING TEST

Use material from Rey's manual labyrinth test.[1] This consists of four boards 7 x 7 inches square, each with nine round pegs. These pegs are arranged in rows of three. On each board one of the pegs is fastened to the board; the others are loose. The boards are made of aluminum (or of wood). All pieces are painted black.

The boards are piled on top of each other. On each board the child has to find the fastened peg by which he can lift the board. On each board this peg is located at a different spot. It looks exactly like the rest of the pegs, so the child has to explore each board separately to find the fastened peg among each group of nine. Then he has to remember its location. He is bound to make mistakes during this first exploration, unless he finds the right one immediately by chance. After all four boards have been handled in the first run, the child is asked to do the task over again and to find the proper location of the fastened pegs without making errors. If he cannot remember, he continues until he remembers all positions without fail.

If the pegs were numbered from 1 to 9 (going from right to left and from top to bottom), the location of the fastened pegs would be as follows (see Figure 16): first board, 1; second board, 5; third board, 3; fourth board, 8. An alternate to this order is: first board, 7; second board, 2; third board, 8; fourth board, 6. (The first series is marked with a black circle in Figure 16, the second with a cross.) Only

---

[1] André Rey, "D'un procédé pour évaluer l'éducabilité," *Archives de psychologie* 24:287–337, 1934; *Six épreuves au service de la psychologie clinique* (Brussels: Bettendorff, 1951).

FIGURE 16. Positions of fastened pegs in Rey's nonverbal learning test

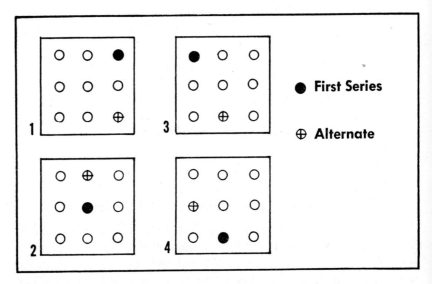

From André Rey, "D'un procédé pour évaluer l'éducabilité," *Archives de psychologie* 24:304, 1934.

the first three boards (instead of four) are used for children from five to seven years of age, or for those with obvious retardations.

1A—STANDARD PRESENTATION. Place the pile of boards in front of the child and say, "Here on this board are nine pegs; one of them is fastened so that it cannot come off. You can take it and lift the board. The other pegs do not hold, they are loose, they come off. You cannot tell the peg that holds just by looking, you have to try to find it. Try the pegs with one hand and see whether you find the one that holds. Once you have found it, remember where it is so you may know it later."

Let the child explore the first board; let him put back any pegs that come loose. If by chance he picks the correct peg first, show him that the others are loose, and do not come off. (If he does not start because he has not understood or because he is too timid, show him how one of the pegs comes off. It is useful to have an extra board on hand for this purpose.) When he comes to the second board, he may pick the peg that is located in the same spot as the one fastened to the first board (as happens frequently). If he does this, say that "each board has a different peg fastened." Have him continue until he finds the correct peg; then continue with the rest of the boards. Once all are done, pile the boards in the initial order, and say: "Now try to remember which pegs are fastened on each board; let us see whether you can find the right ones right away without making mistakes. If you can't, it doesn't matter if you make mistakes; we will try it again until you do find it, and then you may remember it the next time. We will do it until you know them all. Do not hurry; take your time and just try not to make mistakes." Continue, running through the pile a second time, and keep on repeating the same procedure until in three successive runs the child makes no mistakes.

Record as follows: prepare a sheet with vertical columns. Divide each in four squares representing each of the boards. Divide each square into nine sub-squares representing each of the nine pegs on each board. As the child picks up one peg after another on the first board, put down a number in the first square at a spot which corresponds to the location of the respective peg (number 1 for his first pick, 2 for his second, etc.); the last number in each square designates the fastened "correct" peg. Use the second square in the vertical column to note all trials on the second board, etc. This manner of recording indicates the number of errors made in the first exploration as well as their position and sequence.

The next vertical column shows how the child proceeds in the next run (first repetition), the third column indicates his procedure in the second repetition, and so on until he is certain of the position of all fastened pegs. The record then shows kind and number of errors on each board and in each run. With other added observations, it permits the examiner to retrace the child's working process. It shows the succession of trials and errors and their specific characteristics.

Note: How does the child respond? Does he listen to directions or start touching the set before knowing what to do? Is he hesitant and slow, or rash and impulsive? Does he understand directions and adopt an experimental attitude as children generally do at *eight years,* and often earlier? He may scan the board and try some favorite positions (such as corners or center), or may systematically touch the pegs from right to left or top to bottom. Does he take notice of what he finds out, learn from it, and improve his performance? Does he remember the proper locations on some boards, but still fumble on the others, or does he learn the general location of all the fastened pegs at once, but fail to remember which of the positions belongs to which board? Does he, like the younger children, start each board and each run as if it was new to him, but end up each time with the proper peg, apparently without remembering where he previously found it? Does he seem to be unaware that the same peg on each board will hold every time—as seems common with children of *five to six years of age*—or does he try to remember but clearly find it difficult to retain what he knows he could or should? Does he frequently try a position that was successful on the previous board, even though he "knows" that the positions change from one board to the next? Does he show similar lack of auto-control when, on the same board, he again tries a peg which just an instant before he found to be wrong?

Does he become discouraged, tired, or bored by the length of the task, or is he persistent, tenacious, and stimulated? Does he blame himself, the examiner, or the material when he fails, or does he consider the game a "fair" one? Is he agile or clumsy, careful or apt to spill and upset the boards? How does he respond to the examiner's attitude?

Carefully note any suggestions that are being made to the child. Note whether the examiner can remain detached and be simply a sympathetic but objective recorder, or whether personal intervention with praise, encouragement, or admonishment seems needed at certain moments. Note whether or not and how these social interactions modify the child's performance.

This test is designed to study adaptation to a new, unstructured situation in a nonverbal, active, sensory-motor setting. Its author thought of it originally as a "manual labyrinth." As in the classical labyrinth experiment, successful orientation does not depend on any given sign but on structurization of a neutral field through experience and memory. Genetic studies with the same material show that children learn more and more to profit from their experiences as they progress in age. The quicker they appreciate the spatial (Y-shape of the pattern) or temporal (sequence of positions) relationships involved, the more speedily they succeed.

The accompanying chart shows (in percentiles) the number of trial runs (up to the last three totally successful ones) found in groups of Swiss children from five-and-a-half to sixteen years of age.

These norms may help the clinician to appraise a child's performance. Their author warns that even with a Swiss population they

T:VIII:1.   Rey's age norms, based on number of runs needed for success for nonverbal learning test

	Percentile												
	Abnormal		Inferior		Normal						Superior		
Age (years)	0	10	20	25	30	40	50	60	70	75	80	90	100
	First three boards												
5 to 6	20	17	15	13	12	10	9	6	5	4	4	3	3
6 to 7	20	16	14	12	10	9	6	5	5	4	3	3	2
7 to 8	20	15	10	7	7	6	5	4	4	3	3	2	2
	All four boards												
8 to 9	17	14	13	13	11	10	9	8	6	6	5	3	1
9 to 10	17	14	12	11	11	8	7	6	5	5	4	3	1
10 to 11	16	11	10	10	9	7	7	6	5	4	4	2	1
11 to 12	16	11	10	9	9	7	7	6	5	4	4	2	1
12 to 13	14	12	8	7	6	5	5	3	2	2	2	1	1
13 to 16	12	10	8	7	6	5	4	3	2	2	2	1	1
Adult	10	8	7	4	3	2	2	2	1	1	1	1	1

Adapted from Rey, *Six épreuves au service de la psychologie clinique.*

should not be considered rigid statistical measurements, since they are established on a relatively small number of subjects. To the clinician Rey recommends the following norms only: an *abnormal* performance is one that falls below the tenth percentile; an *inferior* performance is one that comes between the tenth and the twenty-fifth percentiles; a *normal* performance may range between the twenty-fifth and seventy-fifth percentiles; whereas a *superior* performance would come between the seventy-fifth and one hundredth percentiles.

Besides these quantitative differences in the number of trials, qualitative differences may be partially evaluated through comparison of learning curves. The number of errors for each run may be plotted on the ordinate, while the successive runs are registered on the ab- scissa. The varied shapes of the curve may be significant for the clinician: a regularly descending curve with steadily decreasing number of errors indicates a normal learning process. A curve that at first descends rapidly but later continues to hover around a low number of mistakes shows that the child has been able to adapt relatively speedily, but has been un- able to consolidate his gain for reasons which may vary. A grossly ir- regular curve with many important ups and downs is characteristic of serious learning difficulties which most frequently are due to cerebral difficulties. These may occasionally be seen also in children with serious emotional disturbances. Besides evaluating the curve as such, the clinician must ascertain from the record how its fluctuations came about. A large number of mistakes on only one board may mean less than a few mistakes made consistently on all boards.

A series of supplementary variations of this test may prove revealing. Choose one or several of the following, once the initial series of positions has been learned thoroughly.

1B—Say, "Now this is fine, this is the way you know them. Now watch me carefully and see what I am doing." While interchanging the first and the second boards, say, "Now I take the first board and put it where the second was, and now I take the second board and put it where the first one was. Do you think you can still find the right pegs right away?" Have the child proceed on all four boards, but do not repeat.

1C—Re-arrange the boards in the initial order. Let the child do them over again once; then leave the boards piled with the fourth one on top, and say, "You see what I am doing; I am just leaving them the way you left them, with your last one on top." Proceed as before.

1D—Rotate the pile 90 degrees.

1E—Line the boards up in a row instead of presenting them in a pile.

1F—Ask the child to indicate the succession of the four positions on only one board or on a penciled schema that represents the square with the nine pegs.

These variations can show how well the previously learned set of positions has been integrated. If it is solidly rooted, the child will be able to remanipulate its relationships to suit the new conditions. However, if the position of the fastened pegs has been only more or less passively registered, the child may find it more difficult to locate them again in their new order.

Rey's nonverbal learning test proves to be a most satisfactory tool in many clinical situations. In general, the material is attractive to children; therefore it can be used to good advantage in many cases of learning difficulty, even with those children who seem much sensitized to their own academic shortcomings. The procedure may allow one to distinguish between those who are genuinely unable to learn and others who have school problems caused by specific emotional or educational circumstances. The test may show certain peculiarities of the learning process, which, if pointed out to them, may be helpful to teachers and therapists. It permits the examiner to distinguish between children who learn through comprehension and gradual structurization of material, and those who learn mostly by rote. Certain fluctuations of attention common in some neurological conditions can be shown.[2] However, the clinician must be sure of the persistence of her findings and guard against mistaking temporary boredom or other lack of motivation for neuropathological signs. In some children with speech difficulty the procedure can help to show the presence of learning abilities that may otherwise not be immediately apparent.

To some degree the procedure may also be adapted for use with children with motor impairment. A child with a weak and awkward grasp may be able to pick up the pegs lightly, although he must be helped to put the loose ones back in place. To avoid spilling the pegs, he should not be asked to lift the board up by the fastened peg. He may occasionally indicate which peg he would like to have the examiner try for him. However, these modifications, if carried too far, may alter the intent of the test and may obscure its sensory-motor and practical components. They must, therefore, be practiced with some discretion. The procedure is unsuited for children with serious difficulties in the use of their hands.

2—AUDITORY-VERBAL LEARNING TEST

Material for this test consists of lists of words read slowly to the child with instructions to repeat afterwards all words he remembers. The following words are used:

List A: Drum, curtain, bell, coffee, school, parent, moon, garden, hat, farmer, nose, turkey, color, house, river

List B: Desk, ranger, bird, shoe, stove, mountain, glasses, towel, cloud, boat, lamb, gun, pencil, church, fish

2A—LEARNING FIFTEEN WORDS.[3] Say, "I am going to read a list of words to you. After I have finished, I want you to say them back to me. Try to listen carefully and to remember as many as you can. You do not need to say them in the order I read them. Here I go. Listen carefully." Read List A clearly and slowly, with intervals of about one second between words. Then say, "Now you go ahead, tell me all

[2] Edith Meyer and Marianne Simmel, "The Psychological Appraisal of Children with Neurological Defects," *Journal of Abnormal and Social Psychology* 42:193–205, April 1947.

[3] This test is adapted from André Rey, "L'examen psychologique dans les cas d'encéphalopathie traumatique," *Archives de psychologie* 28:21, 1941. Recently the procedure has been described and discussed in more detail and with some modifications in André Rey, *L'examen clinique en psychologie* (Paris: Presses Universitaires, 1958), pp. 141–193.

the words you can remember." Get ready to record in a first column all the words the child quotes. If he says a word twice, put it down, but observe, "You said that one before." Make no comments to any other words he says.

Note: How does he take to the task, how does he start? Does he begin by repeating the last words which he has heard, does he start with the first words, or pick some words from the list at random? Does he at first give a group of words in quick succession, and slow down later, as is common, or does he soon start to grope for words to repeat? Is he inclined to say them in the order they were read, or is any other specific order apparent for instance, by association (farmer—turkey, school—bell)? Does he give only words from the list, or does he make substitutions (sun instead of moon) or additions (flower for garden)? Does he say the same word twice, does he check such an impulse (saying, "I said house before") or practice the necessary auto-control mentally only?

Is he cooperative, confident, and cheerful, or is he apprehensive or put upon? Does the task seem reasonable to him; does he keep on trying to find more words, or is he inclined to give up easily? Is he interested or not in the fact that his responses are being recorded? Does he supervise and control what is being put down? Does he seem to talk slowly in order to give the examiner time to write, or, on the contrary, does he speed up to make the task hard for her?

Once the child indicates that he does not know any more words, encourage him gently to keep on trying, but avoid pressure. Say, "This is fine; it is hard to remember many of them the first time. I will read them again, and you say again all the ones you know. I will read them all again as I did before, and you say them all again also with the ones you said before." Proceed as before, reading the same list and having the child recall the same words later. Do this over again until the list has been read and repeated *five* times in all, regardless of whether or not the child knows the fifteen words before the fifth repetition.

Note: How does he react to repetition? Does he seem relieved or bored by it? Is he equally attentive, or does his interest in the task change as time goes on? Does he start to repeat the same words he knew before, or begin with those he missed? Does he in all subsequent repetitions have the same order, or does he modify his method and perhaps improve on it? Does he seem to develop a system? Does he say as many words twice as before or does he do this more often as he becomes

T:VIII:2a.   Rey's age norms, based on number of words repeated,
for learning fifteen words

Age (years)	Percentile				
	0	25	50	75	100
First repetition					
Adult	5	7	8	10	14
11 to 13.6	2–3	6	7	9	12
7 to 9	1–2	4	5	6	10
6 to 7	1	2–3	4	5	8–10
Third repetition					
Adult	10	13	13	15	15
11 to 13.6	10	12	13	14	15
7 to 9	4	8	11	12	14
6 to 7	1	8	9	11	14
Fifth repetition					
Adult	12	14	15	15	15
11 to 13.6	12	13	14	14	15
7 to 9	7	12	13	14	15
6 to 7	5	11	13	13	15

Age (years)	Percentile				
	10	25	50	75	100
5	18	26	34	38	46
6	26	32	42	46	54
7	32	34	36	44	58
8	36	38	46	52	58
9	47	51	53	55	59
10	42	46	52	58	66
11–12	50	54	56	60	64

The norms presented in the top part of this tabulation are those originally established and used by André Rey and his Geneva group with a potentially equivalent list of French words. In the new edition procedure and norms have been revised. The bottom part of the tabulation presents the new norms, adapted from André Rey, *Examen clinique en psychologie*, p. 152. These norms are based on the sum of correct words for all five repetitions, allowing one minute for the first recall and 1 1/2 minutes for all following recalls.

tired? Does he stop giving substitutions as he comes to know the list better, or does he give more irrelevant words as the task lengthens and the novelty wears off?

This procedure is designed to study the way in which a relatively unstructured set of auditory stimuli may be reproduced verbally. In general, a certain number of such stimuli can be retained after one hearing. Some initial meaningful grouping may take place immediately and facilitate recall. Or sequences of words may be reproduced more or less by rote. After the first reading, recall is based on "immediate memory." After repeated readings, however, reproduction of the list becomes a matter of greater psychological complexity and involves in-numerable theoretical questions (not to be discussed here) concerning the multiphasic character of memory and learning.

Normally, a larger number of words is reproduced by children and adults after several readings. Norms established on a Swiss popula-tion with words probably equivalent to those listed here show that a normal *seven- to nine-year-old* may give four to six words after the first reading, eight to twelve words after the third reading, twelve to fourteen words after the fifth reading. *Adults* learn the same words in a shorter time: they are apt to produce seven to ten words after the first reading, thirteen to fifteen words after the third, and fourteen to fifteen after the fifth (see tabulation on page 425).

However, there are considerable individual variations which may be determined by many different factors. Modes of learning may vary from person to person, aside from other intervening factors such as motivation, degree of confidence, fatigue, well-being.

Some children may tend to do best, that is, to reproduce the largest number of words, at the beginning; after subsequent readings they may not be able to add much to their original list; they may remember new words but lose some they knew before. This may happen when the sound of the words rather than their meaning is registered. Other chil-dren may adapt slowly to the task but gradually add more and more words without losing previous ones. This becomes increasingly possible the more the child seems able to organize and manipulate what he learns. Others again may find increasing numbers of correct words during the first two or three readings, but flag in their effort as time goes on. Others again may perform irregularly and show their levelling-off of interest or attention through more words said twice, more associa-tions, etc. There may be various causes of this.

All characteristic ways of functioning in this task may be of interest to the clinician. She can substantiate her observations by plotting the findings of the record in a curve, the ordinate indicating the number of words correctly reproduced, the abscissa representing the sequence of readings. The number of twice-named words and words substituted may be separately marked for each reading. The examiner also can com-pare the number of words given for the first, third, and fifth repetitions with the norms given in the chart on page 425. This may help her to determine gross variations from what appears to be normal and may also be of value for comparison with future performances of the same child, even though the norms' limitations, their Swiss origin, and the inadequate distribution are obvious.

The procedure often provides data about a child which, if confirmed and corroborated by other findings, may help to explain certain of his difficulties. Frequently, it can be made the basis for advice to teachers, etc. The test allows the examiner to observe the child throughout a prolonged working process. From his behavior demonstrated under the specific circumstances some conclusions can frequently be drawn about behavior in similar learning situations. While the test does not rely on factual knowledge beyond that of the words themselves, it requires of the child a certain amount of mental and emotional discipline; it demands attention, resistance to outside stimuli, and attempts at organization. It may, like many other learning situations, not particularly appeal to some children. In spite of this, it seems to most of them a legitimate task of the kind often imposed on them by adults.

When used as a clinical tool, this procedure warrants some precautions: before she decides to give it, the examiner must make sure that there will be no interruptions while it is in progress. The child should not yet be tired or near the point of wanting to be free altogether, yet it may in many cases not be suited for a first test, since its somewhat academic and demanding character may spoil a child's mood for subsequent phases of the examination. Frequently, it depends on the examiner's skill as well as on the particular child, to make the procedure interesting and challenging, but not threatening, in order to obtain the best results.

2B—ADDING SECOND WORD LIST. After List A has been read and reproduced five times, one may introduce List B. Say, "Now I am going to read another list of words to you. But this one I am going to read only once; we are not going to learn it as much as we did the other one. Let us just see what words you remember if I read it just once. You try to get as many as you can, but you know of course that you cannot get them all right away. Here we go." Read List B.

Have the child say all the words he remembers from the list. Record as before. When he has finished, say, "That is fine; now let us say the other ones just once more, the ones you had so many times before. But I will not read them again—you say them as you remember them now."

Note as before. Note whether List B is equally difficult for him, or whether through his experience with List A he gets a smaller or larger

number of words for immediate recall. Note also whether he gains or
loses on what he knows of A after the reading and reproduction of B.
Note whether or not he brings words from List A into List B, and *vice
versa.*

Interference of this kind between the two lists is very unusual for
normal children. They distinguish without difficulty between the words
that belong to the first familiar list and those that belong to the new
one. Such interference, however, is not unusual in children with difficulties in organization and is seen in many cases of brain injury. Similar
phenomena have been described by Werner.[4]

3—VISUAL-VERBAL LEARNING TEST

This test consists of learning fifteen pictures and is adapted from the
previous procedure.[5] A series of pictures of objects is shown to the
child, one by one, and he is told that he will later be asked to enumerate
the pictures he remembers. Use fifteen of the picture vocabulary pictures
from the Revised Stanford-Binet Scale, Forms L or M.[6] (See also II:7.)

From Form M: Automobile, hat, key, airplane, ball, knife, block, flag,
  horse, foot, coat, boat, can, pitcher, arm (omit telephone, soldier's
  hat)
From Form L: Shoe, clock, chair, bed, scissors, house, hand, fork,
  basket, glasses, gun, tree, cup, umbrella, pocket-knife (omit table,
  stool, leaf)

Say, "I have here a lot of pictures. I am going to show them to you
one after the other. I want you to look at them and to try to remember
them. Later, when I am through showing them to you, you want to tell
me all the ones you can remember. You do not need to say them in
order, just try to remember as many as you can. When I show them to
you, you tell me each time what they are; that makes it easier for you
later. Here we go. This is a. . . ." Show the first picture. Avoid having
the child handle the picture.

Do not ask the child, "What is that?" If the child does not name the
picture at once, provide the word for him. Avoid any impression that this
may be a picture-naming test. Accept any name he gives without correcting it.

[4] Heinz Werner, "Abnormal and Subnormal Rigidity," *Journal of Abnormal and Social Psychology* 41:15–24, 1946.

[5] Meyer and Simmel, *op. cit.*

[6] Lewis H. Terman and Maud A. Merrill, *Measuring Intelligence* (Boston: Houghton
Mifflin, 1937), pp. 77, 195, 136, 328.

Present all pictures at one-second intervals, each time covering the preceding one with the next. When all fifteen pictures have been shown and named, remove the pile, get ready to record, and invite the child to "go on, tell me all you know."

Record in columns as in 2. Note as in 2.

When the child stops, or says that he does "not know any more," prod him gently to try to say some more, but do not insist. Say, "I will show them all to you again, and you tell me all of them again, and also the ones you said before." Proceed as before. When the series has been shown a second time, have the child again enumerate all the pictures he remembers. Continue in the same manner until the series has been shown five times (see 2).

The results of this procedure are used and evaluated in ways similar to those described in 2. Learning curves can be established by plotting the results of each repetition. As in 2, the shape of the curve may help to distinguish the slow learner from the speedy one, the impulsive, intuitive one from the slowly plodding one. It may also show up the irregularities of unsteady and disturbed processes of acquisition. The number of pictures named twice and of substitutions or their lack may indicate whether or not the child is able to control his impulse to say what first comes to his mind and to organize his performance so that it suits the task.

A comparison with the norms of the chart on page 425 may allow some tentative judgements about the speed with which a child learns. The clinical impression is that the procedure is somewhat easier for most children than the purely verbal method described under 2, for which the norms were established. It seems that the combination of pictorial and verbal stimuli facilitates recall for most children. However, it would be desirable to establish precise norms for this test and also to study the range of individual differences which seems to prevail. Even in its present rudimentary form this procedure proves useful in clinical work. It furnishes valuable information on how children of various ages learn a set of factors presented to them repeatedly. It is in general more interesting to most children than orally presented words alone. Therefore, the clinician may sometimes find it easier to use than the previously described learning test. With visual aids becoming more and more popular in teaching, the picture learning methods may resemble learning situations the child has encountered in school.

4—RECALL OF FACTS

Use printed card material from the Revised Stanford-Binet Scale: (1)
The Wet Fall (Form L, VIII-year level); (2) The School Concert
(Form M, X-year level); (3) A Distinguished French Acrobat (Form
M, XIII-year level).[7] See also XI:7.

    4A—STANDARD PRESENTATION. Present as directed. Ask the
child to listen to the story read aloud to him, to follow it on a printed
copy while being read to, and to prepare to answer questions later. Score
as directed.

    Note behavior of the child. Note whether he seems to read along
with the examiner, or whether he seems baffled by the printed page
in front of him. Does he seem to listen to what is read, or to read
by himself, or both? Record all the child's responses; note all his
answers to the questions regardless of whether they are correct or
not.

    The procedure is designed to measure memory for facts. It allows
a certain amount of freedom about how to reproduce these facts since
it does not require verbatim repetition of the words read. Comprehension
of word meanings and of the events described seems to facilitate the task.
Those children to whom the facts are clear seem to be at an advantage
in this test. Occasionally, however, one finds a child who gets a satisfactory score because he remembers the words even if he does not understand all their implications. Another child, on the contrary, may have
understood the over-all situation but be inexact in his memory for facts.
Of two responses gaining minus scores, one may show better comprehension than the other. In 2, for instance, to the question, "When was
the concert held?" one child may answer, "I do not know; I think it was
June," whereas another may say, "Around Christmas." Either one of
the children may later be found to know that there was a Christmas play
involved, but the first child obviously failed to relate the facts properly.
The ability, or its lack, to memorize heard facts with or without comprehension may have varied clinical significance and may in individual cases
throw light on other observations relating to memory and learning.

    4B—AFTER TIME ELAPSED. One may want to vary the pro-
cedure. After an hour, or even several days, have passed, one may again
ask the child to answer the same questions, or to tell what he remembers
of the story. This may help E to form a judgement about what happens
after an interval to the material the child has previously learned.

    [7] *Ibid.*, pp. 100, 233, 164, 376, 171, 389.

4C—OTHER VARIATIONS. One may present the story orally only, without giving the child a text to follow and/or compare his performance under these conditions with that under standard conditions. Or one may let him read the selection aloud or by himself without reading it to him and judge memory and comprehension of facts through this method of presentation alone.

These methods of eliciting memory for facts are useful clinical tools, among many others. They raise questions concerning memory in general and its evaluation. Much scientific discussion has been centered around the character and meaning of what is ordinarily called "memory." Claparède many years ago formulated some of the questions that should occur to the practicing clinician who tries to evaluate the memory of school children (or candidates for professional orientation).[8] Among some of these questions are the following: Does the child learn slowly or quickly, does he retain for a long time or forget easily? How does he use what he knows? Are facts recalled easily, or do they come back to him but slowly? Does he remember best when asked direct questions, when shown some clues, or when he remembers spontaneously? Are his memories strong or weak, vague or certain? Has he registered them passively and rather mechanically, or are his memorizations logical and seemingly the result of a more or less voluntary constructive activity?

5—REPEATING SERIES

A series of numbers of varying length is presented to the child orally, with one-second intervals between numbers. He is instructed to repeat each series after the examiner has finished saying it. Say, "I am going to say some numbers. Listen carefully, and when I am through I want you to say them right after me. Now listen."

5A—REPEATING DIGITS FORWARD. Use a series of digits between 1 and 9, avoiding any numerical order. Present in succession one to three series of three digits, four digits, five digits, etc. (Give only two series of each length when planning to use Wechsler standards for scoring.)[9] Continue until it is clear that the child is unable to repeat a series longer than the one last presented to him.

[8] Edouard Claparède, *Comment diagnostiquer les aptitudes chez les écoliers?* (Paris: Flammarion, 1924). See also André Rey, "L'évolution de la mémoire," *Etudes pédagogiques,* 1948, pp. 7–33.
[9] David Wechsler, *The Measurement of Adult Intelligence* (Baltimore: Williams and Wilkins, 1944), p. 176; *Wechsler Intelligence Scale for Children* (New York: Psychological Corporation, 1949), p. 70.

Note: How does he respond to the task? Is he interested in it, or does he find it difficult, boring? Does he become discouraged, or is he stimulated by the increasing length of the series? Does he try regardless of difficulty? Does he notice his errors, or does he seem to think that he is doing all right even while he is making mistakes?

If he seems frustrated by failure or ready to give up, one may try to boost his morale by interspersing shorter series among the longer ones. Note whether he does as well with these as he did before, or whether fatigue and/or discouragement gradually impair his performance.

The presentation described here is similar to the one used in both the Wechsler series[10] and also to the one described by Gesell.[11] In the Revised Stanford-Binet Scale[12] the series are not all presented at once. Each group of digits series appears as a separate test on one or the other age levels. Between repeating digits forward a child may have to repeat others backward (see below). This may alter psychological conditions, but does not seem to have significant influence on the results. Stanford-Binet age levels and the age norms mentioned by Gesell agree that in general children *four-and-a-half years old* are capable of repeating one out of three series of *four* digits. At *six-and-a-half* (according to Gesell, and at age *seven* according to the Revised Stanford-Binet, Form L), they repeat one out of three series of *five* digits. At *ten years of age* the majority of children are able to repeat *six* digits forward.

This procedure is generally used for testing an individual's "rote memory." Its somewhat limited value seems greatest in the work with children, since a certain minimum of rote memory is essential in learning; however, outstanding achievements in rote learning usually have but little relationship to general comprehension. While poor performances may be significant in clinical work as signs of defective functioning, very high performances may, in some cases, be equally worth an examiner's notice. If combined with poor results in comprehension tasks, they may point toward dominance of passive auditory registration over constructive learning.

The test can be used to detect gross auditory difficulty. One may change intensity and pitch of voice, and thereby test whether or not the

---

[10] *Ibid.*
[11] Arnold Gesell, *The First Five Years of Life* (New York: Harper, 1940), p. 177.
[12] Terman and Merrill, *op. cit.*

child is better able to respond accurately to a loud rather than to a soft tone of voice.

One may introduce the following variations.

5B—INTERSPERSED NONSENSE SYLLABLES. Intersperse one or several nonsense syllables in the series of numbers, as, "Five, two, lee, nine," or, "Six, nu, fi, tee."

Note whether or not the child seems to notice the difference between the numbers and the nonsense syllables. Does it alter his efficiency, does he repeat an equal number, or less, or even more of these syllables than he does numbers?

5C—ROUTINE SERIES. When presenting the series of numbers, give some or all in numerical succession; or give other routine series, such as even numbers, or successive numbers in reverse.

Say, "Six, nine, two, three, four," or "Two, four, six, eight, ten," or "Five, four, three, two, one."

5D—GROUPED SERIES. Instead of presenting numbers at intervals of one second, present them in groups of two or three. Say, "Six, nine, two—three, two, five."

These variations may give added information and show whether or not the child is functioning like other children of his age. For all subjects, young or old, grouping and accenting facilitates the task.[13] Also, it is usually simpler to reproduce previously automatized series (numerical sequences, telephone numbers) than it is to recall new sequences of numbers. A child to whom the common automatized series (number sequences, even numbers) do not sound familiar may not be helped when such a series is substituted for a standard unstructured number series. Also, most people are able to retain familiar elements (numbers, letters, words) in larger units than nonsense syllables. To a child who only passively registers sounds, a nonsense syllable interspersed between numbers may pass unnoticed and not increase the difficulty. However, to one who tries to group actively the stimuli which he receives in order to retain more of them, nonsense syllables may be disturbing.[14] An overapprehensive child, again, may find all tasks

---

[13] *Ibid.*, p. 213. See also Lewis M. Terman, *The Measurement of Intelligence* (Boston: Houghton Mifflin, 1916), p. 194.

[14] In an experiment with adults, Rey told his subjects to expect within the series of numbers a "foreign element" (a number said in an "unknown" language). This element reduced the number of correctly repeated syllables wherever the series was long enough to require mental effort rather than passive registration. The unknown word was usually repeated correctly, but some of the familiar numbers were missed instead. Where the series was easy enough to be recalled passively, the foreign element did not produce any change

equally difficult and may show tension and anxiety with simple as well as with difficult series.

6—REPEATING SERIES IN REVERSE

Say, "Now I am going to say numbers, but this time I want you to say them backwards. For example, when I say seven, one, nine, you say nine . . . (wait for the child to say the next figure, but say it for him if he does not), one, . . . seven. Let us try another one." If the child does not seem to understand, demonstrate with a second sample. Then present another series of three, proceed to series of four, five, and possibly six. Repeat each series up to three times (only twice if scoring by Wechsler standards, see previous procedure).

Note: How does the child respond, does he understand that the task is different from the previous one and know immediately what to do, or only after delay? Does he respond correctly, or does he make errors? What are his errors at the beginning of the task, or later? Do they show that he understands the principle but makes errors either immediately or as the series get longer? Does he start with the middle number instead of the last one (repeat "three, one, five" as "one, five, three"), or does he reverse some elements but not all of them (repeats "four, one, seven, three" backwards as "three, seven, four, one")? Does he fail to understand what to do, and instead produce the series forward, as it is told to him? Does he persist in the same kind of error, or does the type of error change as the series get longer and the task more difficult? Is he aware of his errors, does he try to improve, or is he oblivious of them?

Does he become stimulated and encouraged, or more tense and anxious as the test proceeds? Does he do better on easier series or on more difficult ones?

This procedure is more demanding than the previous one and seems to call for a different kind of mental activity. Not only does each series have to be memorized as before, but it also has to be remanipulated and reorganized. Passive registration and auditory recall no longer are sufficient for success, not even in the short series. They must be supplemented by a more active mental process which, through a predetermined mental set, transforms the initially perceived order of the numbers.

---

in efficiency, but was repeated within the series as if it was a regular number. See André Rey, *Monographies de psychologie clinique* (Paris: Delachaux et Niestlé, 1952), p. 200.

The Revised Stanford-Binet Scale, which presents the "digits backward" items interspersed between other tasks rather than in succession (see above), places "three digits in reverse" (1 of 3) on the *seven-year level* (M); "four digits in reverse" (1 of 3) on the *nine-year level* (M, L); "five digits in reverse" (1 of 3) on the *twelve-year level* (M, L); "six digits in reverse" on the *Superior Adult level* (M, L).[15]

This procedure can be of value in clinical work. It helps E to detect difficulties in comprehension and in concentrated effort. Since it is short and easy to administer, it can be used in an examiner's early attempts to get first clues which she may be able to substantiate through further evidence from other procedures. The test may be interesting in itself, or else in comparison with the preceding "digits forward" task. In general, children are able to repeat two more digits forward than they can backward. In some cases the clinician may find greater discrepancies which may prove to have diagnostic significance: some able but neurotic child may do better with digits in reverse than with digits forward (just as he may do better with the longer series of digits forward than with short ones). The fact that the task "in reverse" is admittedly more difficult and demands more active effort and attention may help to relieve his fears that he might fail where he should succeed.

It is a well-known fact that children (and adults) suffering from brain injury may do better with digits forward than digits backward.[16] In the first task they may be able to depend on their auditory memory, whereas they may fail in the second because of difficulty in organizing and re-manipulating mentally what they have memorized. Also, after trauma or illness a child may not be able to sustain the effort and attention necessary for the more demanding task, but still may be able to repeat some digits forward accurately. Significant and consistent discrepancy between both digit tasks may, as a sign, help to detect organic involvement. Where this question arises, the findings must always be corroborated by others before a diagnosis can be considered valid. The examiner must keep in mind that digits in reverse may also be failed through lack of attention stemming from other causes. Also, in all children, brain-injured or not, lack of attention may produce low performances in digits forward as well as backward. A lack of discrepancy between these

---

[15] Terman and Merrill, *op. cit.,* p. 157.
[16] F. L. Wells, *Mental Tests in Clinical Practice* (Yonkers, New York: World Book Company, 1927), Chapter VIII.

two tests only would not necessarily exclude the presence of organic involvement.

7—Memory for Sentences

Use material from the Revised Stanford-Binet Scale, Form L, IV- and V-year levels, and Form M, IV- and VII-year levels.[17]

7a—standard presentation. Say, "Listen, be sure to say exactly what I say."

Note: How does the child respond; does he seem willing, embarrassed, attentive? Does he wait to repeat the sentence until the examiner has finished it, or does he try to repeat in unison? Does he understand what he is to do, or does he respond to the content of the sentence with personal remarks ("I like chocolate ice cream," or "We have a puppy at home"). If he repeats the words, does he seem to understand their meaning, or does he repeat sounds only? Are the sounds correct, or are distortions and omissions present? If he makes errors, misses words, or substitutes others, does he try to reproduce the sense of the sentence correctly, or do his errors indicate that he misunderstands the meaning ("a pity" for "pretty" dress)?

This procedure is primarily a device to test rote memory (similar to repeating digits). It also permits the study of a child's familiarity with words, his facility in reproducing them, his enunciation, and his auditory acuity. It can also show whether or not the child is able to pay attention, to concentrate on a short sequence of stimuli, and to respond to them appropriately as he has been asked to. Though the procedure seems easy to administer, it is not always a popular one with normal children. Many find it somewhat embarrassing. However, occasionally the task seems to be reassuring for a child who is accustomed to get emotional reward from repeating obediently what is said to him. The clinician may find the procedure interesting when it helps her to confirm a hypothesis that she may have formed through other observations. Adequate repetitions of the spoken sentences may prove to be significant in a child who otherwise produces poor responses. One may in some such cases of discrepancies find that the child can repeat what is said to him without being able to understand more demanding verbal tasks, which call for a greater amount of thinking. A child who distorts some words, who drops consonants, or who omits prepositions and other connecting words may

[17] Terman and Merrill, *op. cit.*, pp. 88, 147, 93, 156.

have a hearing difficulty that should be investigated further. A child who looks bland and fails to respond may be one who dislikes the task, or he may be one who does not hear what is said to him.

7B—COMPREHENSION OF CONTENT. One may vary the procedure and add questions about the sentences. Or one may ask the child to say the sentence in his own words. Say, "What is it all about? What does Jack do? Where are the puppies?" Through these questions, one will find out whether or not the child has understood what has been said. Occasionally this may be useful with a child who has speech difficulty and therefore cannot be expected to repeat all words without much strain.

8—MEMORY FOR PICTURES

For description and discussion see II:8.

T:VIII. Most suitable procedures for various age ranges

Procedure	Age
(1), (5a), 7, 8	Two to six years
1–3, (4), 5–7	Six to ten years
1–6	Over ten years

Parentheses around number indicate that the procedure is suitable only for the older children in the age group.

IX

Judgement and Reasoning

VERBAL REASONING

1—DIFFERENCES BETWEEN TWO THINGS

Use material from the Revised Stanford-Binet Scale, Form M, VI-year level.[1]

Say: "What is the difference between a bird and a dog?" Or, if the child does not seem to understand, say, "You have seen dogs and you have seen birds. What is the difference between them?" Score as directed.

Note: Does the child understand immediately? Does he give an essential difference (bird flies, dog runs) which distinguishes both items in terms of a common factor (motion), or does he mention characteristic features of each item which bear no relationship to each other (dog runs, bird is small)? Does he choose for both items a common category that includes the whole species of each (dog has four legs, bird has two), or does it apply to some of each species only (bird is brown, dog is white)? Does he give some characteristic differences for each pair, or does he fall into a stereotyped form of response (bird is small, dog is big, slipper is small, boot is big)? Note also the thematic content of some specific responses (dog may hurt you, bird does not; you have to wear boots outside; you can smash glass when you are mad, but wood won't break).

2—SIMILARITIES BETWEEN TWO THINGS

Use any of the material from the Revised Stanford-Binet Scale,[2]

[1] Lewis M. Terman and Maud A. Merrill, *Measuring Intelligence* (Boston: Houghton Mifflin, 1937), pp. 154, 348. For older children use material from Average Adult level, pp. 180, 400.
[2] *Ibid.*, pp. 158, 357, 97, 228, 126, 291.

the Wechsler Intelligence Scale for Children, and the Wechsler-Bellevue Intelligence Scale.[3] (For example: mosquito—sparrow; apple—peach; pound—yard.)

Present and score as directed.

Note: Does the child understand what he is asked to do, and does he know the words? Does he give differences and have to be reminded to give likenesses instead? Does he need to be given examples and further explanations?

Note all responses, whether scorable or not. Is he slow and deliberate and does he search for the good answer, or is he quick and impulsive and has the answer in a flash? Does he give any common denominator, or does he mention differences only (see 1)? Does he express likenesses immediately in terms of a common concept (both food), or does he first describe one item and then talk about the other in similar terms (as, "You must peel the orange, and you must also peel the banana," or "Bread you use for sandwiches, and meat you put in the sandwiches")? Note quality of responses. Do they seem to be determined by essential concepts or by seemingly unessential qualities (color, use, shape)? Do his categories include all species of an item, or do they apply only to some ("Both have wood and glass" for window—door)? Or are they factually wrong ("Both bite you" for mosquito —sparrow)? Does he give the same kind of response for all items, or does he vary from one to the other, depending on his interest or experience with the items? Note also stereotyped responses and emotional content (as in 1).

3—Similarities and Differences between Two Things

Use material from the Revised Stanford-Binet Scale, Form L, VII-year level, and Form M, IX-year level.[4] (For example: honey—glue; ocean—river.)

3A—STANDARD PRESENTATION. Say, "I'm going to name two things, and you tell me in what way they are the same and in what way they are different." Score as directed.

Note: Does the child understand immediately, or does he need to be

---

[3] David Wechsler, *Wechsler Intelligence Scale for Children* (New York: Psychological Corporation, 1949), pp. 66, 95; *Measurement of Adult Intelligence* (Baltimore: Williams and Wilkins, 1944), pp. 85–87, 177–178; *Measurement and Appraisal of Adult Intelligence* (Baltimore: Williams and Wilkins, 1958), pp. 72–74. All but two of the W–B 1 items are included in the WAIS.

[4] Terman and Merrill, *op. cit.*, pp. 162, 372, 101, 239.

reminded to give differences also, or likenesses? Do these reminders need to be given for the second pair (see directions) or also for those following (see 3b)? Does he, in orderly fashion, give similarities (or differences) first, and then proceed to the other ("Both write, but one has lead and one has ink"), or does he without order produce some differences and some similarities ("Pencil is long and has a point, the pen has a point too, but it is metal and you use ink to write but the pencil writes with lead")? Does he keep track of his own procedure ("They are different because the one has lead and they are the same because they both write"), or does his response develop into a satisfactory solution as he goes along ("Pencil is long and you write with it, the pen you write with too, but you write with ink and the pencil is lead")? Note also as in 1 and 2.

3B—SUGGESTIONS. If the child cannot remember that he has to give both similarities and differences, vary suggestions systematically. Ask such questions as, "What else did you have to do?" or "Now you told me in which way they are different (or alike). What do you need now?" or, "That is right. They are alike because (repeat his statement). How are they different?" Note all reactions to these suggestions.

3C—ADDED ITEMS. Use any pair of 1 or 2 in the manner described in 3a or 3b.

4—SIMILARITIES AMONG THREE THINGS

Use material from the Revised Stanford-Binet Scale, Forms L and M, XI-year level.[5] (For example: snake—cow—sparrow.)

Present and score as directed.

Note: Does the child find any over-all concept (see also 2) or does he proceed to name differences only? Does he first name a characteristic trait of one or two items of one group and then fit it to the remaining ones ("The cow is alive, the snake is alive, and the sparrow is alive," or "The cow and the snake eat and the sparrow eats too") or does he name differences first (see 1) and mention a common factor later only ("The cow walks, the snake crawls, the sparrow flies—they can all move")? Does he find similarity among all three items, or does he succeed in finding it only between two and find no acceptable way of including the third ("The cow and the snake live on the ground, and the sparrow is on the ground sometimes when it does not fly")?

[5] *Ibid.,* pp. 109, 168, 265.

Does he remember all three items of the group, or does he forget the third item while working on two?

By giving procedures 1 through 4 in succession, the examiner may study a child's capacity to shift from one mental set to another. Children who are able to adjust without difficulty to the directions of the new procedure and respond just to what they are being asked show better learning ability than those who, repeating what they did before (in 4, for instance), give not only similarities, as requested, but also differences.

The tasks described here are based on studies of mental processes which in the normal child develop gradually with age and experience. The young child learns early in life to appreciate some similarities or differences on the perceptual level or to recognize differences or similarities on the reflective level. However, the ability to verbalize such distinctions develops later in successive stages. The Stanford-Binet standards seem to reflect this gradual development. In the tasks described above, normal children of *six years of age* are expected to describe familiar absent objects in terms of some distinctive features. They may not be able to express similarities before the ages *seven to eight*. They are not expected to select essential rather than superficial likeness, from the adult's point of view, before *nine to ten years* of age.[6] Groupings by function, shape, or color prevail (as in their nonverbal groupings, see Chapter VI). The highest level of conceptualization—which is that by abstract concepts—may be reached earlier with some of the simpler items than it is with some more difficult ones. Wechsler states that practical and concrete categories are also found in a large number of adult responses.[7] A person's major interests and background, together with intellectual habits, may determine whether he prefers practical or more abstract categories.

In the above tests the normal child passes through various stages of partial solutions as he gradually develops the ability to verbalize differences (1), similarities (2), or similarities and differences at the same time (3); qualitative analysis of these partial (unscorable) solutions may show how his reasoning processes become increasingly mature.

A young child who deals with differences (1) may mention some single dominant distinguishing feature ("The birds say peep, the dog

[6] *Ibid.*
[7] Wechsler, *The Measurement of Adult Intelligence,* p. 86.

runs") but may not necessarily choose common criteria ("Bird says peep, the dog bow-wow"). Or he may mention a common factor (color), but since he may be thinking of individuals (a special dog or a special bird) and not of species, he chooses too narrowly ("Dogs are white, birds are brown"). When he tries to find similarities (2) he may try to think of a common category to fit both items and refrain from describing differentiating features only. He seems ready to use the correct reasoning pattern, but still does not use it "right" from the adult's point of view. His choice of category may be unsatisfactory; it may be wrong, in fact ("Both are insects" for mosquito—sparrow), or not descriptive enough ("Both are straight" for window—door)[8] or not exclusive enough ("Both are glass and wood" for window—door). In spite of these limitations, his reasoning ability seems more mature than that of a child who does not try at all for a common category. In trying to find similarities among three things (4), a child may perform on various levels of competence before he reaches the stage at which correct solutions are common (usually at *ten to eleven*). Children who no longer show tendencies to describe differences only may find common factors for two of the three items only. To deal effectively with all three at once a child must be capable of testing and discarding various hypothetical solutions. As the items become more difficult, they demand more flexibility and also more factual knowledge. Again, those children who try for any over-all category are more mature than those who, faced with this more difficult task, revert to descriptions of differences.

Dealing with similarities and differences simultaneously (3) demands a higher level of reasoning than either differences (1) or similarities (2) alone. Each pair of items must be considered in two terms. The child must keep these in mind and must reflect on his work process to remember what part of the task has been done and what remains to be done. This requires detachment, flexibility, and comprehension of reversibility.[9] Children *under eight to nine years of age* may find it difficult in this procedure to view the same facts from various angles at the same time and to coordinate the multiple relationships involved. Before reaching the stage at which such problems can be solved con-

---

[8] How different the meaning of such a word (straight) may be from the child's point of view and the adult's has been shown by Piaget, Werner, and others. See Heinz Werner, *Comparative Psychology of Mental Development* (New York, Harper, 1940), p. 286.

[9] Jean Piaget, *The Psychology of Intelligence,* trans. (New York: Harcourt, Brace, 1950).

sistently, children may give partial solutions showing varying degrees of competence: one child may be capable of remembering both—the items and the different parts of the task—but make mistaken statements. He may thereby show more ability to organize complex problems than another child who, though he ends up with factually correct solutions, first had to be reminded what to do next because he forgot, became confused, and could not remember how he started out.

The series of test procedures described above proves valuable in clinical work with children. The Revised Stanford-Binet norms help to determine the level of reasoning in an individual case. Experience confirms statistical evidence that the level of achievement in these tests correlates highly with total scores of mental competence.[10] Highly intelligent children score high on these tests. Low performances are seen in children who do not function adequately in other areas of reasoning and organization even though they may score high in other verbal tasks like vocabulary (XII:1), immediate memory (VIII:5,7 and XI: 2,3), or information (XI:10). Up to *ten years of age,* at least, maturity of reasoning is determined by the degree of skill in manipulation of relationships rather than by degree of concreteness or abstractness in responses.

Scoring standards of all scales agree on this point: even though the WISC has a one- and two-point system, norms show that up to *ten years of age* a one-point score on each of the first five pairs (in addition to the introductory items) represents a satisfactory performance. This stresses again the fact mentioned previously that concreteness in similarities is normal in children up to that age, and after that age may be a pathological sign only under certain circumstances. Of more diagnostic significance seems to be the failure of some brain-injured children to find common exclusive categories and their persistence in successively mentioning individual traits, as younger children do. They are also often irregular in their performances, forget parts of the directions, display erratic thinking habits. Some may combine impulsiveness or perseverance with reasonably good factual knowledge.

5—Opposite Analogies

Use material from the Revised Stanford-Binet Scale, Form M, IV-, VIII-, and Average Adult levels,[11] and the Wechsler Intelligence Scale

---

[10] Terman and Merrill, *op. cit.,* p. 228.
[11] *Ibid.,* pp. 146, 340, 160, 362, 178, 398.

for Children, under similarities.[12] (For example: brother is a boy, sister is a . . . ; the dog has hair, the bird has . . . ; lemons are sour, but sugar is. . . .)

5A—STANDARD PRESENTATION. Present and score as directed.

5B—VARIATION. Introduce the task as follows: Say, "Let us play a game with words. I start and you finish it. Listen to me now. I say, 'A brother is a boy; a sister is a. . . .' " Indicate by gesture that it is the child's turn to produce a word to end the sentence. Accept any word he gives and proceed to the next item. If he does not respond spontaneously, produce the correct word for him. Present items from all Stanford-Binet levels in succession.

Note all responses whether correct or not. Does the child immediately understand what is asked of him, or does he look blank? Does he produce the correct words immediately in response to the key words, or does he search for a response and hesitate at first as to what to answer? Is his answer correct but poorly enunciated, or does he talk clearly but repeat one of the key words only? Does he produce words that seem improvised out of the blue? Do they seem to have meaning for him, or are they words given at random with the hope that they may be acceptable? Do his responses seem emotionally revealing? Does he seem to like the task because it allows him to answer briefly? Or does he try to find several answers, embroider on them, become conversational, and have to be reminded to stick to his task? How does he manipulate material as it increases in difficulty? Does the child cling to methods which were successful at first, or is he able to shift to new methods as the need arises? Does he stop trying to use easily activated verbal patterns when these no longer suffice to solve the more difficult problems?

Varied mental functions seem to be involved in these tasks. Analogies have been popular in psychological investigations of language ability, vocabulary, reasoning, etc., and can also serve as projective techniques. Werner reports the findings of genetic studies with analogy tests.[13] When given a multiple choice of terms from which to choose the correct one, young children revealed their diffuse mode of thinking through their choices and subsequent explanations. It was found that the higher the age level, the more marked was the increase of frequency of well-differentiated and unequivocal relations. Often responses which

[12] Wechsler, *Wechsler Intelligence Scale for Children,* p. 66.
[13] Werner, *op. cit.,* p. 314.

are wrong from the adult's standpoint may be meaningful for the child, and therefore of much interest. Werner's point of view here agrees in many ways with that expressed frequently in Piaget's writings.

The items described in the above test procedure vary in difficulty. Depending on the age of the child, some of these items may be easy and demand very little active effort. The answer can be found almost instantly if it forms part of a child's stock of previously acquired verbal patterns. For the *four- to five-year-old,* as for all ages after this, the obvious opposite pair to boy—girl is man—woman; he finds the fourth word as soon as he hears the third. As the items become more diffi- cult, they require more constructive thinking. Proper relationships have to be understood and, in order to produce a correct answer, must be precisely and not merely vaguely understood. When the child tries to an- swer to "dog—hair, bird—?" the word "wings" may come through handy association or through global diffuse perception. But a correct answer comes only after the first impulse has been rejected and the content of the first pair and its relationship to the third word has been analyzed. For an older child, after *eight years of age,* as for the adult, this particular item generally needs little analysis; the necessary opposite pairs are already part of the available stock of automatized patterns.

Depending on his age, the child may have to shift to a more constructive active method after the first two or three items, or after five or six. He must be able to realize when his own verbal automa- tisms no longer suffice and must be able to shift to the more demanding way of solving the problem.

Seen from these and many other angles, the test procedure, simple as it seems, may be of considerable help to the clinician. Through it she may collect additional clues about a child's level of reasoning, his stock of verbal automatisms, his ability to use these appropriately, his ability to shift from one working method to another. Also, she may be able to learn something about a child's responses to the spoken word, about his inclination to stick to a well-defined task.

With young children, the task may have additional merits: often it may serve as a bridge between nonverbal and verbal tasks. A child who is at first reluctant to talk may warm up to this well-structured task. Since he has to answer with only one word, he may feel that this compels him less to a personal and emotional involvement than do other verbal tests. In the opposite case of a child who is unusually talkative and unrestrained, the procedure, because more constricted and well defined, may make a welcome transition to the more structured verbal reasoning tasks (1 through 4).

The Stanford-Binet and WISC scoring standards are useful at least as gauges against which to compare an individual child's performance, even though the variation in presentation described and recommended in 5b obviously makes the rigid use of these norms invalid.

6—Verbal Absurdities

Use material from Revised Stanford-Binet Scale, Forms M[14] and L,[15] VIII-, IX-, X-, and XI-year levels. (For example: (A) A man had flu twice. The first time it killed him, but the second time he got well quickly; (B) I saw a well-dressed young man who was walking down the street with his hands in his pockets and twirling a brand new cane; or, A soldier on the march complained that every man in the regiment was out of step except himself; (C) In the year 1915 many more women than men got married in the United States.)

Present the procedure toward the end rather than at the beginning of an examination. Introduce the task saying, "I am going to read some stories to you. They all are quite silly and foolish. Let us see why they are foolish. Now listen. What is foolish about this one?" Read the story.

Use discretion in the selection of stories. Avoid some of the sickness, mutilation, and death stories with anxious and handicapped children.

Score as directed.

Note: How does the child respond to these stories? Does he enjoy them, or does he seem uncomfortable about them? Does he seem amused, challenged, and superior, or is he baffled, defensive, and uncertain? Note and scrutinize all responses, whether correct or not. Does he understand that he is to find an incongruity within the facts presented, and is to verbalize it explicitly, or does he accept the adult's judgement that the story is "foolish" or "funny" without wondering why? Does he try to discover any logical absurdity, or is he set to find fault with morals, customs, or manners? Does he judge the full story, or only parts of it? Does he understand and know all the words read to him?

Add varying questions ranging from, "How is that?" or "Tell me more about it" to leading suggestions.

[14] Terman and Merrill, *op. cit.*, pp. 159, 358, 161, 368, 165, 377.
[15] *Ibid.*, pp. 101, 235, 103, 244.

Note: Do suggestions and questions have any effect, and if so, what effect? Do they change his ideas, do they help him to express previous ones more clearly, or do they make him use new words only? Does he see new connections between the statements because the questions lead him to a different emphasis, or do they cause him, in general, to pay more attention and to be more interested?

This procedure investigates judgement and reasoning: the thought process involved may vary in kind and in degree of difficulty, but all the stories demand quick, over-all comprehension of a situation rather than gradual construction of a solution. Some findings from studies of children's thinking provide a frame of reference for qualitative evaluations.

Young children's reasoning has been described as realistic and egocentric. It deals with immediate facts one at a time. Young children do not mind logical contradictions, either in their own statements or in those of others.[16] They accept stated facts at face value and judge them as true. As they grow older, they gradually learn to reason with assumed premises, to coordinate multiple facts, and consequently to notice or avoid contradictions. These facts no longer are judged from an absolute point of view only, but are perceived in their multiple relationships with other facts.

Responses to the verbal absurdities may show varied aspects of this development toward mature objective reasoning. At the earliest levels, *seven years and under,* a child may accept, without questioning why, the adult's statement that the story is foolish. If at that age, or when somewhat older, he attempts to find a reason, he may concentrate on one dominant part of the story only. He may judge proprieties, as "He should not have his hand in his pockets" (B), or use immature concepts, as "It could not have happened in 1915. There were no people in America then" (C). Another somewhat more mature child may connect various parts of the stories and try to see relationships, but fail to see crucial ones, "He (the soldier) should walk like the rest of them" (B), or "He got well the second time. He did not have it so bad then" (A).

Some of the stories require a more elaborate vocabulary than others; some are more dependent than others on practical experiences. All are more or less independent of school learning. Terman and Merrill

---

[16] Jean Piaget, *Judgement and Reasoning in the Child,* trans. (New York: Harcourt, Brace, 1928), Chapter IV.

find that this procedure is one of "the most valid and serviceable of our tests" and yields consistently high correlations with total scores.[17] They find that verbal absurdities are an excellent tool to determine reasoning ability. Experience shows that these stories, with their definite scoring system and age-level placement, are of considerable practical use in many cases where quick appraisal of reasoning ability is called for. Their most conspicuous limitation is their morbid content with its preponderance of sickness, accident, and death. This makes their use impractical, if not embarrassing, in many clinical cases, particularly with children with emotional or physical difficulties.

7—REASONING PROBLEMS: ORIENTATION

Use material from the Revised Stanford-Binet Scale, Forms L and M, XIV-year level.[18]

7A—Say (while pointing), "If this is west, where is east (and north, south)?"

Note: Does the child point correctly or not? Does he know that east is opposite to west and north opposite to south, or does he point haphazardly in any direction? Does the question make any sense to him, or is he at a loss? Does he get confused momentarily only, and is he able to correct his error spontaneously, or does he persist in his errors, reverse west and east, etc.?

Proceed to next question.

7B—Say, "Which direction would you have to face so that your right hand would be toward the east?"

Children vary in accordance with their experiences in their skill to think in compass directions. Usually those who have been campers or scouts are at an advantage over those who lack similar outdoor experiences. There also may be some regional differences: in the eastern part of the United States such directions seem less often referred to in daily life than in other parts of the country.

Discontinue if the child makes errors in both 7a and 7b. With children who have succeeded in 7a and 7b, proceed to the other questions of the series.

7C—"Suppose you are going west, then turn to your right, which direction are you going now?" or "Suppose you are going north, then turn left, then left again, then turn right, then right again, which direction are you going now?"

---

[17] Terman and Merrill, *op. cit.*, p. 235.
[18] *Ibid.*, pp. 119, 279ff.

Note: Does the task seem easy or difficult for him? Does he seem to solve it by reflection, or does he use concrete points of reference? Does he perhaps point in one direction and say to himself, "If this is north . . ." and poise his body as if turning? Is he capable of solving all items by one or the other method, or does he have increasing difficulties as more turns and more frequent changes in direction are demanded? Note changes with varied instructions. Allow him to use paper or pencil, suggest to him that he use his body; or, on the contrary, explain that he is not to use any concrete help but must do it all "in his head." To appraise imaginary rotations in space in terms of an assumed system of reference requires highly developed reasoning processes.[19]

According to Revised Stanford-Binet standards, adolescents of *fourteen* are expected to solve three or four out of six of these questions. These norms do not distinguish between those individuals who seem to solve the problem by reflection only and those who also use their own body movements in their efforts at finding solutions. Adolescents and adults with severe motor handicaps frequently have considerable difficulty in these tasks, even if they do not show any other signs of disturbances in reasoning or perception. The intriguing yet unsolved question arises as to whether their lack of body experiences may influence or delay such spatial orientation.

8—REASONING PROBLEM: THE BURGLARY

Use the following material from the Revised Stanford-Binet Scale, Form M, XIV-year level.[20]

My house was burglarized last Saturday. I was at home all of the morning but out during the afternoon until 5 o'clock. My father left the house at 3 o'clock, and my brother was there until 4. At what time did the burglary occur?

Wait for an answer. When it is found, ask the child to explain it. Ask whatever questions are necessary to make it clear how the child reached his solution.

Note: Does he try to find an answer immediately, or does he think that he is faced with a guessing game or a trick question? Does he seem to visualize the events and try to go carefully over the facts again, or does he try to guess? Does he know the word "burglary"; does he assume that

[19] Jean Piaget, *The Psychology of Intelligence*, trans. (New York: Harcourt, Brace, 1950), p. 153. Also Jean Piaget and Bärbel Inhelder, *The Child's Conception of Space*, trans. (London: Routledge, 1956), Chapters XVff.
[20] Terman and Merrill, *op. cit.*, pp. 174, 392.

nobody was home when it occurred? Does he understand that the timings of the family's goings and comings are important and interrelated? Does he know that he must consider the given hours, and also the length of a person's absence and presence at the house, or does he declare that the burglary must have taken place at "two," and explain that this is the only time left since "three, four, and five were taken"?

This problem uses time relationships as a system of reference, as the previous ones (7) used spatial relationships. A multitude of such relationships have to be coordinated in order to find the correct answer.

Norms of the Revised Stanford-Binet Scale place this test at the *fourteen-year level*. These norms give credit for any correct answer. Since the Stanford-Binet examiner does not inquire into the method that leads to the solution, some few children may receive credit for an intuitive guess rather than for an adequate mature solution.

9—REASONING PROBLEM: INGENUITY

Use material from the Revised Stanford-Binet Scale, Forms L and M, XIV-year level.[21] (For example: A mother sent her boy to the river to bring back exactly *two* pints of water. She gave him a . . . pint can and a . . . pint can. Show me how the boy can measure exactly two pints of water using nothing but these two cans and not guessing at the amount. You should begin by filling the . . . (larger) can first. Remember you have a . . . pint can and a . . . pint can and you must bring back exactly two pints of water.)

With each problem, wait for an answer, then ask the child to explain.

Note his method of approach. Does he mentally lay out the given facts carefully and then proceed to peruse them, or does he try to find an answer impulsively? Does he accept as helpful the suggestion that the larger can should be filled first, or does he consider this an added complication and wish he could start with the other can? Does he seem to visualize the cans as containers to be manipulated, or does he think of them mainly as arithmetic figures which he tries to add or to subtract? Does he declare the task impossible and, disregarding the instructions, suggest compromises?

If the child finds a proper solution for the first problem, does he try to apply the same principle to the second and third problems but find out that some further imaginary steps have to be taken? Does he

[21] *Ibid.*, pp. 118, 279, 175, 395.

modify the pattern of operations to fit the new circumstances, or does he keep clinging rigidly to the formula of the first problem?

If it becomes clear that the child will not spontaneously find a solution to the first question, the examiner should try various suggestions: remind the child that "there is plenty of water in the river, and there would be no harm in wasting some."

Note whether this leads him to a more realistic approach to the problem.

Or, explain to the child how the first problem can be solved; then either introduce another equivalent problem and then note whether the principle of the solution has been understood. Or introduce the second problem.

Note whether the explanation has been understood enough so that it can be applied and properly modified to fit the more complex second problem.

Like the preceding reasoning tests (6 through 8), this procedure requires thought processes involving manipulation of multiple relationships. Familiar arithmetic facts have to be applied to a realistic, properly visualized situation. An element of enterprise and ingenuity is part of the solution which has the form of an imaginary sequence of actions. This test procedure is, in various ways, similar to arithmetic reasoning problems common in school mathematics.

According to the norms of the Revised Stanford-Binet Scale, adolescents of *fourteen years of age* are expected to pass one of the three problems, whereas two and three successes are passes on the *Average Adult* and *Superior Adult* levels, respectively. Experience shows that individuals seem to vary some in their ability to solve this task with ease. Familiarity with problems of this kind helps. Certain aggressive, practical children, with a "know how" for puzzling problems, seem to have an advantage over the more passive, contemplative ones.

All reasoning problems described under 7, 8, and 9 demand a minimum of previously learned information. Thought processes in themselves, rather than their results, are the subject of interest. Mature, flawless solutions are based on well-elaborated systems of reversible operations. Normal children develop with age the ability to manipulate more and more complex systems of operations. Not until in early adolescence are they ready to solve intellectual problems of high order, since it is only then that they are capable of understanding and performing all the necessary mental operations.[22]

For the clinician, these tests are valuable from various angles: they are short and relatively simple to give; the norms provided with them may serve as a helpful gauge; the qualitative observations described above add to their significance and offer further clues by which to judge a person's mental competence or deviations from normal. Most children enjoy these tasks and accept them as fair and interesting challenges. Some overmeticulous, neurotic children may be absorbed in and anxious about some of the details (the burglary itself, the danger of spilling water), but still be able to get to the nucleus of the problem and proceed correctly. Children with distortions of reasoning of the kind seen in some forms of brain injury may also cling to practical details. Whether they do or do not, they generally have many difficulties in seeing all aspects of each problem at once. Most of them remain unable to coordinate multiple relationships. They may cling to any one or several aspects of the problems, solve them partially, but be unable to see all of them in their correct relations to the others.

PICTORIAL REASONING

10—PICTURE ARRANGEMENT

Use the following material from the Wechsler Intelligence Scale for Children and the Wechsler-Bellevue Intelligence Scale:[23]

From WISC:
Scales, Fight, Fire, Burglar, Farmer, Picnic, Sleeper, Gardener, Rain

From Wechsler-Bellevue Scale:
Nest, House, Hold-up, Elevator, Flirt, Fish, Taxi

10A—STANDARD PRESENTATION. Present and score as directed.

Note all responses whether correct or not. Note also all trials and spontaneous changes. Watch the child's manner of work: does he look the cards over and come to some decision, but reassess it while he places each card? Or does he proceed quickly without verifying his decision, once it is made? Does he fail to look at the pictures in detail but inter-

---

[22] Piaget, *The Psychology of Intelligence,* Chapter V.
[23] Wechsler, *Wechsler Intelligence Scale for Children,* p. 74; *Measurement of Adult Intelligence,* pp. 87–89, 179–181; *Measurement and Appraisal of Adult Intelligence,* pp. 74–77. Six of the seven W–B 1 series are included in the WAIS.

change them only because he thinks he should? Or does he start to describe one picture after another in the order in which they were put down for him?

10B—TELLING THE STORY. When his arrangement is completed, ask him to "tell the story" or to "tell what it is all about."

Note carefully all of the child's descriptions. Does he name an over-all theme first, then describe the events in detail, or in broad terms only? Does he read off each card successively as if each one was a separate picture story, or does he consider the interrelationships between any or all of the pictures?

10C—SUGGESTIONS AND QUESTIONS. Add various suggestions and questions. If the order has been correct but the story not explicit enough, cross-examine the child to determine whether success came partially by accident or was based on full comprehension (Burglar: did he consider the different sizes of the window openings?). Interchange the two window cards. Ask whether this wrong solution would be acceptable too. If so, recheck the reasons. He may find nothing wrong with the proposed solution, but he may also accept it only out of respect for the examiner. If the solution or story is inadequate or incomplete, the examiner may suggest a second try at another arrangement and note any change. Or the examiner may produce the correct arrangement and ask, "Could you tell the story this way?" or "Does that make a story?"

Again note all responses. Does the proposed order modify his original solution? Does he accept it, reject it, or prefer it? Does he try to adapt it to his own solution, or does he give up his original version altogether?

Note, in all arrangements and stories: Do they fit together in a continuous, logical, and plausible story and make "sense" from the adult standpoint? Are the stories infantile, bizarre, original, or do they tend to follow conventional patterns? Do they show significant emotional attitudes? Are wrong stories based on incorrect perceptions of the pictured details, on neglect of some details, or on lack of experience of the events pictured? Did the child consider all relationships that were involved, or did he fail to coordinate multiple relationships that were necessary for the right solution (concerning Fish, did he see the fish in the bucket and also the position of the line in relation to the water level? or concerning Sleeper, did he see the hands on the clock and relate the time to the events?).

This procedure is of considerable psychological interest. The mental

processes that are involved are fairly complex. They develop gradually
as the child gets older. In an early study with similar materials, Piaget
and Krafft described and discussed in some detail the characteristics
of the reasoning process underlying young children's solutions and differentiating them from those of adults.[24] For the older child and adult,
a "sensible story" is a plausible and logical story with a single action
and certain consequences or morals. All parts of the story go together,
and events follow one another chronologically. Inconsequential details
are excluded as irrelevant. According to Piaget, the young child up to
seven years of age does not have the same criteria for a "sensible story."
He does not care whether a story is likely or not. He adds events in chain
succession without needing interrelationships between them. There is
no rigorous chronological sequence of events. When he thinks or talks
about them, he can have them go in any order and still be satisfied
with his story. For him there is no distinction between what is relevant
and what is not. Frequently, he describes each picture separately because it is too difficult for him to coordinate all events and personalities
into one story. Also, contrary to the adult's procedure, he cannot
easily revise his own solution. Once he gets an idea for a story, he tries
to fit the circumstances to it because he cannot use ideas hypothetically
only and test or reject them later.

As the child gets older, he gradually learns to organize his stories
in a more adult manner. The timing of this development varies with
the complexity of the stories (as the Wechsler scoring standards
show). Seen from this angle, all solutions to the picture arrangement
tests gain added significance. Correct and faulty solutions become means
to evaluate a child's developmental level in reasoning, aside from the
numerical scores which are based on success, failure, and speed only.
Correct arrangements may prove to be accidental successes when the
accompanying story shows that they were not based on full comprehension. However, not all faulty solutions are due to basic difficulties
in logical reasoning; some may be caused by inattention (concerning
Sleeper, failure to see the time on the clock), or poorly structured perceptions (regarding Flirt, she has a big hat on). Some reveal a child's
lack of experience with common events (concerning Hold-up, prison
picture before court session, or concerning Gardener, failure to connect the worm in the garden with fishing), or his emotional attitudes

[24] Helen Krafft and Jean Piaget, "La notion de l'ordre des évènements et le test
des images en désordre," *Archives de psychologie* 19:306–349, 1925.

or preoccupations (Hold-up, "He is in prison. Here he got out again. He holds up a guy. Then he tells the judge that he did not do it").

From *eight years on* normal children may be expected to abandon infantile thought processes. They have less and less difficulty with the simple series and also find increasingly mature forms of solutions in the more complex ones. Even though children from that age up may still lack comprehension of some of the stories, they are more apt to try for plausible and logical arrangements. They may distort some aspect, overlook details, or press the facts to suit their needs, but they show increasing concern with logical necessity and begin to avoid contradictions. If distorted infantile arrangements persist with regularity in a child of *nine to ten years of age,* one must suspect some abnormality in the reasoning processes. These may be found in children with general mental retardation or in those with distortions of mental functioning due to brain injury. These latter have difficulties in coordinating multiple facts here, as in other reasoning tasks (see 6 through 9).

Children with emotional disturbances are apt to produce stories that hold together from the logical point of view. This can frequently be of great diagnostic importance, since it proves that the child's mental development is essentially intact. Whether correct or wrong from the scoring angle, the arrangements of these children may be often conspicuous and unusual. Details are apt to be neglected for the sake of a dominant theme which may reveal anxious preoccupations and may result in bizarre solutions.

11—Picture Absurdities

Use the picture material from the Revised Stanford-Binet Scale, Forms L and M, VII- and XIV-year levels and Form M, XII-year level.[25] (For example: (A) a man in a tree sitting on the limb he is cutting; (B) a man on scales carrying books in his arm; (C) a man sawing a log with an inverted saw; (D) a dog chasing a rabbit the wrong way.)

11a—standard presentation. Say, "What is funny about this picture?" Score as directed.

Note all responses, whether correct or not. Note how the child understands the question. Does he accept the examiner's statement that this is a "funny" picture and simply describe the picture and declare it funny? Or does he seriously try to discover an incongru-

[25] Terman and Merrill, *op. cit.,* pp. 156, 351, 97, 226, 170, 388, 118, 278.

ity and either find it or declare that there is nothing funny or that he is unable to find it? Does he look for a fault with the artist or with the picture or with the actions of the persons that are shown? Does he think the pictures are humorous, or stupid, or morally wrong ("He should not cut the tree")?

Wherever possible note on what evidence the child bases his judgement. Does he notice all important factors and consider them all, or does he see parts of what is shown? Does he know scales (B), see the rabbit tracks (D), or the teeth of the saw (C), or does he mistake the scales for a lamp or a gas pump? Are such errors due to poor eyesight, to hasty scanning, or to lack of experience with scales and saws?

11B—QUESTIONS. After the child has given his first responses, question him further regardless of whether or not his answer was "correct." An insufficient response, though unscorable by Stanford-Binet standards, may conceal proper comprehension because it is not well expressed. A "good" response, however, may be produced without complete comprehension. For example, to Man in Tree (A), he may say, "He is going to fall" (a plus response); he may know the danger in climbing trees without even considering that the man must fall with the limb he is cutting. Or he may answer, "He is going to fall because he is cutting the tree." When asked, "He needs to cut the tree, so how should he do it?" the same child may say, "He should do it from the ground." He fails to see that this solution is impossible because the limb is too high for the man to reach.

One may add varied questions about the pictures. These can furnish interesting clues to some of the child's notions about spatial relationships, relations of weight and height, physical causality, and also about his stock of information and his feelings. Some questions may lead to others. For instance, after the picture showing cat and mice, one may ask, "Why don't they like each other? What other animals don't get along well, and why? Who might chase whom, and who would win? How many mice?"

The pictures vary in their content, and therefore in their demand. Some depend on knowledge (cat and mice, books and scales), others more on common sense and observation (rain, umbrella); others again seem to call predominantly on some form of sensory-motor experience and/or on anticipation of physical events (Man in Tree).

Varied methods can lead to solutions: one child may immediately see the most important factor and state it correctly, another may first light upon an irrelevant detail but in so doing notice another one and try (or not try) to relate it to the first one. Others may immediately see what seems most relevant, but before stating it scan the picture again in order to substantiate their finding and to coordinate all factors. In general, the latter procedure may be considered the most mature one.

Tests on picture absurdities involve many questions in the area of development of thought. They would lend themselves to careful genetic qualitative analysis. Such a study would improve understanding of responses of individual children. Even without such information the material is a useful tool for the clinician. In general, normal children are able to understand the absurd pictures mentioned at the age levels at which the test scales place them. Caution is required in work with handicapped children: there one must often try to distinguish between failure which may be due to lack of experience and that caused by faulty reasoning.

12—PICTURE COMPLETION (MUTILATED PICTURES)

Use material from the Revised Stanford-Binet Scale,[26] the Wechsler Intelligence Scale for Children, and the Wechsler-Bellevue Intelligence Scale.[27] For example: from the Revised Stanford-Binet Scale, Form M, V-year level, table (leg missing), coat (sleeve missing); from the Revised Stanford-Binet Scale, Form L, VI-year level, rabbit (ear missing), glove (finger missing); from the Wechsler Intelligence Scale for Children, coat (buttonholes missing), rooster (spur missing), cow (cleft in hoof missing); from the Wechsler-Bellevue Intelligence Scale, card (ninth diamond missing), crab (leg missing), and mirror (reflection of arm missing).

Present as directed. Say, "What is gone?" or "What is not there?" for the younger age levels (see Stanford-Binet), or say "I am going to show you pictures in which there is a part missing" etc. (WISC). Revised Stanford-Binet directions call for verbal responses; pointing is not scorable. Both Wechsler tests accept as a solution pointing to the

[26] *Ibid.*, pp. 152, 347, 95, 223.
[27] Wechsler, *Wechsler Intelligence Scale for Children*, p. 72; *The Measurement of Adult Intelligence*, pp. 89–91, 178–179; *The Measurement and Appraisal of Adult Intelligence*, pp. 77–78. Eleven of the fifteen W–B 1 pictures are included in the WAIS.

part missing instead of naming it. However, the meaning must be clear and the response not spoiled by an inadequate verbal response.

Note all responses, whether correct or not. Does the child understand what to do? Is he interested in finding the right answer, or is he content to find anything to say? Does he name the whole picture, or some detail? Does he care whether or not his response is correct? In case of failure, does he find fault with himself or with the picture? Does he declare that he does not recognize the picture or the missing part? Does he look for a clearly visible missing part, or does he expect it to be minute, hidden, and hard to find? Does he prefer the finer, less obvious details to the grossly visible ones?

This procedure involves a variety of psychological processes: first the picture must be recognized, then its incompleteness must be appreciated and determined. With the simpler items, the most important missing part is easily recognized. With some other pictures, close inspection and attention is demanded, along with familiarity with similar objects, a decision on what is essential and what is not. A score of problems regarding perception, cognition, etc., enter in and are too complex to be discussed here.

Young children (until *five or six years of age*) have difficulty analyzing the pictures enough to see missing details.[28] When a picture is familiar to them, they may recognize and name the whole at once, but they do not necessarily notice the imbalance of the parts. When presented with a less familiar or larger picture, they may fail to see the total picture because they are attracted by some dominant detail. As they get older, the parts and the whole become more thoroughly integrated and therefore more open to analysis. The more complex pictures of the series depend more on experiences with the objects shown. They also demand selective judgement of what are essential, and what nonessential, details.

The clinician may find in some cases that items which involve small details like the cleft in the hoof of the cow or the spur of the rooster are solved with greater ease than some others with more obvious incongruities like the slit in the screw. Such attention to small detail may be found in brain-injured children. Similar tendencies were described by Werner and Strauss[29] and can occur also in many other procedures (see Chapters II and VII).

[28] Terman and Merrill, *op. cit.*, p. 223.
[29] Alfred A. Strauss and Heinz Werner, "Disorders of Conceptual Thinking in the Brain-Injured Child," *Journal of Nervous and Mental Diseases* 96:153–172, 1942.

13—WOOD PICTURE COMPLETION TEST[30]

Use a series of eleven colored pictures mounted on two plywood boards. In each picture an inch-square piece has been cut out. Accompanying the boards are sixty inch-square pieces. From these, the subject has to choose the piece which best fits into the cutout of each picture. For each of the pictures there is a correct solution and several alternates representing imperfect but not totally erroneous solutions. The test was developed as a companion piece to the Healy picture completion test II.[31] It has been recommended as a substitute, if not a true alternate, for the Healy test.

The pictures show a succession of activities illustrating a schoolgirl's day (in contrast to the Healy boy).

Begin by showing the pictures to the child. Point out that all the pictures show the same girl in different situations throughout her day. Place the box with the sixty pieces neatly arranged at one side of the child. Use the first picture for demonstration. Show that of the three possible insets only one can be entirely correct. (For example, in the first picture it is morning; shadows show on the floor. The correct inset has to be one with a window with sun shining brightly; the inset with a window showing a moon at night is as wrong as another inset showing rain on the window.) After this demonstration, the child is to fill all the cutouts as he chooses. No further comment is made by the examiner except that the child may make any changes he wishes.

Note how the child proceeds. Note his trials, hesitations, intermittent choices, changes. Note his manner of work. Does he study one or all of the pictures first and then decide what he needs? Does he inspect the box with insets first, and then decide where one or another may fit? Does he study all available insets, looking for some specific one? Does he, when he is working on one picture, first systematically pick out all possible solutions for it, and then make a choice among them, or does he first come by chance on one suitable inset, place it, and only later come upon another which he thinks may fit better, and therefore must then be tried? Note what his choices are. Do they, even if incorrect, make some inherent sense, or do they seem to be picked entirely at random? Does he, for instance, try to place all blank insets or all animals? Does he try to match the color of some of the objects

[30] Louise Wood, "A New Picture Completion Test," *Journal of Genetic Psychology* 56:383–409, 1940.
[31] W. Healy, "Picture Completion Test II," *Journal of Applied Psychology* 5:225–239, 1921.

in the pictures, or does he pay attention to proportions between objects? Do his choices indicate general comprehension, but a tendency to overlook details? Does he, not noticing all the elements of the pictured scenes, tend to make his own interpretations and choose accordingly?

When the child has finished and has been invited to look over his work for a check, proceed to question him about all his choices which are correct. This is necessary because it may often happen that a correct solution was reached accidentally. Indicate the alternates for each of the correct choices and ask whether or not either one of them would do equally well.

Note the child's reactions to these questions. Does he take them as suggestions that he was wrong and should choose again, or does he stick by his first choice? Does he do so from a desire to resist, or to be through with the task, or because he has valid reasons to believe that his choice is best? If he changes to another inset, ask him why.

Like the Healy test, this procedure involves innumerable aspects of psychological functioning. It demands attention and sustained interest for a prolonged task to be done independently without help. It requires recognition of the pictures, familiarity with the situations shown; it calls for analysis and comprehension of what is seen, for decision and choice of what might fit, for consideration of temporal, spatial, and causal relationships, for appreciation of what may be plausible and what may not be. In short, it calls for active and constructive reasoning processes with inherent demands for imagination, initiative, and social sense.

At different ages children meet the requirements of the test in varying ways, depending on their level of maturity, their personalities, experiences, etc. In general, the quality of their performances increases consistently with age, as can be seen in the quantitative norms.

Qualitatively descriptive norms have not been made available by the author of the test, who studied children and adolescents *between seven and seventeen*. Experience shows that younger children tend to make their selections on different grounds than older ones. Some of the younger ones may be interested in simply filling spaces, and therefore pick insets at random, as they come upon them. Some try to place an especially interesting inset (a cat or a dog), some are careful to fill all the available places with animals. Others match object to object (seeing a house in the picture, they place another one in the nearby empty space). Others try to match one or another color that they perceive in a picture and in an inset (a purplish squirrel matched to a shadow of similar color).

In general, it seems that younger children either consider one whole picture without attention to important details or concentrate on some group of details and are unable to coordinate all factors involved. Also, they consider each picture separately, jumping haphazardly from one to the other without taking notice of the continuity of the story. As they get older, they attach more and more importance to meanings and facts underlying the pictured events; they coordinate more factors and make finer discriminations. Also, they feel more and more obligated to find the one objectively correct solution. For the younger children, on the contrary, a solution is satisfactory as long as it seems right to them for reasons of their own; they feel less compelled than older children and adults to have these reasons meet generally accepted standards.

The procedure can be of considerable interest to the clinician— equal at least to the Healy test that until now has been extensively used by several generations of psychologists.[32] It is not only most popular with children of all ages, it also furnishes interesting results within a wide age range. It gives the examiner opportunity to observe the child during a prolonged working process in which she may follow him step by step with a minimum of words and questions. This may lead to many significant clues to working habits, level of reasoning, personality characteristics. For instance, one may see overcautious, anxious behavior when a child picks a blank inset only because he may be afraid to commit himself to more complex and demanding decisions. Or one may notice a child's lack of regard for inherent relationships when he persistently matches color to color or object to object without comprehension of the meaning of the pictures.

14—Reasoning in Mechanics: The Bicycle

This procedure is adapted from Piaget.[33] Say, "I guess you know about bicycles. Have you got one (or does your brother have one)? Do you know what it is like? Could you draw one for me?" If the child seems

[32] Compared with the older test, it seems to have two distinct advantages: though developed in the 1930's, its pictures seem less dated, with clothing and furnishing still less outmoded than those in the Healy test. Its scoring system permits more gradings in performance, with consideration given to negative responses in general and to the character and degree of a child's errors in particular. Unfortunately the manufacturer (C. H. Stoelting, Chicago) has discontinued this test material.

[33] Jean Piaget, *The Child's Conception of Physical Causality*, trans. (New York: Harcourt, Brace, 1930), Chapter IX.

uncertain, encourage him, saying, "I know it is difficult, but you could try. Do the best you can." The drawing should not be less than four to five inches. If the child is very young, or is overly hesitant in getting started, draw for him the outlines of two wheels, expecting him to continue on his own. When the picture has been finished, start questioning him. Say, "How does the bicycle go; how does it work?" To the answer, "On wheels," say insistently, "Yes, but what happens? How does it get going when you get on it?" Do not suggest answers, but keep on trying to find out what the child knows about the problem. When this is clear, check once again by pointing to each part of his drawing, asking each time, "What is that one for?"

Note all his answers, but make sure to understand not only what he *says* but what he *means*. Note whether he answers readily because the problem seems simple to him, or whether, taken by surprise, he thinks about it and gradually arrives at some answer. Note whether or not he remains puzzled. Does he first give a solution, then revise it by another, but know that neither is satisfactory, or does he produce his responses with assurance and aplomb? Note carefully the content of his responses and check on them through further questioning. Does he correctly describe the action of one part on another ("The pedals turn a little wheel, that wheel turns a chain, the chain is attached to the rear wheel . . .")? Does he mention several, or only one, of the parts as agents of the movement ("It goes because it has wheels" or "handlebars" or "because it has spokes," or "a seat"), but seem unaware of any interaction between parts? Or does he give answers that seem to fall in between these two: for instance, does he see that two parts influence each other, but disregard any cause-and-effect relationship ("The pedals turn the little wheel," and a little later, "The little wheel makes the pedals go")? Or does he know already that there must be irreversible relationships, but is unable to define them accurately ("The chain makes the rear wheel turn—it is attached to the tire")?

This procedure was originally designed to study children's reasoning. Like other of Piaget's studies, its results show how children come gradually as they get older to understand causal relationships among observable events. A sequence of stages could be outlined for the bicycle problem, as for others. Each child is thought to go through the same series of stages at some time of his development. In his study on children in Geneva and Paris in the 1920's, Piaget found that most boys of *eight years of age* can explain intelligently the mechanics that make a bicycle go; (since girls vary but are consistently behind boys, Piaget reports on boys only). Before they reach this stage they may give partial explanations only. They may notice the interaction of some of the parts, but remain uncertain about what is cause and what effect. They may draw any one of the important parts without relating them properly. *Up to five years of age* the boys in Piaget's study gave irrational explanations. While they might draw some wheels and perhaps one or another detail only, they might, if questioned, declare that any other interesting detail (the seat, lantern) might be responsible for the motion of the vehicle.

The clinician who is interested in using these techniques must do so with some care: the test is not a drawing test but a procedure to appraise comprehension and quality of thought process. The drawings serve only as a concrete basis for the discussion, which must be handled delicately. All resemblance to a quiz or any other question-answer type of task is to be avoided. Reliable results are obtained only if the child's own beliefs and way of reasoning can be brought out in a pleasant, unpressured conversational exchange between him and the adult.[34]

The procedure can help the clinician to determine a child's maturity of reasoning. Children with developmental deviation in reasoning ability may give responses typical of younger age levels. Those whose thought processes seem distorted by brain injury may frequently be unable to accurately analyze the relationships involved in the bicycle problem at the proper age. Even if they seem up to their age level in other respects (such as verbal ability), they may understand only partially the interaction of parts and the cause-and-effect relationships, and be unaware of the logical contradictions in their stated beliefs.

15—REASONING IN ARITHMETIC

For description and discussion see I:7–9 and XI:5.

T:IX. Most suitable procedures for various age ranges

Procedure	Age
(1), (5), (12), (15)	Two to six years
1–3, (4), 5, 6, 10–12, (13), (14)	Six to ten years
2–7, (8), (9), 10–15	Over ten years

Parentheses around number indicate that the procedure is suitable only for the older children in the age group.

[34] For a discussion of Piaget's "clinical method," see Jean Piaget, *The Child's Conception of the World,* trans. (New York: Harcourt, Brace, 1929), p. 8.

X

Everyday Sense, Common Knowledge, Comprehension

1—QUESTIONS TO PARENTS

Ask the parents of the young child whether he seems to know them, whether he recognizes other members of the family when he sees them or hears them. Does he respond even when he hears them mentioned, or only when he is specifically asked about them ("Where is Daddy?")? Does he notice when he is handled by less familiar persons? Ask whether he "knows his bottle," has likes and dislikes in food. Does he recognize food which he does not like as soon as he sees it, or only after he has tasted it again? Does he recognize other signs when he sees or hears them? Does he, for instance, know that his bib means a meal, that his outer clothing means a ride, or the sound of the refrigerator door, food? Does he anticipate that his father will come in when he hears his car in the driveway? Does he know certain routines (getting dressed or going to bed), does he know what comes first or next, does he seem to notice any variations in these routines? Does he know who sits where at the supper table, and does he miss somebody who is absent? Does he mostly pick up objects that he happens to see, or does he purposefully go to look for things? Does he go for them on request or on his own initiative? If he is sent for something, can he find anything he is asked for ("my pocketbook on the dresser"), or does he understand requests only when they are related to the immediate situation (an ashtray when mother has lit a cigarette)?

Use wording which suits the family's individual situation. Introduce names of siblings, places, etc. Avoid suggestions. Start with general questions which later can be elaborated and made more precise, as "What happens at mealtime?" "What things does he bring?"

Note whether a mother or father responds with ease and confidence or whether such questions lead to doubts, hesitations, and defensiveness. Does a parent answer proudly and enumerate many specific examples, or is his reply, "I think so," or, "I do not know; we have never tried this." Note whether a single sample of behavior is finally mentioned which, when further described, may turn out to be a doubtful bit of evidence. Note whether a mother can state with certainty, "I know he could not do this." Try to check carefully but tactfully whether examples are true illustrations of what was asked for.

Questions about daily happenings in a young child's family obviously have considerable psychological and developmental significance. The experiences which the baby has with people and things in his immediate environment are the material by which he comes to understand relationships among objects, people, and places in general, and to learn to see himself as part of them.[1] The *four- to five-month-old* baby who recognizes his mother or his bottle has established his first points of reference.[2] The *seven-month-old* baby becomes aware of strangers;[3] he also refuses certain foods when he sees them. His ability to discriminate has increased, and his responses become more differentiated. By the *first half of the second year* he has acquired innumerable "schemata" and understands more and more signs.[4] The above types of questions all refer to situations which normal children master within the first two years.

The clinician can get much useful information from such questions. All refer to situations which are common in the lives of most children; all can yield information about a child's responses, his comprehension, and his social relationships. The fact that they are independent of the examiner, the test material, and the strange testing room is appreciated by most parents. They are pleased and often relieved that the examiner shows interest in life at home.

All topics of this nature are best approached naturally during free

---

[1] Jean Piaget, *The Origins of Intelligence in Children*, trans. (New York: International Universities Press, 1953).

[2] Arnold Gesell and C. S. Amatruda, *Developmental Diagnosis* (New York: Harper, 1941), pp. 39ff.

[3] *Ibid.*

[4] See Piaget, *passim.*

conversation rather than in an overly structured interview. Usually they should be reserved for some time during or after the examination and should not be started before the parents seem to be at ease. Once the examiner has played with the child, the burden of proper representation no longer rests on the father and mother alone. Therefore, they may be able to talk more freely. The examiner also then may be more confident of asking the proper questions. In work with handicapped children particularly, embarrassment can thus be avoided, because a first impression of the child's potentialities and physical and mental limitations has been gained. This also helps E to evaluate a parent's attitude and to judge whether he seems reasonably objective or too pessimistic, optimistic, or defensive.

The list of questions asked of parents obviously can be extended indefinitely. When a child is about *two years of age and older,* one may ask about more situations in daily living and about the child's comprehension of these. Does he know where things are kept? Does he know the cookie box only when he sees it, does he go to the refrigerator and point toward the milk bottle, or would he, if he had to, even know how to get himself a sandwich or a lunch? Could he direct a new babysitter where to find things (as can many children over *three years of age*)? Does he recognize cereal wrappers, know his own clothes, know generally what belongs to whom? Does he know where things go; does he put things away only when told where, or does he, for instance, himself know how to separate spoons from forks and how to put them in their own places in a drawer? Does he, when he sets the table, go for each spoon separately, or does he realize in the beginning how many he needs for a certain number of people (as a *four- to five-year-old* may do)? Does he find his toys accidentally, or can he go look for a missing object, knowing where he might have left it?[5] Can he find his way home from the next corner, or from a point farther away? Could he go to a nearby store on an errand and would he know if he was not given the right thing? If he frequently visits a supermarket, does he know where certain things are to be found, and does he know how to get there and find his mother again?

2—Questions to the Child

2A—ABOUT HIS FAMILY, HIS TRIP, HIS MEALS, HIS DAYS. Ask the child all kinds of questions: for instance, "How did you get here?"

[5] See also Chapter V.

"Who drove the car?" "Where did you sit?" "Where did Mummy sit?" "Who came with you?"

Ask, "Do you have boys and girls (brothers and sisters) at home? What are their names? Where are they now? What does the baby eat? What do you eat for breakfast? What kind of cereal? What does it look like? What do you put on your cereal? Why sugar? What does sugar taste like, and salt? Do you know a dog, a cat? Does he have a name? What does he eat? When do you feed him?" Or, "How do you get your milk? Who brings it? In what is it? What else is in your refrigerator? What do you need to make toast? What is it made of? What are scrambled eggs made of? What is orange juice made of?"

These questions have varied factors in common: they relate to observations of daily living often not especially talked about in the child's day. He has to reflect on certain aspects of his experience, single them out from others, report on them. Most *four-year-olds* find some answer to most questions of this group; some questions may be within the range of normal *three-year-olds*.

2B—ABOUT MATERIALS, MONEY, PRICES. For questions of this kind, see the Revised Stanford-Binet Scale, Forms L and M.[6] Ask what things are made of, as "What is a house (book, window, chair, dress, shoe) made of?" These questions are placed on the *four-and-a-half-year-old* level in the Stanford-Binet Scale. Ask older children what bread or cake is made of (or hammer, picture frame).

Ask, "Do you know money—like nickels and dimes, etc.? Which is more money? How many pennies in a nickel,[7] in a dime? How many nickels in a dime, in a quarter? What can you buy for a nickel, for a dollar, for ten dollars?"

Show various coins; show five pennies and a nickel. Ask what he can buy for one and for the other. Note whether one means "more money" than the other to him. Note what he knows of values. Does "more" mean more coins or greater value (ten pennies more than a dime, for instance)? Ask how much he would need to buy a bicycle; if he replies that it "costs a lot" note whether or not he thinks in terms of only a dollar or two, which may be "a lot" for him.

While normal children of *seven years of age* usually can tell how many pennies are in a nickel or in a dime, they may not yet be

[6] Lewis M. Terman and Maud A. Merrill, *Measuring Intelligence* (Boston: Houghton Mifflin, 1937), pp. 90, 214, 150, 343.
[7] David Wechsler, *Wechsler Intelligence Scale for Children* (New York: Psychological Corporation, 1949), p. 61.

able to transform quarters into nickels or a dollar into dimes. This inability may be due not only to lack of experience but to lack of comprehension of notions of quantity. Piaget discusses the well-known fact that young children only gradually learn to understand the "conversation" of quantities. At *five* they may feel that five single pennies are "more" than a nickel. Up to about the age of *seven,* the term "as much" does not necessarily mean that two items are interchangeable with regard to quantity. Only gradually do children learn the relativity of such terms as "a lot." Not until *ten or eleven years of age* do they count with the knowledge that "a lot of money" means different things for different people.[8]

2C—ABOUT SPORTS, TELEVISION PROGRAMS, CURRENT EVENTS, POLITICAL FIGURES. Ask many other types of questions, all designed to discover how the child comprehends what goes on around him. Note whether a child who watches television or sits at a window most of the day takes in what he sees. Does he recognize familiar names, can he place or identify them, does he know world events, local events, or the color of his neighbor's house? Can he name a series of vegetables he eats, of animals he meets in the neighborhood, of cars belonging to different houses nearby? What does he think of the news, of the weather, or the prospects of his favorite baseball team?

Such questions have a definite place in clinical examinations. Psychiatrists are accustomed to using them freely to get some idea about a patient's mental status and competence. Psychologists find them especially appropriate in examinations of severely handicapped children *over the age of ten.* For such patients they are frequently more relevant than standardized tests of comprehension which may call for factual experiences common for normal people but removed from those who are unable to get around. These children's level of comprehension can best be tested on their own ground. With their daily experiences, their hobbies, and their interests as test material, one may be able to judge their maturity of reasoning by the manner in which they have understood what comes their way, regardless of how seriously limited it may be in scope. Even in the absence of accurate norms, the examiner with some general knowledge about other children equally handicapped or not, can arrive at a reasonable estimate of a child's understanding. For instance, the baseball fan may refer to certain phases and events of the

[8] Jean Piaget, *The Child's Conception of Number,* trans. (London: Routledge, 1952), Parts I and II. Also Alina Szeminska, "Essai d'analyse psychologique du raisonnement mathématique," *Cahiers de pédagogie expérimentale et de psychologie de l'enfant,* Number 7 (Geneva: Institut des Sciences de l'Education, 1935).

games he has ardently followed in the World Series, or, like some younger child, he may know just the winning team or the names of one or two players. One television viewer may have picked up various bits of information about places and their inhabitants, whereas another may not know the difference between Disneyland and the White House; he may know only that both may be seen on the screen.

3—COMPREHENSION TESTS

Use material from the Revised Stanford-Binet Scale,[9] the Wechsler Intelligence Scale for Children,[10] and the Wechsler-Bellevue Intelligence Scale.[11] (For example: (A) from the Revised Stanford-Binet Scale, What must you do when you are thirsty? (Form L, III 6), Why do we have books? (Form L, IV), What's the thing for you to do if another boy (or girl) hits you without meaning to do it? (Form L, VII), What should a man do if he finds he is earning less money than it takes to live on? (Form M, VIII); (B) from the Wechsler Intelligence Scale for Children, What's the thing to do when you cut your finger? What would you do if you were sent to buy a loaf of bread and the grocer said he did not have any more? What should you do if you see a train approaching a broken track? (C) from the Wechsler-Bellevue Intelligence Scale, What is the thing to do if you find an envelope in the street that is sealed and addressed and has a new stamp? What should you do if while sitting in the movies (theatre) you were the first person to discover a fire? Why are laws necessary?)

Score as directed.

Note all responses, whether acceptable for scoring or not. Note whether the question itself was understood. If not, try to determine whether the child does not know the meaning of one or another word ("less money," A) or whether he does not understand the implication of the phrase ("a train approaching a broken track," B). Instead of giving an answer, does he only repeat part of the question? Does he respond to some part of the question only ("If you find an envelope, you might use it again," C), or does he respond to the whole? Note emotional overtones in his answers: is he inclined to be moralistic ("He should not hit you," A; or "You should be more careful and not cut your finger,"

[9] Terman and Merrill, *op. cit.*, pp. 85, 88, 98, 144, 150, 158, 102, 206, 212, 232, 339, 345, 355, 241.

[10] Wechsler, *Wechsler Intelligence Scale for Children*, pp. 63, 91.

[11] David Wechsler, *The Measurement of Adult Intelligence* (Baltimore: Williams and Wilkins, 1944), pp. 80, 173–174; *The Measurement and Appraisal of Adult Intelligence* (Baltimore: Williams and Wilkins, 1958), pp. 67–69. Eight of the W–B 1 questions are included in the WAIS.

B)? Is he defensive ("I would not fight," B; or "I would not keep the money," B), or unrealistic ("I would tell the trainmen; perhaps I would telephone," B; or "I would find some water and put it out," C)? Is he, or does he want to appear, independent and self-sufficient, or does he express his need for help ("I would tell my mother"). Does he seem objective, see various possibilities, and only after consideration choose the best way ("I would probably like to shout 'fire'—but that would not do," C)?

The comprehension questions discussed here vary considerably in content and therefore in demands on those who reply to them. Some of the questions refer to everyday events and common sense; some require experience and knowledge which may be more or less foreign to young children but common to adults and older children. Some of the questions involve unusual situations unlikely to happen to a young child. Others may be common experiences of many normal children but not of other groups. The wording of some of the questions may cause more personal emotional involvement than that of others; some may cause frightening thoughts. Most children can answer some of the questions from immediate experience with similar situations; some questions, however, need activation of previously learned facts and can be solved only by those who have acquired these facts. Many of the situations call for imagination and for the ability to work with hypothetical premises. The "comprehension questions" may be heterogeneous in the reasoning processes they involve. In practice they prove of considerable value to the clinician. The richness of clinical data they supply can often lead to a quick and pertinent over-all appraisal of a patient.[12] When dealing with children, one should tend to avoid the atmosphere of a quiz and therefore try to choose carefully the moment for introducing the test. It may also be necessary to drop one or the other of the questions if they seem too flagrantly inappropriate for an individual child.

T:X.   Most suitable procedures for various age ranges

Procedure	Age
1, 2a	Up to two years
1, 2a, (2b), 3	Two to six years
2b, 2c, 3	Six to ten years
2b, 2c, 3	Over ten years

Parentheses around number indicate that the procedure is suitable only for the older children in the age group.

[12] See *ibid.*, p. 80.

XI

Automatisms, Academic Tools
Factual Information

1—AUDITORY SERIES AND ASSOCIATIONS

1A—NURSERY RHYMES AND JINGLES. Ask the child, "Can you say rhymes?" or ask him directly, "Do you know 'Jack and Jill went up the . . .'?" Pause between words. Note whether the child recognizes the familiar words immediately and tries spontaneously to supply the next word. Note whether he seems to expect the examiner to produce it, or whether the line does not seem to mean anything to him. If so, try other familiar verses, or ask his mother about any favorite jingles.

1B—BABY TRICKS. Try some of the common baby tricks, such as "pat-a-cake," "bye-bye," "how big is the baby?" Ask, "Where is your nose (mouth, ear, eyes)?" or more difficult questions, such as "Where is your chin (elbow, knee)?"

Inquire of mother about favorite stunts and try them.

Note whether the child will produce them also if a strange rather than a familiar voice gives him the proper cue.

The majority of children in our culture are exposed to material of this kind: baby tricks (pat-a-cake, bye-bye) are commonly in the repertoire of the *ten-month-old* baby. Around *two years of age* and often earlier most children know some parts of the body (mouth, nose, eyes, hair). By the same time they become interested in jingles; by *two-and-a-half to three years of age,* they start adding words or gestures to rhymes spoken to them.[1]

The procedures investigate previously acquired patterns of responses

---

[1] Arnold Gesell, *The First Five Years of Life* (New York: Harper, 1940), p. 447.

to certain verbal clues. They depend on the child's experience. They allow one to judge how in a given situation the child may be able to reproduce what he has learned. Though such conditioned responses are among the earliest manifestations of learning ability, they alone cannot be relied upon to judge ability for future learning in more complex situations. The significance of these responses as a measure of mental competence diminishes rapidly with age. However, in early childhood they permit some insight into a baby's social attitudes and skills. Frequently, they also reveal some facts about the people surrounding the child; some parents or siblings put too much, others too little, effort into teaching the baby new tricks. In some families, social games are part of an easy-going, affectionate atmosphere. In others, they are occasions for strain. Some proud parents use them to show off their baby, while other anxious ones need them to convince themselves that all is well.

2—Automatic Series

2A—saying number series (counting). (See also I:7.) Say, "Do you know how to count?" or say, "Let us say 'one . . . two . . . three.' " Wait for the child to supply the next number.

2B—saying abc. Introduce as above. Frequently, children of preschool age spontaneously initiate either one of these series during the testing interview. The examiner has to be alert to pick up the cues and to encourage the child to go on with whatever series he may have started.

Note: Is counting *per se* meaningful to him, or are number words a rhythmic accompaniment to his actions only? Does he rattle off a long series correctly, or does he just get up to a certain number and from then on improvise haphazardly, repeating numbers without order? Is he content to show his ability to count only once, or does he try to repeat the same performance whenever he can, whether the occasion is appropriate or not?

Most normal children gradually learn to count through casual contact with number series and some help by parents or siblings. By *four years of age* they ordinarily know how to count up to ten.[2] (The ABC's are frequently acquired in the same way, though perhaps with less consistency.) The clinical examiner may be interested in determining whether or not the child of preschool age has responded to such normal opportunities. His failure to do so may be a sign that he is not yet ready for academic training beyond the kindergarten level.

[2] *Ibid.,* p. 172.

More notable for the clinician, however, may be a child who knows how to count (or to say some of the alphabet), but fails in many other important areas of functioning. Such discrepancy may occur in varied types of abnormal behavior: some children learn best by rote, but have difficulty in situations that depend on the comprehension of inherent relationships. Others prefer formalized, structured material such as numbers and letters because they require a minimum of personal involvement. The predominance of auditory skills over cognitive ones is common in varied types of brain injury. The tendency to stay aloof from contents that demand decision or personal judgement is found in neurotic children. Though both may be good at repeating numbers, there are important differences between them. Neurotic children frequently not only repeat numbers and letters automatically, but, contrary to brain-injured children, may be able to manipulate and reorganize them, often with considerable skill (see below).

2c—MANIPULATING NUMBER AND LETTER SERIES. If a child is fluent in 2a or 2b and reproduces the series without error, ask him: (1) "Start from six (or twelve), or from the letter m." (2) "What number comes after seven (after ten), before five (before eleven)?" (3) "Say numbers backwards from ten (or twenty)."

Normal children of school age are able to manipulate in this manner series which they know automatically. "Before" and "after" questions are common in the number work of first-grade children. *Eight-year-olds* are expected to count backwards from twenty to one.[3] Series which were learned by rote during the preschool days become better integrated and more flexible as development proceeds. The child learns to dissect, reorganize, and restructure them. Such manipulation of previously acquired patterns is essential in constructive learning.

2D—SAYING AND MANIPULATING "DAYS OF THE WEEK." Use material from the Revised Stanford-Binet Scale.[4] Say, "Can you say the days of the week?" Then ask, "Which day comes before Friday? before Tuesday? after Monday?" Score as directed.

This procedure (2d) examines on a higher level series similar to those presented before (2a to 2c). It tests again the child's ability to manipulate them.

Note whether the child who fails does so because he does not understand what "days of the week" are; note whether, when reciting the series, he omits days or reverses their order, whether he confuses "before" or "after," or is unable to manipulate and dissect automatic series in these terms.

If a child gives no response or volunteers to say, "April, March," suggest, "I mean like 'Monday, Tuesday, . . .' " The child who responds immediately to this suggestion and makes no errors either in recitation of the series or in the "before" and "after" questions may fall below the Revised Stanford-Binet standards for the VIII-year level. However, his ability to recite and manipulate the series of days after suggestions marks him as superior to those children who cannot handle the notion of "before" and "after" at all, or who cannot recite the days in order. His failure may have been due to lack of vocabulary rather than to lack of reasoning ability or knowledge.

2E—SAYING AND MANIPULATING "MONTHS OF THE YEAR." Use other series such as the "months of the year" in the same way.

3—ARITHMETIC FACTS

3A—AUTOMATIC SERIES AND VARIATIONS. Say: "One and one is . . ."; "Two and two is . . ."; "Three and three is. . . ."

If the child seems able to respond quickly and correctly, but appears to rattle problems and answers off like another automatic series, introduce the following variations: ask in the same tone of voice and at the same speed as before, "One and one is . . . ; Two and two is . . . ; *Three* and two is . . . ; Four and four is . . . ; Four and *six* is. . . ."

Note: Is the child startled, yet does he adapt himself properly and give the correct answer? Does he fail to notice the change of pattern and instead keep on rattling off answers such as: "One and one is *two,* two and two is *four,* three and two is *six,* four and four is *eight,* five and four is *ten,*" etc.? Or does he notice the "trap," search for the proper answer, but not "know"?

Addition of numbers within ten is usually well within the limits of *seven- to eight-year-olds,* who in most school systems learn these facts in the first grade.

3B—ONE TIMES THREE, TWO TIMES THREE. If the child is able to recite multiplication tables in sequence, ask individual problems: "Four times three, seven times three," or, "Eight times three," then, "Three times eight."

Note whether he can produce these answers immediately or with some delay. If the latter, watch his silent procedures. Does he murmur to himself, "One times three, two times three," until he reaches the problem which he is trying to solve? Does he use his fingers three at a time, adding them up as he goes along, or does he ask for paper and pencil and make marks in groups of three so that he can count them afterwards? Does he know "eight times three" right off, but not know "three times eight" because he has not yet "had" the "eights"?

These problems are within the limits of normal *eight- to nine-year-olds,* who generally in the third grade become familiar with multiplication tables which they also use in written multiplication. Elementary arithmetic may be taught in various ways, depending on educational principles. Some school systems begin with drill; first-grade children may be taught to memorize series of "additions within ten" (one and one is two, two and two is four). Other teachers drill individual arithmetic facts (two and one is three, five and seven is twelve). Once these number combinations have been memorized by rote, children can draw on this stock of facts and learn to dissect them, to restructure them, and to manipulate them to fit the more complex problems of the following school years.

The more progressive school systems postpone drill until the children have an understanding of the number system. They are taught to manipulate concrete quantities first; then they learn to combine these with numbers abstractly. Only when this stage has been reached do they memorize number facts so that they may recall them speedily for use in compound problems. Many schools seem to have adopted teaching programs in arithmetic that include both the concrete, meaningful approach to numbers and some drill. Individuals vary widely in their skill for mathematical thinking; some are more dependent than others on how they are being taught. Sooner or later, however, most normal children come to understand the basic system underlying arithmetic processes enough to use simple arithmetic facts as tools in more complex operations. Children whose mental development is impaired by brain injury may have success in arithmetic as long as only memorization of factual material is asked for. They may succeed well in automatic series or learned arithmetic facts, but often they are unable to isolate a problem from the context in which it was learned.[5]

[5] Alfred A. Strauss and Laura E. Lehtinen, *Psychopathology and Education of the Brain-Injured Child,* Volume I (New York: Grune and Stratton, 1947), Chapter X.

4—Serial Use of Arithmetic Facts

4a—ADDING THREE UNDER REPEATED DIRECTION. Say, "Let us do additions, like 'two and *three* is . . .' "; wait for the answer, then say, "And *three* . . . , and *three* . . . , and *three*. . . ." Do not correct any errors.

4b—ADDING THREE WITHOUT REPEATED DIRECTION. Say, "Now you do it all on your own; you add three to your last number until you get high up in the 30's." Say, "Start with one and three . . . , and three." Let the child proceed on his own; do not correct any errors.

Repeat with seven, or with other numbers *ad lib*.

Note the child's methods (as in 3b). Does he use his fingers? Does he seem to count mentally, or does each solution come to him immediately? If he makes errors, does he notice them and correct them? Do errors seem due to inattention or speeding, or do they seem to show that the child is not familiar enough with the number system? Note any significant difference between the quality of performance in 4a and 4b. More mental control is demanded in 4b: the child must state his own problem by keeping track both of his last sum and what number to add.

4c—ADDING ONE, THEN TWO, THEN THREE. Say, "Now let us make it a bit harder: two and *one* is . . . , and *two* . . . , and *three* . . . , and *four* . . . , etc." Do not correct any errors.

Say, "Now you do the same thing on your own. You always add one more to your last number. First you add *one,* then *two,* then *three,* etc., just as we did together. Now, start with three and *one* . . . , and *two* . . . ; now you are on your own. What is next?"

Let him proceed on his own. Do not correct any errors.

Note: Does he understand immediately or with delay? Does he keep adding the same number instead of the next higher one (as in 4a and 4b—three and *one* equals four, and *two* equals six, and *two* equals eight), or does he lose track of his last sum (three and *one* equals *four,* and two equals *six,* and three equals *four,* and five equals *six*)? Does he know how to proceed correctly, but start to make mistakes? Is he aware of them, and does he try to correct them? What are his errors? Does he use the wrong procedure, or does he add wrong? Do other familiar series interfere (three and *one* equals four; and *two* equals *six;* and *six* equals twelve)?

This task demands considerable mental control. Two progressing series must be kept in mind and coordinated at each step. Experience shows that this (still unstandardized) test is well within the abilities of normal *nine- to ten-year-old* children. However, those who have poor mental control can be spotted by their difficulties. Though they may have the necessary addition facts handy, they get confused and come to neglect progression in one or the other series. Others may be completely unable to coordinate both series. The clinical examiner may suspect some difficulty in the learning processes if this task is consistently failed. Anxiety, fatigue, difficulty in organization, or any combination of these may be the cause.

5—ARITHMETIC PROBLEMS AND ARITHMETIC REASONING

Use materials from the Wechsler Intelligence Scale for Children and the Wechsler-Bellevue Intelligence Scale.[6]

5A—STANDARD PRESENTATION. Present and score as directed.

5B—VARIATIONS. Let the child continue beyond the time limit if he seems to need more than the time allowed. Proceed to the next problem only after it becomes clear that he will not produce an answer. Note all answers whether correct or not. Try to discover how the answer came about. Ask him about it, "How did you get that?" and let him try again. Note whether or not he chooses correct operations, correct computations, etc. Does he find the answer in the simplest way, or does he use cumbersome, roundabout methods?

5C—SUGGESTIONS TO THE CHILD. If the child is unable to decide what operation to use, one may suggest that "this is multiplication," etc., and note whether the suggestion is taken and used to advantage. The problems vary in their demands and in the psychological processes which they involve. Direct counting of concrete quantities and comprehension of the meaning of "except" is required in some (WISC, 1, 2, 3). Simple addition and subtraction within ten is required in others (WISC, 5, 6, 7, and Wechsler-Bellevue 1, 2). Both groups of problems are within the abilities of most *seven- to eight-year-olds*. Some (WISC 10, 11, and Wechsler-Bellevue 4, 5) involve small divisions which are usually within the capacity of *eight- to nine-year-olds*. In these problems the subject is asked about certain combinations of numbers. The answer

---

[6] David Wechsler, *Wechsler Intelligence Scale for Children* (New York: Psychological Corporation, 1949), p. 64; *The Measurement of Adult Intelligence* (Baltimore: Williams and Wilkins, 1944), pp. 82, 175; *The Measurement and Appraisal of Adult Intelligence* (Baltimore: Williams and Wilkins, 1958), pp. 69, 70. The ten W–B 1 items are included in the WAIS.

comes intuitively to persons experienced with number facts. However, it requires reflection and mental operation from a child who has not yet automatized simple arithmetic facts.

Some of the more difficult problems (WISC 12–16 and Wechsler-Bellevue 6–10) demand more subtle operations in addition to automatized number facts. For instance, problem 7 in the Wechsler-Bellevue Scale: "If seven pounds of sugar cost twenty-five cents, how many pounds can you get for a dollar?" Here the subject is required to see the relationship between the terms "twenty-five cents" and "a dollar." The figure that results (4) has to be applied to a third term (7). Unless the subject is clear about all relationships involved, he may make various mistakes: he may try to multiply 25 x 7, or add twenty-five cents to one dollar. Or he may immediately see twenty-five cents and one dollar in the proper relationship and come up with a 4, but then deal with it in the wrong way: he may find that 4 is the answer he has been asked for, or he may come up with the answer 21, explaining that he had to subtract 4 from 25, or he may say the answer is 11 and explain that he added 4 to 7 because one gets 4 more for a dollar than for twenty-five cents. In order to find the correct answer, the subject might see the relevant relationships immediately at a glance; if he is less experienced, he may have to think about successive steps to take; often he may do so by trying to make a mental picture of the concrete situation.

Many theoretical thinkers of various creeds have found mathematical reasoning processes a gold mine for the study of thought processes.[7] Aside from theoretical considerations, the clinician can get important information about her patient by analyzing the reasoning processes which he uses in arithmetic problems. She may be able to differentiate between patients who use the proper steps and those who do not. This may frequently tell more about an individual's mental competence than the fact that the end result was correct or incorrect. A wrong answer may be the product of a more mature reasoning process than a correct one arrived at by the wrong operation. For instance, in the above example a child may say that the answer is 21 because he multiplied 7 x 4 (but made a mistake in computation), while another may come up with the

[7] See E. L. Thorndike, *The Psychology of Arithmetic* (New York: Macmillan, 1922). Also Max Wertheimer, *Productive Thinking* (New York: Harper, 1945). Also Jean Piaget, *The Child's Conception of Number,* trans. (London: Routledge, 1952). Also Alina Szeminska, "Essai d'analyse psychologique du raisonnement mathématique," *Cahiers de pédagogie expérimentale et de psychologie de l'enfant,* Number 7 (Geneva: Institut des Sciences de l'Education, 1935).

correct answer, 28, but explain that he got this by adding 4 to 25. This latter child may have hit on the correct answer even though he defaults in computation as well as in reasoning.

6—COMBINING WORDS

Use dissected sentences from the Revised Stanford-Binet Scale.[8] (For example: Form M, IX-year level, "a have dog I fine"; Forms L and M, XIII-year level, "for the started an we country early at hour.")

Present and score as directed.

Note whether the child is confident or apprehensive when presented with printed material. Does he go about it as if he expected to read the words with ease; does he concentrate on finding the right order in which to put the words, or does he try painfully to read word after word? Note which words, if any, seem difficult for him.

With children who seem to have difficulty reading the words, one may ask them to point out those words they know and help them with others. This test may serve as an initial gauge by which to judge reading. Often this task seems to be less threatening than an ordinary reading test because attention is directed toward the sense of the sentence rather than toward reading skill.

These procedures involve reading comprehension and ability to manipulate words meaningfully. Some children may be skillful in only one of these aspects. They may have some intuitions about proper words in the right context even though they may have difficulty deciphering an individual word. Others may be able to read single words but lack the comprehension and flair to combine them.

7—FOLLOWING AND READING STORIES

Use the following material from the Revised Stanford-Binet Scale, Form L: The Wet Fall (VIII-year level); Form M: The School Concert (X-year level); and A Distinguished French Acrobat (XIII-year level).[9]

Present and score as directed as tests to evaluate "memory for stories" (see also VIII:4).

Note also: Does the child seem to follow the lines of his copy while the story is being read to him? Does he seem to read, to listen, or to do both?

The material can be used as a gauge to evaluate reading ability and

[8] Terman and Merrill, *op. cit.*, pp. 161, 368, 172, 276.
[9] *Ibid.*, pp. 100, 233, 165, 376, 171, 389.

reading comprehension. Ask the child to read the story aloud and to try to remember what he has read. Note how he reads, where he hesitates, substitutes, etc. Watch his method when he stumbles over a word. Does he try to study it, sound it out, guess it, or give up?

8—READING SINGLE PRINTED WORDS, LETTERS, NUMBERS
Print individual words. Have the child read them or let him match objects to them (see VI:11c).

Investigation of reading ability by the few methods mentioned under 6 to 8 is obviously incomplete and rudimentary only. Often these procedures may suffice to show, however, whether or not the child has problems in this area and whether they seem more prominent in word recognition or in reading comprehension. In the great majority of cases, symptoms in reading are closely correlated with manifestations in other areas of functioning which are investigated in the psychological examination.

9—SPELLING AND WRITING WORDS
Ask the child to write his name and address (see III:2c). When it is done, ask him to spell it. Ask for other words, ranging from difficult ones ("The Children's Hospital") to simple ones ("go," "to," "mother"). Ask him to write or to spell any other words which he may know.

Note whether he is accustomed to writing fluently or whether he stumbles over certain letters. If the latter, try to see or ask whether he is uncertain about how to make a letter, or whether he does not know which letter should come next. Note his procedure with familiar words and compare it with his approach to unfamiliar words. Note whether he spells orally as easily as he writes, or *vice versa*.

School methods vary considerably in their approach to spelling. Therefore, the clinical psychologist may find it difficult to use performances in spelling as a gauge of efficiency without knowing more about how the child was taught. There are children who seem to have special skill in spelling and are able to rattle off very difficult words. Others have great difficulty with simple words. Some know only words they have learned; others try to guess at new ones. Normally children can also write or print the words which they can spell orally. Occasionally they can only spell, not write, the same words. This may be of special interest to the clinician. It seems that these children have memorized by rote a sequence of letters which remains otherwise meaningless to them and which they cannot transfer to the medium of written letters.

10—FACTUAL INFORMATION

Use information questions that largely refer to material learned in school and/or through books or other educational media. (It seems legitimate to distinguish this type of information from that acquired mostly through experience and everyday contacts. See Chapter X.) Certain of the questions from the Wechsler Intelligence Scale for Children and the Wechsler-Bellevue Intelligence Scale seem to fall into the factual information category more than do some others.[10] (For example: from the Wechsler Intelligence Scale for Children, How many pounds are there in a ton? What is the capital of Greece? How far is it from New York to Chicago? and from the Wechsler-Bellevue Intelligence Scale, Where is London? What is the capital of Japan? Who wrote *Hamlet?*)

10A—STANDARD PRESENTATION. When an accurate score is desired use all items of one scale and score as directed.

For adults most of the items may involve information which has been acquired in a lifetime of average opportunity.[11] However, in children command of similar material may depend more on the teaching they may have received. Their responses may show what education they have had and what use they have made of it. If they fail in some of the items, they may have not had the opportunity to learn about them, or they may not have been able to profit from their lessons. Some may succeed because they have learned by rote, others because they have found out through comprehension. Wealth of factual information and good performances in answering such questions may not necessarily be an indication of mental efficiency and competence; occasionally these tests may be deceiving.

Facts perceived in proper relationships build up a stock of information on which the individual may draw for new use in the future. Material which has been learned without comprehension, by rote or drill only, becomes stale and will soon be unproductive. A normal person is apt to forget such facts more easily than material which has become meaningful. One may find exceptional individuals who have many iso-

[10] Wechsler, *Wechsler Intelligence Scale for Children*, pp. 61–62; *The Measurement of Adult Intelligence*, p. 172; *The Measurement and Appraisal of Adult Intelligence*, pp. 65–67. Eighteen of the twenty-five W–B 1 items are included in the WAIS.
[11] Wechsler, *The Measurement of Adult Intelligence*, p. 78.

lated items of factual information at their disposal and reproduce them under certain stimuli but not under others. They may be unable to reason about these facts and unable to apply them to new circumstances.

The clinician may find it interesting to make these distinctions, especially in the case of children. Added questions can help to determine not only what has been learned, but also what has been understood.

10B—QUESTIONS. Many of the above information items lend themselves to further questions which can test comprehension. For instance, after questions about London, or the capital of Japan, ask for other capitals; ask for the relationships between capitals and states and continents ("What is England? Is it like Paris or like Europe or like France?"), or ask for further comments on the word "capital."

With questions about distances between New York and Chicago (WISC) or Paris and New York (Wechsler-Bellevue) ask about other distances (from Boston to Cambridge, or New York to San Francisco). Whether or not the answer to the original question was a correct one, one may get an impression about the child's frame of reference and the reasoning processes which help to elaborate it.

In some of his earlier studies, Piaget put similar questions to children of various ages.[12] He found confused notions even among those children who had learned about countries, states, etc., and who could properly answer direct questions about them. He discovered that children up to *nine and ten years of age* might assert that Geneva is in Switzerland, that Switzerland is larger than Geneva, but at the same time deny that one could be in Geneva and in Switzerland at the same time and that an inhabitant of Geneva could be also Swiss. These statements—easily duplicated in other young children—show their lack of understanding of the relationships between parts and wholes; here, as in other areas, the child thinks of various units with various names side by side rather than in the proper relationships, which are understood only when a certain level of maturity of reasoning is reached.

When seen from such angles, the child's ideas about things he has learned gain significance for the clinician who tries to evaluate mental competence and maturity.

Adding discussions to information questions may be especially helpful with some older children who, because of physical handicaps,

[12] Jean Piaget, *Judgement and Reasoning in the Child,* trans. (New York: Harcourt, Brace, 1928), Chapter III.

have not had the opportunity to acquire the facts. Even though they may not know the actual answer to the question, they may reveal in conversation how they understand what they are being asked about. This may lead to a more reliable estimate of their potentialities than the answer itself. For example, a person may not know the capital of Greece, and say so. But he may know where Greece is in relation to other countries, may know some of its history, and remember some of its city names. Obviously, in spite of his failure on the particular item, he would seem better informed than another child who may have memorized all the capitals of many countries and thus knows Athens, but not know whether or not its inhabitants are Greeks, Romans, or Athenians, and whether it takes more time to fly from Boston to Athens or to New York.

10c—COMPREHENSION OF FACTS. In practice one may find the borderline between information and comprehension to be rather fluid. Both WISC and Wechsler-Bellevue "information" series contain items that might belong in one or the other category. The same is the case with "comprehension" questions (see Chapter X).

T:XI.   Most suitable procedures for various age ranges

Procedure	Age
1	Up to two years
1, 2a, 2b, (2c), (8), (10)	Two to six years
2–5, (6), (7), 8–10	Six to ten years
3–7, 9, 10	Over ten years

Parentheses around number indicate that the procedure is suitable only for the older children in the age group.

XII

Vocabulary

1—PICTURE BOOK, PICTURE VOCABULARY, OBJECT NAMING

For younger children use the material discussed in II:1,6,7,11 and VI:8.

2—ORAL VOCABULARY

For older children use material from the revised Stanford-Binet Scale,[1] the Wechsler Intelligence Scale for Children,[2] or the Wechsler-Bellevue Intelligence Scale[3] as directed, or say, "Let us see how many of these words you know. I'll say a word and you tell me what it means. What is an orange?" Give plenty of time, but do not insist if it becomes clear that the child does not know what to say. Explain, saying: "Well, we could say all kinds of things; we could say that we could eat it, or that it is a fruit, or that it is orange color, or anything like that."

Proceed to the next word. In this procedure the examiner might do well to keep up a certain speed and verve. Avoid dragging the test out too long. Often it may seem best to skip some word if it seems clear that the child would give a correct answer.

(For example, from the Revised Stanford-Binet Scale, Form L (vocabulary), "orange, envelope, straw, lecture, Mars, skill," etc.; from the Revised Stanford-Binet Scale (abstract words), "pity, curiosity, com-

[1] Lewis M. Terman and Maud A. Merrill, *Measuring Intelligence* (Boston: Houghton Mifflin, 1937), pp. 302–323, 165, 380, 109, 261, 112, 269.
[2] David Wechsler, *Wechsler Intelligence Scale for Children* (New York: Psychological Corporation, 1949), p. 68.
[3] David Wechsler, *The Measurement of Adult Intelligence* (Baltimore: Williams and Wilkins, 1944), pp. 98, 196–207; *The Measurement and Appraisal of Adult Intelligence* (Baltimore: Williams and Wilkins, 1958). The list of forty-two words in the W–B 1 has been replaced in the WAIS by forty new words.

pare, conquer, envy, authority," etc.; from the Wechsler Intelligence Scale for Children, "bicycle, knife, hat, letter, umbrella, cushion," etc.; from the Wechsler-Bellevue Intelligence Scale, "diamond, nuisance, nitroglycerine, stanza, pewter, ballast," etc.)

Score as directed.

Note all responses, whether correct or not. Note whether the child is familiar with the word or whether he knows only about in which area it might belong. If he explains a word, does he try to find one description or definition only, does he try to be precise and brief or does he embark on lengthy explanations? Does he keep it objective or does he get involved in relating personal experiences? Note whether he thinks he knows the word but confuses it with another that sounds like it to him. If he does not know the word, does he try to guess its meaning? Is he ready to say, "I do not know" and try to shake off further demands, or is he puzzled? Note whether or not showing him the word printed helps him to recognize it.

Watch for possible hearing difficulties; listen carefully how he repeats the word, if he does. Has he heard it correctly or with some distortion? Note how he expresses himself. Does he find it easy or difficult to say what he means? Does he have mechanical difficulties getting words said properly or does he seem uncertain about how best to express what he thinks? Does he use gestures to help him illustrate his statements or does he even depend on them exclusively?

Note the content of his definitions. Does he choose a synonym for the stimulus word (for cushion, a pillow), or does he describe an action ("Cushion"—"you put it under your head")? Does he describe some special feature ("Donkey"—"it has four legs"), or does he try to fit it into some category ("Donkey"—"a living creature that is kept in some kind of enclosure or in a special building called a barn")?

Note any emotional overtones, personal experiences or feelings ("Authority"—"they have the power to do anything to you").

Responses to vocabulary items reflect a person's developmental level in various ways. With advancing age, the number of known words increases. Definitions become more precise and objective and may become more abstract as the person grows older and develops more mature reasoning habits. The developmental processes which underlie children's definitions of words are too complex to be described in detail here. Werner, among others, has pointed out that the young child de-

fines an object by describing it. Children's concepts tend to have a concrete content; even though a term he uses may seem abstract from the
adult point of view, for the child it may have a particular, individualistic
meaning, that is based on his concrete experiences.[4] The tendency
toward defining words in concrete terms persists all through childhood,
though it gradually decreases. Aside from developmental differences,
there are emotional, social, educational, cultural, and later, occupational
influences reflected in a person's vocabulary. These may determine its
character, its range, and the type of definitions—whether they are in
purely abstract or in more concrete terms.[5]

The clinician may find vocabulary techniques valuable in more
than one way. Wechsler and other authors before him found that vocabulary tests are an excellent measure of a person's general intelligence.
The numerical results provided by the scoring systems with adults as
well as with children are at least a useful gauge by which to arrive at an
initial estimate of mental competence. The responses one obtains give
clues to a child's level of reasoning, his ability to express his ideas, his
manner of speech, his working habits and personality traits.

The popularity of this test procedure varies with children: some
may find it boring or threatening while others may find it exciting and
challenging. For most it means a task in which one is to show what
one knows rather than what one can accomplish. This feature—similar to
tests of academic knowledge and information—makes it more suitable in some cases than in others. Older children are apt to like it better
than younger ones. An examiner may find it easy to propose the test
to children who, for one reason or another, like to show their knowledge;
it is more difficult to present it to children who, used to defeat in other
quiz situations, tend to avoid any task of that kind.

Some children like to deal with words more than others; yet their
vocabulary scores may be either high or low. There are extreme cases:
one may find exceptionally high scores in children who otherwise seem
to lack desire to be communicative. They may give correct and even
rather wordy definitions for each word. However, their manners may
cause the examiner to suspect that words are for them no real means for
social exchange and mutual understanding. Rather they may enjoy assembling an arsenal of weighty words that assures them respect and

[4] Heinz Werner, *Comparative Psychology of Mental Development* (New York:
Harper, 1940), p. 272.
[5] Wechsler, *The Measurement of Adult Intelligence*, p. 99.

admiration of those who hear them. Their wordiness provides them with a collector's pleasure and at the same time protects them from the emotional demands of personal contacts. Such children often are oversensitive and poorly adjusted; frequently there is a history of delayed speech development (with a sudden burst of verbal activity breaking out later on only). In contrast to this group of children one may find others who also enjoy using many words; they may be great talkers, socially responsive, and known for their verbosity; yet, they use many words without knowing what they mean and, therefore also have low scores in vocabulary tests. There are many children who get along in daily life on a small vocabulary: some of them may know and understand many words they never use, others do not. While there may be many factors influencing development of vocabulary—some of them mentioned earlier—facility of speech or its lack are not *per se* necessarily related to level of vocabulary scores, at least not in older children. Patients with severe dysarthria for instance, are often conspicuous for trying and understanding big words. Others with minor speech impairments only may leave hard words alone because they find them too cumbersome or dangerous to use. Yet, they may know them when they hear them or read them. Others again with or without speech difficulty may neither say nor know many words at all.

One may find any of these situations in children with brain injuries, whether these have been present at birth or later on. A clinician does well to consider carefully any conditions that may have helped to determine certain performances in vocabulary tasks and try to see them in the light of other findings. In general it is more tricky to use diagnostically the results of these tests in children than it appears to be in adults. This might be due mostly to the intricate relationships between language development, learning and reasoning ability, sensory-motor development, and environmental opportunity that all vary from age to age.

T:XII.   Most suitable procedures for various age ranges

Procedure	Age
1	Up to two years
1, (2)	Two to six years
2	Six to ten years
2	Over ten years

Parentheses around number indicate that the procedure is suitable only for the older children in the age group.

INDEX

Index